PAIN IN PERSPECTIVE

Edited by **Subhamay Ghosh**

Pain in Perspective
http://dx.doi.org/10.5772/2627
Edited by Subhamay Ghosh

Contributors
Subhamay Ghosh, Jørgen Riis Jepsen, David M. Hallman, Eugene Lyskov, David McBride, Helen Harcombe, Ayse Ozcan Edeer, Hulya Tuna, Julio José Contreras Fernández, Rodrigo Liendo Verdugo, Matías Osorio Feito, Francisco Soza Rex, Mario Pribicevic, Sherif Hosny, W. McClatchie, Nidhi Sofat, Caroline B. Hing, Longinus N. Ebirim, Omiepirisa Yvonne Buowari, Subhamay Ghosh, Kenji Sato, Satoshi Fukumori, Kantaro Miyake, Daniel Obata, Akio Gofuku, Kiyoshi Morita

Published by InTech
Janeza Trdine 9, 51000 Rijeka, Croatia

Publishing Process Manager Vedran Greblo
Technical Editor InTech Prepress, Novi Sad
Cover InTech Design team

Additional hard copies can be obtained from orders@intechopen.com

Pain in Perspective, Edited by Subhamay Ghosh
p. cm.
ISBN 978-953-51-0807-8

For EU product safety concerns:
IN TECH d.o.o., Prolaz Marije Krucifikse Kozulić 3, 51000 Rijeka, Croatia,
info@intechopen.com or visit our website at intechopen.com.

Meet the editor

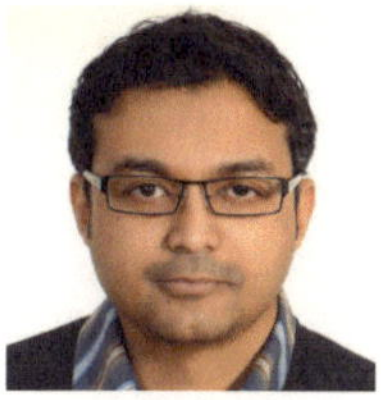

Dr. Subhamay Ghosh graduated as a doctor of medicine from the University of Pécs. Dr. Ghosh is specialist in Anaesthesia and Intensive Care Medicine. He has worked at the Imperial College London's, Lung Physiology Research team at Chelsea and Westminster Hospital, London and has a Ph.D. in 'Physiology of antioxidant modulation of acute organ injury'. He has not only contributed to the understanding of basic science research involving antioxidant organ injury of the lung, liver and heart but has translated bench to bedside scientific ideas into publications of clinical research. Dr. Ghosh currently works as a Senior Lecturer at the University of Pécs, Hungary and as a Consultant of Anaesthesia at Kettering General Hospital, University of Leicester, U.K.

Contents

Preface XI

Chapter 1 **Introduction to Pain, Religion and Analgesia 1**
Subhamay Ghosh

Chapter 2 **Work-Related Upper Limb Pain and Its Diagnosis: Contribution from the Neurological Examination 11**
Jørgen Riis Jepsen

Chapter 3 **Autonomic Regulation in Musculoskeletal Pain 35**
David M. Hallman and Eugene Lyskov

Chapter 4 **Work Related Musculoskeletal Pain and It's Management 63**
David McBride and Helen Harcombe

Chapter 5 **Management of Chronic Musculoskeletal Pain in the Elderly: Dilemmas and Remedies 93**
Ayse Ozcan Edeer and Hulya Tuna

Chapter 6 **Shoulder Pain in Swimmers 119**
Julio José Contreras Fernández, Rodrigo Liendo Verdugo, Matías Osorio Feito and Francisco Soza Rex

Chapter 7 **The Epidemiology of Shoulder Pain: A Narrative Review of the Literature 147**
Mario Pribicevic

Chapter 8 **Knee Pain in Adults & Adolescents, Diagnosis and Treatment 187**
Sherif Hosny, W. McClatchie, Nidhi Sofat and Caroline B. Hing

Chapter 9 **Physical and Psychological Aspects of Pain in Obstetrics 219**
Longinus N. Ebirim, Omiepirisa Yvonne Buowari and Subhamay Ghosh

Chapter 10 **A Novel Application of Virtual Reality for Pain Control: Virtual Reality-Mirror Visual Feedback Therapy 237**
Kenji Sato, Satoshi Fukumori, Kantaro Miyake, Daniel Obata, Akio Gofuku and Kiyoshi Morita

Preface

I admit it is a painful climb, but the pain of it is a positive pleasure for me.
Each step upward makes me feel stronger and fit for the next.

Mahatma Gandhi

Pain has been there since man has existed and whatever the method or technique of its relief, if successful will always lead to a special place in the heart of the person receiving it and also to the person delivering it. 'Pain in Perspective' takes us into a journey of how it all began and then leads us to understand the various concepts of pain relief today. From musculoskeletal pain to complex shoulder pain and from neurological examination to charting out pain, this book describes new ideas and latest descriptions of pain concepts and their treatment.

The origin and genesis of this work evolves from my work as an anaesthetist and daily encounters with pain in individuals. It is very difficult to put down in words the painful experiences patients go through during their stay at hospitals or at home. Equally difficult is the depiction of euphoria upon relief of pain and all the unpleasant experiences surrounding it. The purpose of this book is to describe some areas, if not several, of acute and chronic pain and methods to alleviate it with modern ideas and latest concepts. Since pain is not restricted to any particular sub-specialty or group, this book is targeted to medical students, nursing staff, general practitioners, specialists like anaesthetists, surgeons and residents of all specialties.

'Pain in Perspective' has taken over a year to collect, combine and refine all the chapters. The resources used for this book have been latest articles published in peer reviewed journals and easily accessible on pubmed and other medical databases. I advise readers to brush up the very basic concepts of biology, physiology and anatomy before reading this book.

Writing this book has given me more insight into pain and has chiselled several corners to allow me to see several ideas about pain that I had not dealt with earlier. It has definitely taken me closer to understanding my patients both professionally and psychologically.

I remember an incident while writing the book and I believe sharing it would be beneficial to our readers. During the early stages of writing my chapter, my two year old daughter came running to me that she had bruised her hand and that she was in pain. I could not see any swelling, laceration, cut or any sign of injury. I took her hand and caressed it and put a wet cloth over it. She smiled and said that it didn't hurt anymore.

I hope 'Pain in Perspective' will give our readers the same energy and joy in reading that it has given us as authors of this book in writing it.

I would like to thank all the authors for their dedication and hard work in completing this book and to the publishing team to help us publish our works.

As a special note of gratitude, I would like to thank my wife Boglarka, my daughter Sarolta and my son Samrat for their support, patience, love and understanding which was my motivation for this book.

Subhamay Ghosh
Anaesthetics and Intensive Care
Kettering General Hospital
University of Leicester,
UK

Chapter 1

Introduction to Pain, Religion and Analgesia

Subhamay Ghosh

Additional information is available at the end of the chapter

http://dx.doi.org/10.5772/53922

1. Introduction

1.1. Early history of pain

Human beings have always pondered and tried to understand why they feel pain and how to reduce it. In the past, pain and disease were thought to be consequences of human wrong doing. Whether pain is an independent sensation and the product of dedicated neural mechanisms continues to be a topic of debate [1]. The Western concept of pain has evolved with understanding of the world around it and attitudes toward pain have changed and developed in accordance with the science and religious climate of the period [2]. The 19th and 20th century saw the advent of new anatomical, physiological and biochemical insights and modern pain theories were developed. Modern analgesic drugs were synthesized along with new invasive procedures for pain management strategies. The older traditional beliefs, concepts and attitudes however were not been replaced completely and have survived to some degree in modern patients to this day [3]. The oldest evidence of the 'joy plant' as described in clay tablets by the Sumerians showing the cultivation and use of the opium poppy to bring joy and reduce pain have been found dating back to 5000 B.C. [4] Remains of Neolithic settlements in Switzerland have shown the cultivation of poppy seeds (Papaver somniferum) as early as 3200-2600 B.C. [5]. Opium remnants found in Egyptian tombs and other evidence from Thebes shows its use in the 15th century B.C. 'Theban opium', an alkaloid centuries later called Thebain was used to relieve pain and the Ebers Papyrus from 1552 B.C., describes how the Goddess Isis would sedate her son Horus with opium as a sedative for children [6]. In 800 B.C. Homer wrote in his epic poem Odyssey that a man used opium to soothe his pain and forget his worries [7]. The ancient Greek, Aristotle believed that pain was due to evil spirits that entered the body through an injury seeing pain and pleasure not as sensations but as emotions indicating that the heart was the source of pain rather than the brain. A similar view was shared by Hippocrates who believed that pain was caused by an imbalance in the vital fluids in the body [8]. Persian philosopher, Ibn Sina studied and mentioned relief of pain in his 14 volume book 'The Canon of Medicine' in 1025. The Middle East was well aware of the beneficial effects of opium and traders introduced it to the Far East. In Europe it was reintroduced by Paracelsus [1493-1541] and in 1680 it had reached England.

In 1664, French philosopher, René Descartes wrote Traité de l'homme where he said that the body was more of a machine, and that pain was a disturbance that passed down along nerve fibres until the disturbance reached the brain [9]. This theory changed the perception of pain from a spiritual, mystical experience to a physical, mechanical sensation meaning that a cure for such pain could be found by researching and locating pain fibres within the body rather than a religious view of linking it to the power of God. This also moved the centre of pain sensation and perception from the heart to the brain and changed the idea of pain altogether and paved the way to newer concepts.

2. Religious concepts of pain

Treating patients clinically with significant pain can be extremely difficult. Medicine provides incomplete pain relief for many patients and a significant percentage of them remain in moderate to severe pain, and their lives are drastically changed in areas including relationships, work, and leisure. Patients with chronic pain may turn or return to religion and spiritual practices to help them cope with their pain [10, 11]. Studies have found religion/spirituality to be related to higher, lower or unrelated to pain levels and distress [12, 13]. Different religions have various views on pain.

Acceptance is an important concept which has been studied in detail pain literature and also in Hindu traditions. The rich Hindu culture promotes acceptance of pain and suffering as the just working of karma- ones actions in this life or reincarnation as seen in Hinduism and Buddhism. By accepting one's condition, one becomes less attached to changing or altering it. Acceptance of pain and detachment from any struggle with the experience of pain means that painful or pain-free states would be accepted equally. Detachment from this world, in order to be focused on God or The Ultimate, is a primary goal in Hindu traditions [14]. The Sacred Bhagavad Gita, has conversations in the form of songs where Lord Krishna makes references of pain:

> *Notions of heat and cold, of pain and pleasure, are born, O son of Kunti, only of the contact of the senses with their objects. They have a beginning and an end. They are impermanent in their nature. Bear them patiently, O descendant of Bharata.* (Bhagavad Gita 2.14].

> *That person who is the same in pain and pleasure, whom these cannot disturb, alone is able, O great amongst men [Arjuna], to attain to immortality.* [2.15]

The Gita questions and explains that: What is pleasure for you may be pain for somebody else. What is pain for you may be pleasure for somebody else. Also, what you found pleasurable sometime in the past, you don't enjoy as much now. And what you enjoy now might be something you hated in the past. Pleasure and pain, likes and dislikes, these are just notions of the mind. They appear and disappear. They are impermanent. Even heat and cold are just notions of the mind.

Buddhism explains pain in a deeper perspective by saying that 'Life is a suffering' and that 'Pain and suffering is caused by attachment'. Pain in Buddhism refers not only to physical pain, aging, sickness, and death, and to emotional pain like jealousy, fear, loss and disappointment but also to the existential sense that life is permanently out of joint. Everything is touched by the shadow of dissatisfaction, imperfection, and disappointment. Suffering, in the Buddhist sense, is a pervasive condition. No one escapes it. Even enlightened teachers grow old, suffer the pains of decay, and die. The way out of this pain is following the eightfold path and meditation.

In Islam, the views of pain and suffering resemble those held by its sister faiths, Judaism and Christianity. Pain is either the result of sin, or it is a test meaning that a true Muslim will remain faithful through the trials of life. Pain and suffering also reveals the hidden self to God and is a way so that God may see who is truly righteous by allowing the anguishes and endeavours of life to open up the soul and reveal it to God. God uses pain and suffering to visualise within human beings and test their characters, and correct the unbelievers. According to the Islamic philosophy of life, there is a transcendental dimension to pain and suffering [15].

In Judaism, Just as the Torah describes the pain the women underwent in Egypt, it describes the commensurate joy they felt when they were freed. The Holy Torah describes how after successfully crossing the Red Sea, the Jewish people broke out into song. After recording the song of Moses and the men, the Torah writes:

> "*Miriam, the prophetess, Aaron's sister, took a tambourine in her hand, and all the women came out after her with tambourine and with dances*" (Exodus 15:20].

In Sikhism, suffering is an ingredient of life which has spread through the whole of the world. The Holy Guru Granth Sahib tell us: *"Unto whom should I tie up and give the bundle of my pains? The whole world is overflowing with pain and suffering"* and also *"Wherever I look, I see loads of pain and suffering."* So, across the whole of the globe, pain and suffering are a major part of life which all who have to traverse through this human existence will have to endure to a lesser or greater extend.

In Jainism, pain and violence refer primarily to injuring one's own self, a behaviour which inhibits the souls own ability to attain mokṣa or liberation. At the same time it also means violence to others because it is this tendency to harm others that ultimately harms ones own soul. Furthermore, the Jains have extended the concept of Ahiṃsa or non-violence, not only to humans but to all animals, plants, micro-organisms and all beings having life or life potential. All life is sacred and everyone has a right to live fearlessly to its maximum potential.

Traditional Christian views on pain and suffering suggest that everything about life has its goal or aim in a mystical reality, the Kingdom of Heaven, for which earthly life is a preparation. While neither illness nor health are seen as ends in themselves, both are viewed as proceeding from the will of God for our benefit and have no ultimate meaning or purpose outside of eternal life [16].

Pain and suffering, although mystic in early Christianity has always been considered a not fully understood side of eternity. However, pain and suffering has been described in several places as truths from God's Word in the Holy Bible:

Pain and suffering produces intimacy with God (Job 42:5].

Job, who endured unspeakable suffering, said, "My ears had heard of you but now my eyes have seen you." Intimacy with God is often borne in the furnace of affliction. "During times of suffering, we experience God at a deep, profound level."

Pain equips us to comfort others [2 Corinthians 1:3-5].

Suffering gives us compassion for others who are hurting, enabling us to minister more effectively. People who suffer want people who have suffered to tell them there is hope. They are justifiably suspicious of people who appear to have lived lives of ease. Those who have suffered make the most effective comforters.

Suffering and pain refines us.

We can read in Isaiah 48:10 that "…I have refined you, though not as silver; I have tested you in the furnace of affliction."

The meaning of this verse makes it clear that pain and suffering have a way of bringing our strengths and weaknesses to the surface.

Pain and Suffering produces growth and maturity (James 1:2-4].

If we turn toward God in our pain, He can use our suffering to mature our faith. We see this biblical truth illustrated through the persecuted church. After hearing their testimonies, few would deny that suffering produces beauty and maturity of spirit.

Pain and Suffering conforms us into God's image (Romans 8:28-29].

We may be tempted to read these verses to say that God will bring good out of everything. While He can and does redeem pain in our lives, these verses speak of being conformed to God's image through our suffering.

3. Analgesia, the relief from pain

The modern age has brought along a different concept of pain, quite different to its early historical and religious roots. The definition of 'Pain' is an unpleasant sensory and emotional experience associated with actual or potential tissue damage, or described in terms of such damage [17]. Acute pain is common amongst hospitalised patients particularly following surgery. Postoperative pain, if not treated properly can lead to chronic pain and can be associated with other organ dysfunction as well. There is evidence showing that morbidity and length of hospital stay is clearly affected by the type of pain service available [18]. The importance of post-operative pain management is so high that higher hospital expenditure can be attributed to it as a result of poor patient satisfaction which may translate into pressure on the health system of the nation [19]. Assessment of quality of pain incorporates measuring many dimensions including physiological endpoints, adverse events and psychosocial status. The increasing interest in evaluating quality of pain reflects the overall increased interest in patient-focused assessments. Unlike the traditional outcomes focusing on morbidity, mortality, quality of recovery from pain assesses other non-traditional outcomes focused around patient-oriented endpoints. By influencing the many domains assessed by quality of recovery, postoperative pain may have a general detrimental effect on quality of recovery [20]. Therefore, postoperative pain and relief affects both medical resource use and patients' ability to resume the normal activities of their lives after discharge from the hospital to home [21]. Even though there is sufficient relief with conventional analgesics, postoperative pain interferes with patients' ability to sleep, walk, and participate in other activities. Medications used postoperatively account for a small portion of total expenditures. Satisfaction scores are not a sufficient indicator of analgesic control. These data can be used to help improve pain relief [22].

3.1. Understanding pain

In order to understand *nociception,* it is essential to understand the mechanism behind it and only then is it possible to specifically target the source of the pain stimulus. The several concepts of evaluating and understanding pain are described in the chapters to follow. Here we shall outline the common mediators involved in the mechanism of pain and some of its treatment options.

Pain and inflammatory stimuli result in a series of diverse effects as seen in figures 1 and 2, including pain transduction, sensitisation of central nervous system and peripheral nerve endings [23].

Nociceptors or receptors of pain do not have a continuous function under normal activity but when stimulated upon pain stimuli or when tissue irritation or injury occurs respond with a magnitude relevant to the degree of the stimulus [24].

3.2. Multimodal pain relief

From a clinical point of view the ideal analgesic would provide pain relief, reduce other analgesic associated side effects and improve overall clinical outcome. This as a result would decrease morbidity, mortality and duration of hospital stay and thus reduction in expenditures.

The concept of multimodal analgesia was introduced to combat pain and costs by combining various analgesic techniques [25]. The effectiveness of an analgesic agent can be enhanced by combining effects of various mechanisms to achieve synergistic effects. Paracetamol (acetaminophen) when combined with NSAIDS (non-steroidal anti-inflammatory drugs) provide additive analgesic effect in mild to moderate acute pain [26].

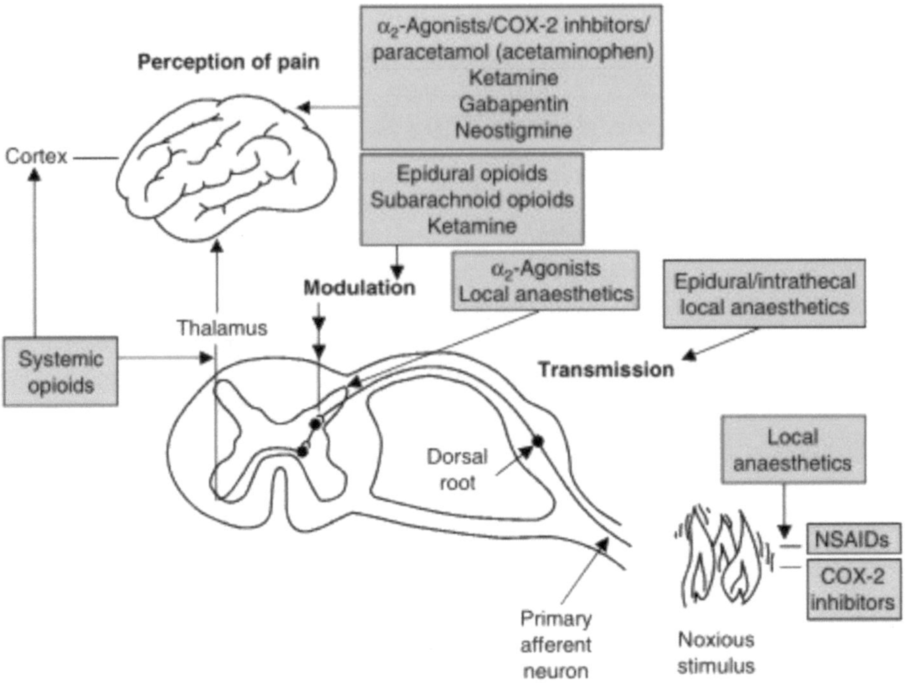

[Taken with permission from Pyati and Gan. Perioperative pain management. CNS drugs 2007; 21: 185-211].

Figure 1. Figure 1 shows the pain pathway and various sites of action of analgesics. COX (Cyclo-oxygenase), NSAIDS (Non-steroidal anti-inflammatory drugs).

The synergistic effects of α-adrenergic and opioid systems has been shown with the effects of clonidine potentiating the effects of morphine [27]. Transcutaneous electrical nerve stimulation (TENS) in an optimal frequency can significantly reduce consumption of analgesics for post-operative pain relief up to 26% compared to placebo [28]. It can even be used to treat phantom pain and stump pain in adult amputees [29]. Epidural analgesia with a combination of local anaesthetics and opioids is an excellent multimodal method for better analgesia and enhanced recovery. Epidural analgesia should not be considered as a single generic entity because many factors like the congruency of catheter insertion location to site of surgical incision, type of analgesic regimen whether local anaesthetic or opioids, and also the type of pain assessment which can be either at rest or dynamical. All these may influence its efficacy. Epidural analgesia, regardless of analgesic agent, location of catheter placement, and type and time of pain assessment, provided better postoperative analgesia compared with parenteral opioids [30]. Continuous perineural techniques have been known to offer the benefits of prolonged pain relief reducing the need for opioids and thus reducing side effects. Studies have shown the positive effects of continuous peripheral nerve blocks over PCA (patient controlled analgesia) with morphine or PCEA (patient controlled epidural analgesia) [31]. Pain relief can be attained by the conventional pharmacological option of administering opioids like morphine or fentanyl. Morphine and Fentanyl have

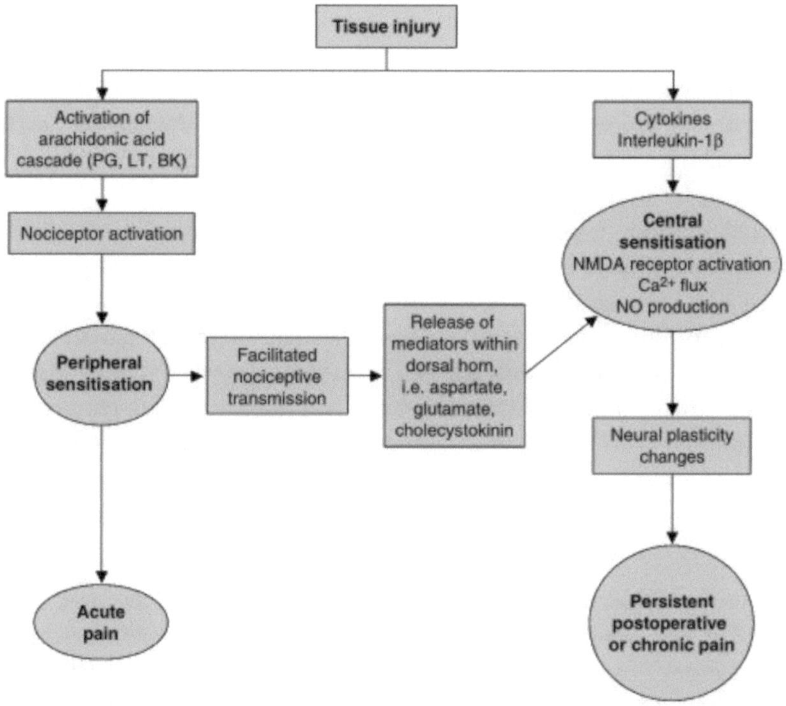

Figure 2. Figure 2 shows the sensitisation of the central nervous system and peripheral nerves. BK (bradykinins), LT (leukotrienes), NO (nitric oxide), PG (prostaglandins). [*Taken with permission from Pyati and Gan. Perioperative pain management. CNS drugs 2007; 21: 185-211*].

been the analgesic drugs of choice for anaesthesia for decades. Transdermal Fentanyl provides a non-invasive opioid pain delivery system for acute pain management. The adverse effects of such opioids are quite common and patients frequently have nausea, vomiting, pyrexia, pruritis and hypotension. Paracetamol is very effective for mild to moderate pain and given along with opioids reduces their requirements by up to 30%. Paracetamol is now regularly used i.v. intraoperatively or for post-operative pain relief. It is found to be particularly useful in paediatrics. Sodium salicylate, discovered in 1763, was the first of the NSAIDS which have been the cornerstone in acute pain relief with their opioid sparing effects. There are now over 20 different NSAIDs, from six major classes determined by their chemical structures, available. Ketorolac is particularly useful in short term management of moderate to severe pain. But as with other non-selective NSAIDS, Ketorolac may trigger allergic or hypersensitivity reactions. Careful patient selection is essential if use of Ketorolac is considered. Contraindications to its use include a history of, or current risk of, gastrointestinal bleeding, risk of renal failure, compromised haemostasis, and hypersensitivity to aspirin (acetylsalicylic acid) or other NSAIDs, labour, delivery and nursing. These can be attributed to cyclo-oxygenase (COX-1] inhibition [32]. Selective inhibition by COX-2 inhibitors like Parecoxib are significantly better and very useful in gynaecological procedures where it can be administered intraoperatively and immediately post-operatively before oral analgesics are tolerated. Ketamine enhances pain relief particularly post-operatively. It acts as an antagonist at the NMDA receptor and can be associated with pathological pain states like hyperalgesia and allodynia. Tramadol acts as a μ-opioid receptor agonist and works through a modulation of serotonin and norepinephrine. Unlike other opioids Tramadol lacks respiratory depressant effects and carries a lower risk for bowel dysfunction. Pain relief by epidural and spinal anaesthesia or combined spinal-epidural anaesthesia have found major success in obstetric procedures because of the major advantage over general anaesthesia and thus the parturient can stay awake during a caesarean section. They are very useful in covering intra and post-operative pain for lower limb, abdominal and thoracic surgery. Although not shown to decrease pain score greatly or need for rescue analgesia, infiltration of the wound with local anaesthetics by the surgeon following a surgical procedure can help for immediate temporary pain relief. A similar technique with conflicting reports is intra-articular injection of analgesics especially following arthroscopic procedures. A systematic review revealed that intra-articular injections provide moderate pain relief for a short duration [33].

A more definite method of post-operative pain relief are peripheral nerve blocks. With the availability of direct visualisation by ultrasound, nerve blocks are becoming very popular for their precision and accuracy for pain relief. Continuous infusion of local anaesthetic agents through catheters provide adequate post-operative pain relief in both hospital and ambulatory settings reducing hospital stay and post-operative complications significantly. As novel analgesic therapies using Gabapentin, naloxone and nalbuphine make their way into therapy of neuropathic pain, newer non-pharmacological techniques like acupuncture, yoga, relaxation techniques, music therapy and hypnosis are becoming very popular.

Adequate multimodal pain relief requires knowledge and understanding of pain pathways and correct application of a combination of various techniques can be very beneficial to the patient, the institution and as a result for the state.

Author details

Subhamay Ghosh
Anaesthetics and Intensive Care, Kettering General Hospital. University of Leicester, UK

4. References

[1] Perl ER. Ideas about pain, a historical view. Nat Rev Neurosci. 2007; 8: 71-80.
[2] Jaros JA. The concept of pain. Crit Care Nurs Clin North Am. 1991; 3: 1-10.
[3] Sabatowski R, Schäfer D, Kasper SM et al. Pain treatment: a historical overview. Curr Pharm Des. 2004; 10: 701-16.
[4] Cohen MM - The history of opium and opiates. Tex Med, 1969;65:76-85.
[5] Booth M - Opium - a History, New York, St Martin's Griffin, 1998.
[6] Baraka A - Historical aspects of opium. Middle East J Anesthesiol, 2000;15:423-436

[7] Booth, Martin. Opium a History. London: Simon & Schuster, 1996.
[8] Bonica JJ. History of pain concepts and pain therapy. Mt Sinai J Med. 1991; 58: 191-202.
[9] Melzack R, Katz J. The Gate Control Theory: Reaching for the Brain. In: Craig KD, Hadjistavropoulos T. Pain: psychological perspectives. Mahwah, N.J: Lawrence Erlbaum Associates, Publishers; 2004.
[10] Ashby JS, Lenhart RS: Prayer as a coping strategy for chronic pain patients. Rehabil Psychol 39:205-209, 1994
[11] Keefe FJ, Affleck G, Lefebvre JC, et al. Coping strategies and coping efficacy in rheumatoid arthritis: A daily process analysis. Pain 69:43-48, 1997
[12] Harrison MO, Edwards CL, Koenig HG, et al. Religiosity/spirituality and pain in patients with sickle cell disease. J Nerv Ment Dis 193:250-257, 2005.
[13] Skevington SM, Carse MS, Williams AC: Validation of the WHOQOL-100: Pain management improves quality of life for chronic pain patients. Clin J Pain 17:264-275, 2001.
[14] Whitman SM. Pain and suffering as viewed by the Hindu religion. J Pain. 2007; 8: 607-13.
[15] Abulfadl Mohsin Ebrahim. Islamic perspective of Euthanasia. JIMA. 2007; 39: 173-178.
[16] Young A. Natural death and the work of perfection. Christ Bioeth. 1998; 4: 168-82.
[17] International Association for the Study of Pain: Pain Definitions [cited 10 Sep 2011]. "Pain is an unpleasant sensory and emotional experience associated with actual or potential tissue damage, or described in terms of such damage" Derived from Bonica JJ. The need of a taxonomy. Pain. 1979; 6: 247–8.
[18] American Society of Anesthesiologists. Practice Guidelines for the Management of Acute Pain in the Perioperative Setting. ASA, 1995.
[19] Wu CL, Richman JM. Postoperative pain and quality of recovery. Curr Opin Anaesthesiol. 2004; 17: 455-60.
[20] Dolin SJ, Cashman JN, Bland JM. Effectiveness of acute postoperative pain management: I. Evidence from published data. Br J Anaesth. 2002; 89: 409-23.
[21] Gottschalk A, Smith DS, Jobes DR, et al. Preemptive epidural analgesia and recovery from radical prostatectomy: a randomized controlled trial. JAMA 1998; 279: 1076–82.
[22] Strassels SA, Chen C, Carr DB. Postoperative analgesia: economics, resource use, and patient satisfaction in an urban teaching hospital. Anesth Analg. 2002; 94: 130-7.
[23] Pyati S, Gan TJ. Perioperative pain management. CNS Drugs. 2007; 21: 185-211.
[24] Sorkin LS, Wallace MS. Acute pain mechanisms. Surg Clin North Am. 1999; 79: 213-29.
[25] Kehlet H, Dahl JB. The value of "multimodal" or "balanced analgesia" in postoperative pain treatment. Anesth Analg. 1993 Nov;77(5):1048-56.
[26] Altman RD. A rationale for combining acetaminophen and NSAIDs for mild-to-moderate pain. Clin Exp Rheumatol. 2004; 22: 110-7.
[27] Spaulding TC, Fielding S, Venafro JJ, Lal H. Antinociceptive activity of clonidine and its potentiation of morphine analgesia. Eur J Pharmacol. 1979; 58: 19-25.
[28] Bjordal JM, Johnson MI, Ljunggreen AE. Transcutaneous electrical nerve stimulation (TENS) can reduce postoperative analgesic consumption. A meta-analysis with

assessment of optimal treatment parameters for postoperative pain. Eur J Pain. 2003;7(2):181-8.

[29] Mulvey MR, Radford HE, Fawkner HJ, et al. Transcutaneous Electrical Nerve Stimulation for Phantom Pain and Stump Pain in Adult Amputees. Pain Pract. 2012 Aug 30.

[30] Block BM, Liu SS, Rowlingson AJ, et al. Efficacy of postoperative epidural analgesia: a meta-analysis. JAMA. 2003; 290: 2455-63.

[31] Singelyn FJ, Gouverneur JM. Postoperative analgesia after total hip arthroplasty: i.v. PCA with morphine, patient-controlled epidural analgesia, or continuous "3-in-1" block?: a prospective evaluation by our acute pain service in more than 1,300 patients. J Clin Anesth. 1999; 11: 550-4.

[32] Reinhart DI. Minimising the adverse effects of ketorolac. Drug Saf. 2000; 22: 487-97.

[33] Moiniche S, Mikkelsen S, Wetterslev J, et al. A systematic review of intra-articular local anesthesia for postoperative pain relief after arthroscopic knee surgery. Reg Anesth Pain Med. 1999; 24: 430-7.

Chapter 2

Work-Related Upper Limb Pain and Its Diagnosis: Contribution from the Neurological Examination

Jørgen Riis Jepsen

Additional information is available at the end of the chapter

http://dx.doi.org/10.5772/50884

1. Introduction

Painful upper limb conditions affect more than 1/5 of the adult population. They have a major influence on the level of functioning and cause significant social costs. Being regarded as frequently work-related, many of these disorders are potentially preventable.

Clinicians are often challenged with respect to the diagnosis, treatment and prevention of upper limb disorders. One reason for this is the lack of consensus on diagnostic case definitions and the unknown or poor validity of many of the applied physical diagnostic tests [1,2]. Diagnostic case definitions are important for epidemiological as well as clinical purposes. Their value lies in their practical utility in distinguishing groups of people with the same symptoms and/or physical characteristics or whose illness share the same causes or determinants of outcome. This means that the best case definition for a disorder may vary according to the purpose for which it is being applied [3]. Never the less, we need valid case definitions for clinical purposes as well as for surveillance and preventive purposes. The prognosis in potential scenarios should also be known, such as with various future work-demands and exposures [4].

We have made little progress with regard to all those issues over the last decades. Ignorance to the role of the peripheral nerves in upper limb pain conditions may be one of the reasons for this inadequacy.

It has been estimated that 75 % of work-related upper limb disorders are not covered by diagnostic criteria [5]. Therefore they are often described as "non-specific", "repetition strain injury" or, e.g. as "mouse arm", which may suggest causation but neither the responsible pathology nor its location.

1.1. The conventional physical approach to upper limb patients

The conventional physical approach to upper limb patients is often insufficient. It is basically based on the traditions in e.g. orthopedic surgery to identify conditions such as tendinitis, epicondylitis, or osteoarthritis and among rheumatologists to relate pain conditions to inflammatory joint and muscle disorders. Unless there are clear and severe pareses or sensory disturbances, neurologists tend to follow the same path and relate upper limb pain to similar disorders of insertions or muscles – in particular when subsequent imaging and electrophysiological assessment have not been helpful.

A few typical examples of common interpretations will be provided:

- *Relating to location of symptoms:* Lateral elbow pain or shoulder pain may be attributed to lateral epicondylitis or rotator cuff tendinitis without meeting the criteria for these conditions. There is often no apparent consideration and mostly no exclusion of potential alternative causes for the pain.
- *Relating to localized soreness:* Pain may in broad terms be attributed to tendinitis or to a myofascial disorder even without the identification of the involved tendon(s) (e.g. "forearm tendinitis") or muscle(s) (e.g. myofascial pain in the neck or shoulders). Alternative causes are rarely considered and excluded. Indications of e.g. tendinitis such as swelling, redness etc. are usually absent in these patients.
- *Relating to the character of pain, or parestesia:* Carpal tunnel syndrome is always considered. When carpal tunnel syndrome is excluded, the next step tends to be a focus on the potential presence of cervical root compression. Following further investigations such as electrophysiological or imaging, the clinician frequently tends to exclude a neurological condition and to leave the patient untreated. In many of these patients the pain is now regarded as deriving from muscles or – in case of being mainly located at the elbow or shoulder – possibly as relating to insertional tendinitis. The intermediate portion of upper limb nerves with an extension of almost one meter tends to be ignored. If laboratory studies do suggest a neuropathic condition, patients may be treated accordingly (e.g. with carpal tunnel surgery). Other patients may still receive such treatment in spite of negative laboratory examinations and with variable results.
- *Relating to weakness or sensory abnormalities:* There is a tendency to attribute muscular weakness to the presence of pain ("pain-induced weakness") even in the absence of pain/pain provocation during testing of a specific muscle. Similarly, sensory abnormalities that involve several dermatomes or the cutaneous innervation-territories of several peripheral nerves tend to be termed "diffuse". With painful testing of a muscle, alternative painless testing of other muscles with the same innervation is rarely done. The possibility of simultaneous afflictions of several upper limb nerves, or of the brachial plexus is also rarely considered in patients presenting with a challenging pattern of sensory abnormalities.

In summary, clinicians examining upper limb patients tend to direct their main attention to tendons, muscles or insertions rather than to the peripheral nerves. Practitioners in occupational medicine tend to follow the same track as orthopedic surgeons, rheumatologists, and neurologists. Consequently patients with work-related upper limb complaints are likely to be diagnosed as, e.g. tendinitis, epicondylitis, or a myofascial condition – even in the absence of objective evidence to support these diagnoses (or patients are not diagnosed at all) rather than being diagnosed with a disorder confined to or involving the nerves.

In addition, there is a tendency to focus on the location where the symptoms dominate (but where the disease is not necessarily located), and to neglect that the disease may be situated elsewhere. This is unfortunate since the location of the disease may well be distant to symptoms – in particular in case of a neurological condition.

1.2. Neuropathic upper limb pain

The pain in many upper limb conditions – including many "non-specific" conditions – is frequently of a neuropathic character. The pain typically worsens following use when the arm is at rest, such as during the night. Another characteristic feature is the tendency for the pain to move from one location to another. The presence of muscle weakness/fatigue, parestesia and/or other sensory disturbances, and the inadvertent loss of handgrip are other common complaints. All these symptoms are compatible with a neuropathic condition such as an affliction of the upper limb peripheral nerves at one or several locations.

Therefore, the conventional physical examination (inspection, movement, palpation of muscles and tendons, etc.) should be supplemented with an examination of representative physical items that reflects the function of the peripheral nerves.

The clinical neurological examination is based on a classical paradigm which is accepted by all physicians. Still, it is rarely applied in a comprehensive manner. While the neurological upper limb examination usually includes an evaluation of items such as handgrip force, fingertip sensibility and the Tinel sign at the volar wrist, the examination does not always represent a systematic and detailed approach to the upper limb peripheral nerves. One example is the bedside examination of strength in representative upper limb muscles. Manual muscle testing seems to be forgotten or discredited – perhaps because of an unjustified confidence in the potentials of electrophysiological assessment of the peripheral nerves [6]. Therefore, patients may be misinterpreted, misdiagnosed and consequently not offered the proper treatment.

A precise diagnosis is an essential prerequisite for treatment as well as prevention, and requires the identification of the involved tissue and where it is located, and of the character of the involved pathology. This task is not always easy but it always requires an examination that reflects the symptoms.

This review describes an easy neurological screening approach to the upper limb patient based on manual testing of nine muscles.

1.3. Studies of upper limb patients and exposed workers

Previous studies have demonstrated the reliability of a comprehensive neurological examination, which included manual testing of the individual and patterns of strength in a representative sample of upper limb muscles. Strength (14 muscles), sensibility to touch, pain and vibration (seven territories), and mechanosensitivity of nerve trunks (ten locations) were predominantly assessed with moderate to very good reproducibility (median κ-values 0.54, 0.69, 0.48, 0.58, and 0.53, respectively). In addition, neurological patterns could be reliably identified (median correlation coefficient 0.75) [7,8].

The examination permitted the classification of each of 82 upper extremities as with or without any of the defined neurological patterns with a high agreement (kappa = 0.75) [7,8]. This is an acceptable reliability, which is in fact superior to that of other parts of the neurological examination that one usually trusts, e.g. the Babinski sign [9]. This examination had a high predictive ability in terms of distinguishing between symptomatic and non-symptomatic limbs (positive/negative predictive values of 0.93/0.90 in limbs with agreement between the two blinded examiners) [10].

Using this approach indicated that upper limb peripheral nerve afflictions were frequently responsible for work-related upper limb pain in the majority of the examined upper limb patients in a hospital based clinic of occupational medicine [10], general practice[11], and occupational groups such as computer operators [12]. The infraclavicular part of the brachial plexus, the posterior interosseous nerve at the edge of the supinator muscle, and the median nerve at elbow level were the most common locations of nerve afflictions, and these locations were often combined in the same limb [7,8,10].

The high frequency of relatively clear neurological patterns in accordance with afflictions at various locations within the brachial plexus is in accordance with a few reports of plexopathy in a work-related context [13-15]. Brachial plexopathy is, however, still regarded by many as a rare condition or as a condition that cannot be diagnosed by a physical examination. The previous studies also indicated that the isolated occurrence of carpal tunnel syndrome and of ulnar nerve entrapment at the elbow level, both of which are generally regarded as the most frequent upper limb nerve entrapments, seem to have less importance as work-related conditions [8].

Exit position for the physical examination	Muscles (Innervation)
Position I (Figure 2)	Pectoral (Ventral thoracic nerves)
	Posterior deltoid (Axillary nerve)
Position II (Figure 3)	Biceps brachii (Musculocutaneous nerve)
	Triceps (Radial nerve)
Position III (Figure 4)	FCR (Median nerve)
	ECRB (Radial nerve)
	APB (Median nerve)
	ECU (Posterior interosseous nerve)
	ADM (Ulnar nerve)

Table 1. The studied muscles and their innervation. The shaded fields indicate the three antagonist pairs of muscles. Abbreviations: See text

These experiences may be useful for others – not least with regard to the many upper limb pain conditions that cannot otherwise be explained by the current diagnostic approaches. Therefore, a review will be provided on the techniques for the manual testing of muscle strength in a few representative upper limb muscles. Manual muscle testing is now an integrated routine in the author's physical examination of patients with upper limb complaints in an occupational context.

1.4. The neurological examination

The upper limb neurological examination is based primarily on a systematic semi-quantitative examination of the following items, of which the first is regarded as the most important:

- Manual assessment of the strength in selected indicator muscles [7,16] (Table 1).
- Mechanosensitivity of nerve trunks at locations where they tend to be compromised. This may be assessed by the demonstration of mechanical allodynia of nerve trunks by mild pressure [8] (Figure 1).
- The sensibility in homonymously innervated cutaneous territories can be evaluated through an assessment of the perception of, e.g. touch, pain or vibratory stimulation with a tuning force (256 Hz).

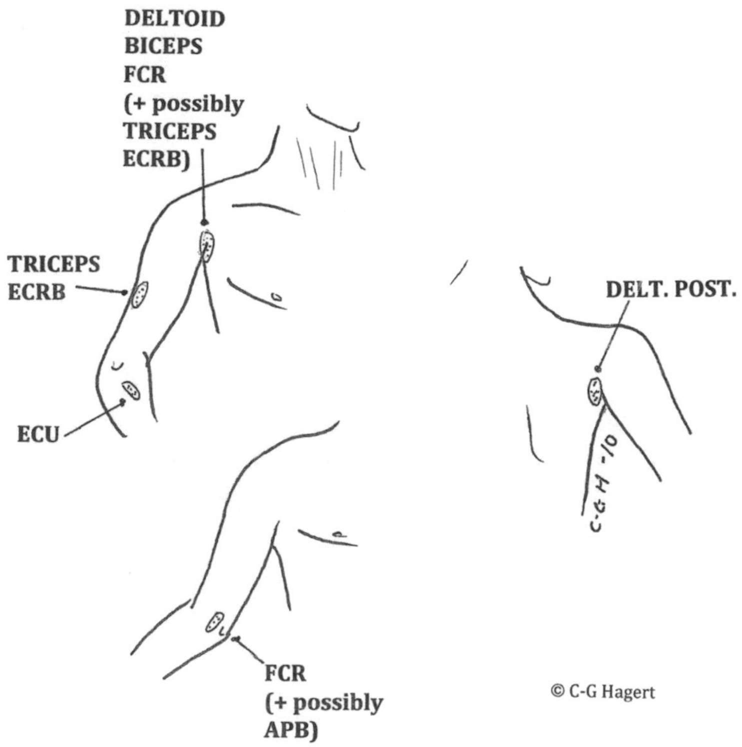

Figure 1. Locations of nerve trunks examined for mechanosensitivity. Abbreviations: See text

The neurological upper limb examination requires a familiarity with anatomy. This acquaintance is not necessarily possessed by all clinicians that meet patients with work-related upper limb complaints. I regard it as essential that the expertise must be maintained by regular lookups in textbooks, since previously acquired knowledge is easily forgotten.

The examiner should know the biomechanical function of the muscles since each of them should be tested in a position that favours its isolated action. The understanding of the neurological patterns and the palpation of nerves also requires knowledge of the motor (and sensory) innervation of each nerve, and of the location of narrow passages, where there is a particular risk of external compromise of the nerve (Figures 1, 3 - 7) [8].

The importance of testing the individual muscle strength is due to the fact that this assessment (in contrast to an evaluation of sensation) permits the examiner to locate a focal nerve affliction along the course of a nerve. Therefore, I suggest that the physical examination should always – in particular in patients with upper limb pain conditions that can otherwise not be explained – include an assessment of the strength in a number of individual muscles. These muscles should be selected to reflect the function of the upper limb nerves taking into consideration the branching and innervation pattern of each nerve. The presence of weakness in one or several muscles – and the occurrence of weaknesses in patterns in accordance with anatomic facts – strongly suggest the presence of a peripheral neuropathic condition and indicate the location along the nerve. At this location one would expect mechanical allodynia of the implicated nerve trunk.

Manual muscle testing and the interpretation of the outcomes may be regarded as complicated. This review aims to make it simple by focussing on a limited amount of muscles.

I will describe how manual testing of these muscles is performed, how the outcome is interpreted, and how this examination can contribute to the diagnosis of upper limb conditions.

1.5. Rationale

The rationale for focal diagnostics based on muscle testing is simple and would be accepted by any neurologist: Muscles innervated peripherally to a focal neuropathy such as following compression are expected to be weak while those innervated from branches leaving more proximally would tend to be intact. The following three examples illustrate the rationale.

1. *Median nerve:* A weak abductor pollicis brevis (APB) muscle but an intact flexor carpi radialis (FCR) muscle suggests a carpal tunnel syndrome. A weak FCR muscle (sometimes along with a weak APB muscle) suggests a more proximal nerve affliction, such as, e.g. of the median nerve at the elbow level (pronator syndrome) [9].
2. *Radial nerve:* A weak extensor carpi ulnaris (ECU) muscle together with intact extensor carpi radialis brevis (ECRB) and triceps muscles suggests an affliction of the posterior interosseous nerve at the edge of the supinator muscle (radial tunnel syndrome). Weak

triceps and ECRB muscles suggest a more proximal affliction, such as, e.g. of the radial nerve at the triceps arcade at the midst upper arm (in which case the ECU tends to be intact).

3. *Ulnar nerve:* A weak abductor digiti minimi muscle (ADM) suggests an ulnar nerve affliction, the level of which, however, cannot be defined without examining an extra muscle, the flexor digitorum profundus to the small finger (FDP V). If that muscle is weak, the affliction will be at the elbow level, cubital tunnel syndrome, whereas, if intact, the affliction will be at the wrist level, Guyon's canal.

When a nerve is focally affected by compressive or tensile forces, one would also expect an abnormal tenderness (mechanical allodynia) on palpation of the nerve trunk at the site of affliction/compression. I therefore search for this phenomenon by palpating the nerves at locations known from experience as critical (Figure 1). The assessment of abnormal nerve trunk tenderness must take into account that nerves located superficially are easily palpated while palpation may be more difficult with deeply located nerves.

1.6. Muscles in the neurological examination

In the upper limb we have 60 muscles. The examination of all of these takes a long time and is not necessary. A previous validation study dealt with 14 muscles [7] but even this number may be regarded as difficult to deal with and time consuming for many clinicians.

Therefore manual testing of the strength in nine muscles only is proposed:

- Six muscles representing three antagonist pairs (flexors – extensors) (Table 1) are tested in the following succession: Pectoral – Posterior deltoid; Biceps – Triceps; FCR – ECRB.
- This is followed by testing of three additional individual muscles: ECU, APB and ADM.

In order to make the examination as comprehensive and accessible as could possibly be, it is additionally proposed to examine for the presence of mechanical allodynia of nerve trunks at the locations indicated in Figure 1.

2. Physical examination

2.1. The technique for manual muscle testing of the three antagonist muscle pairs

The strength in each muscle is manually assessed and compared in between the two sides by simultaneous examination on the two sides. In case of bilateral afflictions, the observed strength is compared with the expected taking into consideration the sex, age and constitution of the examined subject. The patient is examined while comfortably seated in a chair without armrests.

The three individual antagonist muscle pairs are evaluated from proximal to distal, each with a standard position of the upper limbs (Table 1, Figures 2-4) [8]:

Position I (Figure 2)

The patient's arms are elevated horizontally forward, with the elbows kept fully extended, the forearms pronated, the wrists kept at neutral and the hand clenched. Standing in front of the patient, arm adduction (Pectoral muscles) and abduction (Posterior deltoid) is tested by applying force against the patient's wrists from inward out and from outward in, respectively. The preferred exit position for testing of the posterior deltoid is to have the patient keep the arms 30 degrees outward.

Position II (Figure 3)

The patient's upper arms are now kept along the sides of the chest, the elbows flexed at a right angle with the forearms pointing forward and kept at neutral position, the wrists kept at neutral and the hands clenched. Standing in front of the patient, the examiner leans forward toward the patient's wrists, asking the patient to "carry" the examiner (elbow flexion, defined as Biceps brachii). Standing behind the patient, the examiner lifts the patient's wrists upward (Triceps) against the patient's resistance.

Position III (Figure 4)

The patient leans forward, resting the forearms on the thighs with the wrists just distal to the knees. First, the patient's forearms are fully supinated. With the patient's hands clenched and the wrists slightly flexed, the examiner leans forward, pressing toward the proximal interphalangeal joint knuckles of the index and long fingers to extend the wrists of the patient (FCR). Then the patient's forearms are fully pronated. The patient keeps the hands open and the wrists extended while the examiner leans forward and presses against the knuckles of the index and long fingers to flex the patient's wrists (ECRB).

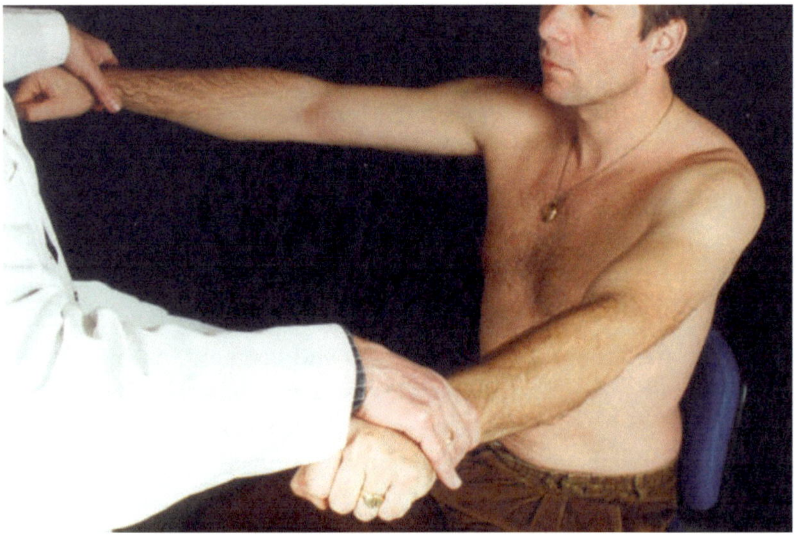

Figure 2. Position I. Testing of the posterior deltoid muscle

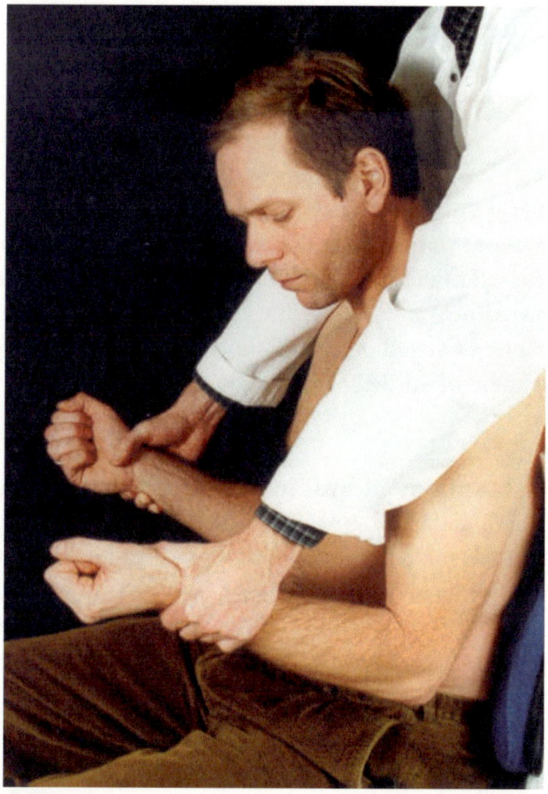

Figure 3. Position II. Testing of the triceps muscle

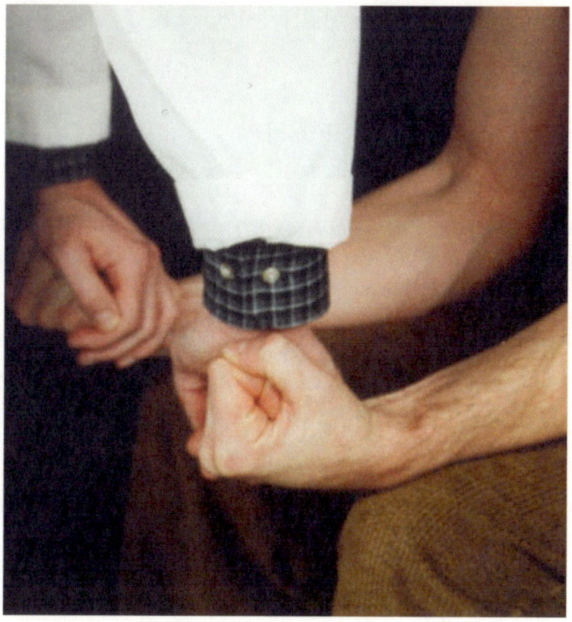

Figure 4. Position III. Testing of the FCR muscle. Abbreviations: See text

2.2. Interpretation of the outcome of the testing of the three antagonist muscle pairs

Position I (Figure 2)

Being innervated through all the cervical roots, the major pectoral muscle is mostly kept intact in cases of peripheral upper limb nerve afflictions. Therefore, a normal strength in this muscle provides evidence on patient cooperation and we can rule out malingering. This is why I prefer to start the examination with testing of the pectoral muscle. A weak deltoid muscle may be due to an affliction of the axillary nerve in isolation or of the brachial plexus (Figure 5). The assessment of whether the C5 and C6 root is involved may rely on other findings, including weakness of additional muscles (Figure 6).

Position II (Figure 3)

Weakness of the biceps brachii or triceps muscle (or of both muscles) may be due to an involvement of the musculocutaneous nerve and/or the radial nerve at upper arm level, respectively, or (more often) of the brachial plexus. The latter is particularly likely if a deltoid weakness has already been demonstrated (Figure 5). A cervical root impingement is less likely with weakness in both muscles, since this would require the involvement of multiple roots (Figure 6).

Position III (Figure 4)

Weaknesses in the FCR and the ECRB muscles may be due to a brachial plexopathy. A brachial plexus involvement may be suspected when a deltoid weakness has already been demonstrated. Weaknesses of any of the two muscles can also occur in isolation. Of particular importance in this context is the weakness of FCR, which indicates a median nerve affliction at the elbow level (Figure 7).

2.3. Examination of three additional muscles

The examination of the three antagonist muscle pairs captures a major part of the upper limb peripheral nerve-morbidity including many upper limb conditions that cannot be identified with a standard physical approach ("non-specific" upper limb disorders, "repetition strain disorders").

However, this examination cannot identify frequent entrapment neuropathies such as radial tunnel syndrome, carpal tunnel syndrome and ulnar nerve compression. This requires study of the strength of the ECU, APB and ADM muscles, respectively.

The testing of these three muscles is also simple. The distal part of the patient's forearm is firmly held by the examiner's one hand while pressing the ulnar-deviated wrist in the radial direction (ECU) (Figure 8). The patient brings the thumbs into opposition and the examiner presses them down toward the palms (APB) (Figure 9). While the patient has the small finger abducted, the examiner applies pressure at the tip of the finger in the radial direction toward the ring finger (ADM) (Figure 10).

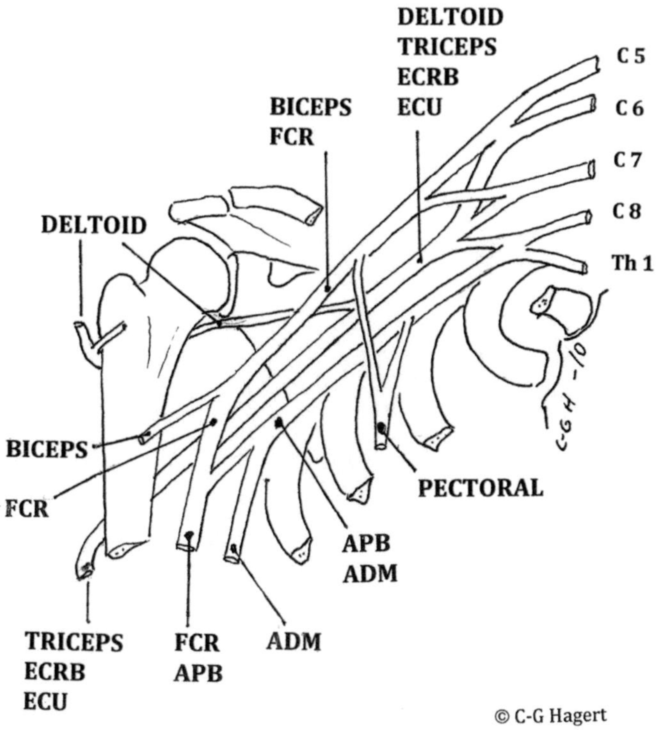

Figure 5. Brachial plexopathy. Abbreviations: See text

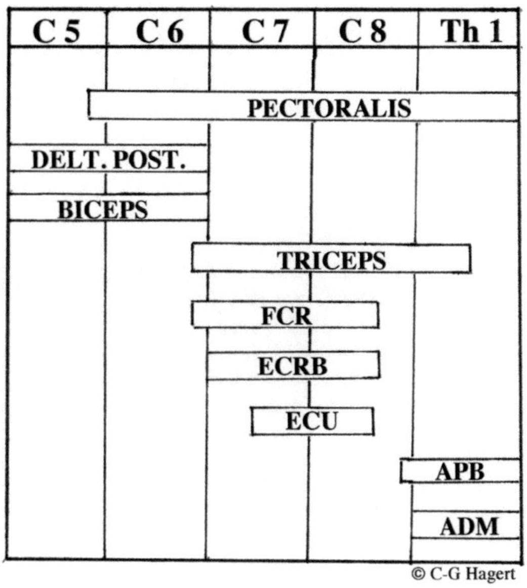

Figure 6. The innervation of upper limb muscles from the roots forming the brachial plexus. Abbreviations: See text

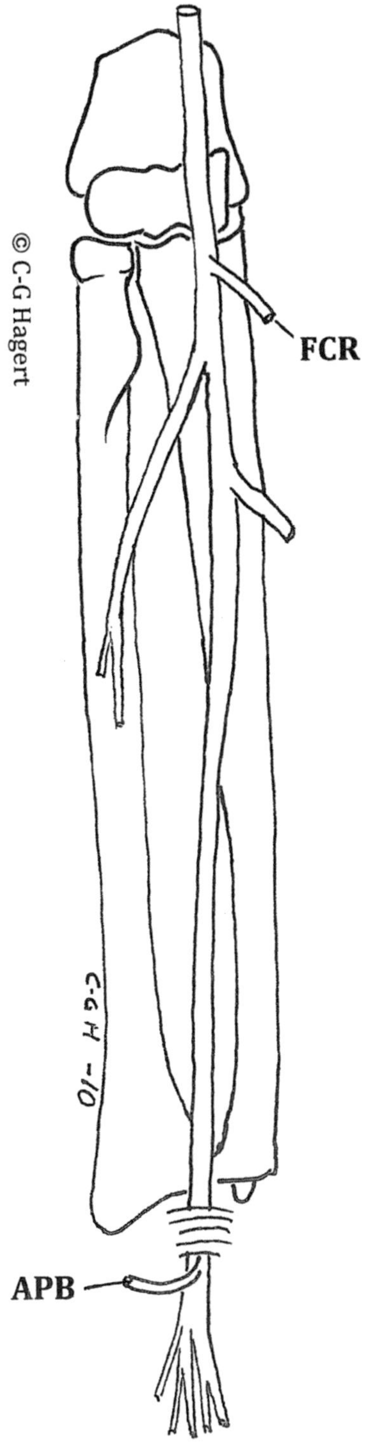

Figure 7. Median neuropathy. Abbreviations: See text

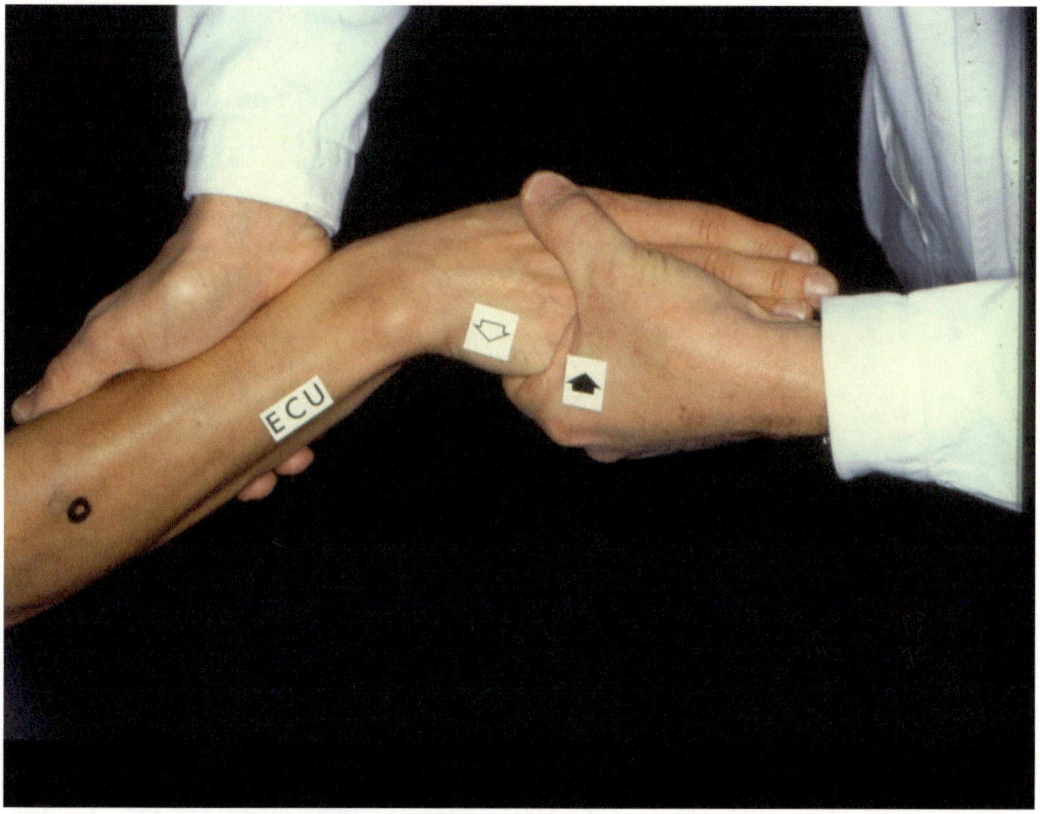

Figure 8. Testing of the ECU muscle

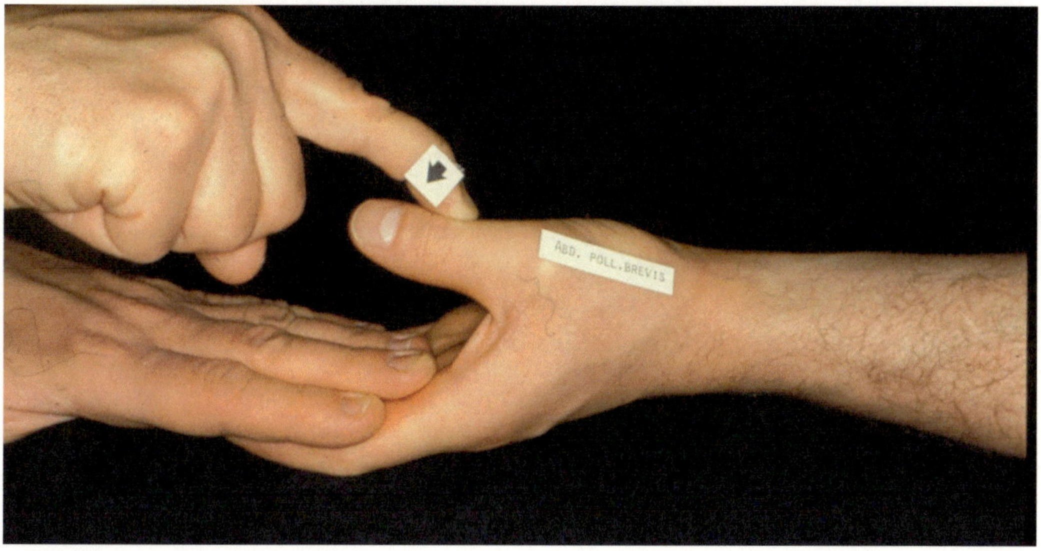

Figure 9. Testing of the APB muscle

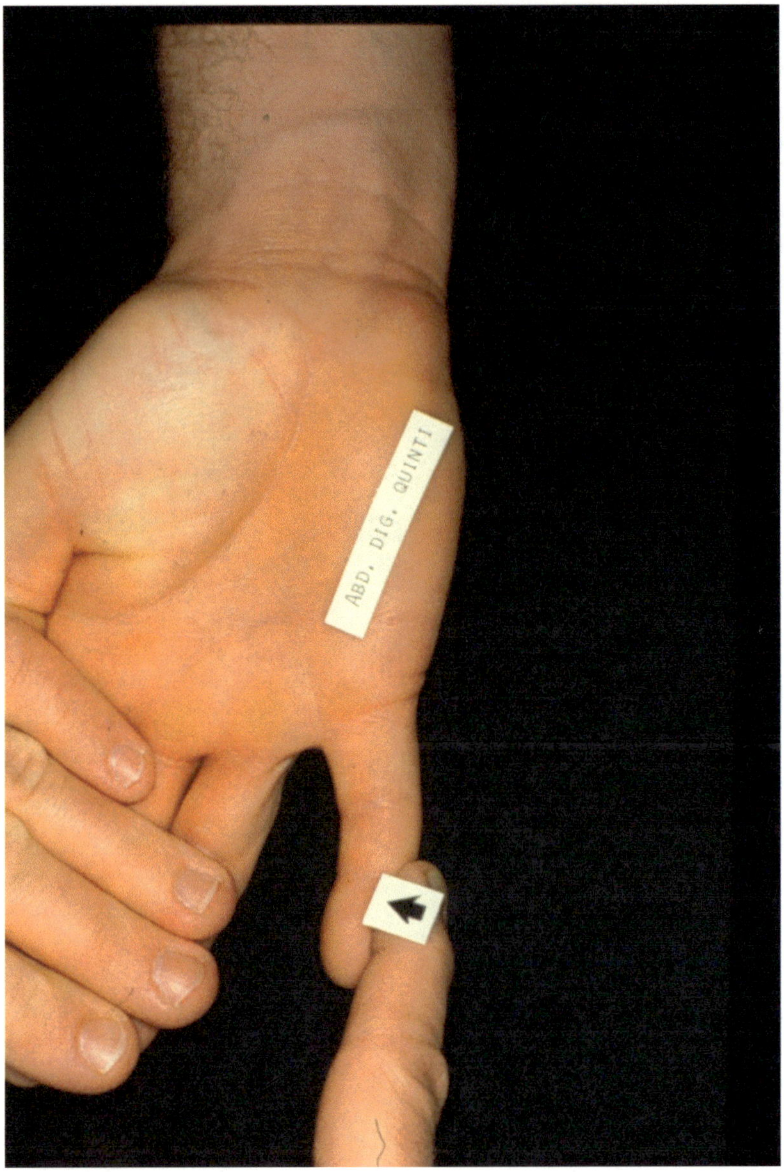

Figure 10. Testing of the ADM muscle

2.4. Interpretation of the outcome of testing three additional muscles

A weak ECU indicates a radial tunnel syndrome (Figure 11). APB weakness indicates a carpal tunnel syndrome. It should, however, be noted that an isolated carpal tunnel syndrome requires an intact FCR (Figure 7). A weak ADM indicates an ulnar nerve involvement, either at the elbow level (in which case the strength in the FDP V will also be reduced) or at the wrist level (in which case the FDP V will be found normal) (Figure 12).

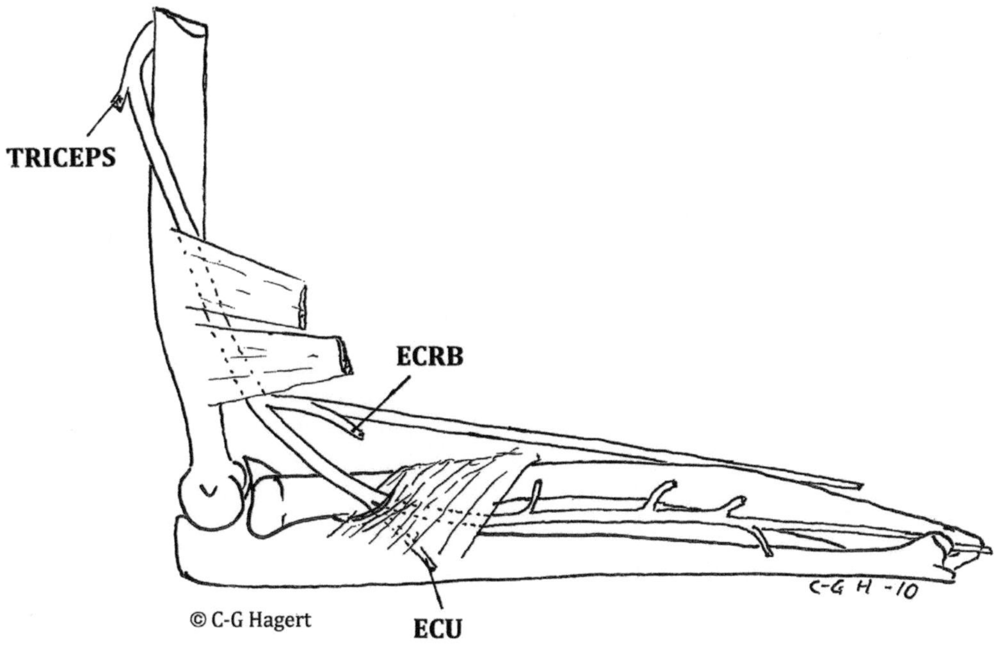

Figure 11. Radial/posterior interosseous neuropathy. Abbreviations: See text

2.5. Consequences of the examination

If weakness is found in one or more of these nine muscles, focal neuropathy cannot be excluded. In this case, further muscles with the same innervation are to be tested. With the identification of individual or patterns of weakness that may reflect peripheral nerve affliction(s), one would expect mechanical allodynia of nerve trunks at the implicated locations and this feature should therefore be looked for (Figure 1).

Due to the rarity of other locations of nerve afflictions of the upper limb, focal upper limb neuropathy can be excluded with a high certainty if all nine muscles are intact and of equal strength bilaterally. Therefore, it is recommended that these muscles are routinely investigated in all upper limb patients.

2.6. Validity of the examination

As previously demonstrated, the strength in these nine muscles can be reliably assessed by blinded manual testing of individual muscles (median κ-value = 0.56 (range 0.33-0.72)). Patterns of weakness (in combination with sensory deviations from normal and mechanical allodynia of nerve trunks at locations appropriate to the innervation and course of nerves) were also reliably assessed (median κ-value = 0.77 (range 0.83-0.70) [7].

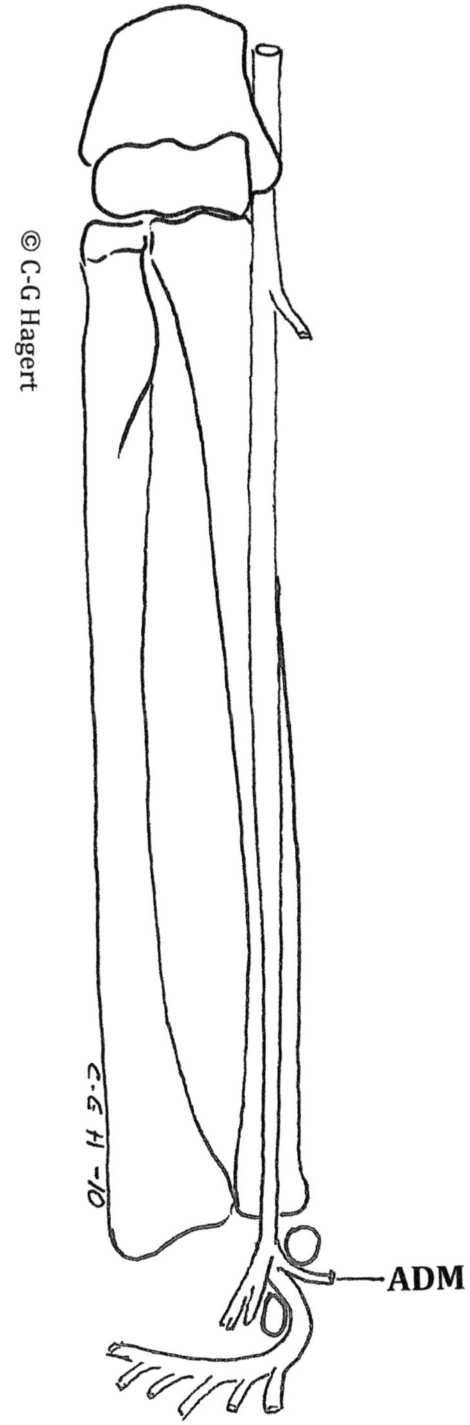

Figure 12. Ulnar neuropathy. Abbreviations: See text

If the examination was limited to just six muscles (the three antagonist pairs, Table 1) the diagnostic sensitivity of the assessment with symptoms (pain, weakness and/or numbness/tingling) by each examiner was 0.92 and 0.84, respectively, but the specificity only 0.70 and 0.50, respectively. The positive/negative predictive values were calculated to 0.73/0.91, respectively, for one of two blinded examiners and 0.59/0.79 for the other. These figures indicate that an examination limited to just these muscles can identify weaknesses in almost all symptomatic limbs, and consequently demonstrate the minimal contribution of the additional examination of the three additional muscles (ECU, APB and ADM) in the studied sample, in which isolated radial tunnel syndrome, ulnar nerve entrapment, and carpal tunnel syndrome was rare [10]. However, the low sensitivity of the examination means that this limited examination cannot stand alone but must be supplemented with an examination of additional neurological parameters, notably of mechanical nerve trunk allodynia.

3. Discussion

To provide our patients with the best management, and to better prevent upper limb conditions many of which are apparently work-related, it is of importance to diagnose them correctly. This chapter presents a simple physical approach to the upper limb nerves that can contribute to do so in a reliable and accurate way.

The research and clinical experiences of our team have suggested that the majority of upper limb pain presented at a department of occupational medicine is of a neuropathic character and is caused by peripheral nerve afflictions with specific locations [7,8,10]. Application of the same physical examination in upper limb patients in the primary health sector [11], and in occupational risk groups [12,17] identified similar disorders displaying the same physical neurological abnormalities.

The locations of neuropathy was dominated by the infraclavicular brachial plexus (behind the minor pectoral muscle – pectoralis minor syndrome), the median nerve at elbow level (frequently just proximal to the elbow joint and also at times more distally, e.g. pronator syndrome), and the posterior interosseous nerve (Arcade of Frohse – radial tunnel syndrome). As also noted among computer operators with severe upper limb complaints, these three locations were often combined [17].

For several reasons, it was not feasible to confirm the observations at the physical examination by electrophysiological studies. In a validation study with multiple outcomes, e.g. nerve afflictions with many locations, it is not possible to perform an extensive bilateral examination of nerve conduction at a high number of locations and of electromyography in many muscles. It takes time, it is costly and it is very uncomfortable for the patients. Furthermore, the electrophysiological examination should always be designed from physical findings at a preceding neurological examination of sufficient meticulousness.

In addition to these constraints, many nerve afflictions including median or interosseous nerve entrapment at elbow level, and brachial plexopathy are frequently quite inaccessible by electrophysiological methods. This is due to a low sensitivity with respect to minor and mixed and partial peripheral nerve lesions that are characteristic to many of these patients [6]. The regeneration of nerve lesions may also complicate the electrophysiological assessment.

The electrophysiological examination of upper limb patients to should take these limitations into account. In the absence for example of a detailed previous physical examination, the electrophysiological examination is likely to target an irrelevant disorder, e.g. carpal tunnel syndrome when the problem is really an entrapment that is located more proximally, e.g. at elbow level or involving the brachial plexus. This is a major problem since many clinicians tend to regard electrophysiological examinations as the golden standard for upper limb focal neuropathies. Consequently, clinicians may be reluctant to trust the outcome of their own physical examination and rather regard that the truth is the outcome of the electrophysiological study, which may well be false negative or false positive. For these reasons, electrophysiological studies are not always of diagnostic help in this type of patients and to my experience may often confuse the clinician.

The presented screening examination of the upper limb nerves is reliable and valid. It consists of an assessment of the strength in nine muscles with the focus on the identification of patterns of weakness and of focal mechanical allodynia of nerve trunks.

The significance of this approach is evident from previous studies [10-12]. As an example, one third of a series of 82 pronator syndromes in 73 patients had previously undergone carpal tunnel decompression without remission and the remaining patients were given various other diagnoses. The average duration of symptoms was three years. On examination, all patients had a weak FCR. Following release of the median nerve at the elbow, 55 out of the 73 patients reported that they were free of symptoms and had regained normal strength. The remaining 18 patients had regained strength, but still complained of elbow pain [18].

Extending the examination of the three muscle antagonist pairs to include three additional muscles would be important with any possibility of a peripheral neuropathy that is not identified by weakness in the first six muscles examined. In particular, this is the situation with radial tunnel syndrome, carpal tunnel syndrome and ulnar neuropathy.

As an example of the first location of entrapment, radial tunnel syndrome, almost all 43 patients in a series of operated cases were previously misinterpreted as lateral epicondylitis because the strength in the ECU was not assessed. The average duration of symptoms in this series was 4.7 years, and the patients were over time given various kinds of treatment and even surgical release of the epicondylar muscle insertion without any positive effects. Following nerve release, 88% of the cases reported that they were symptom-free [18].

Upper limb disorders of a non-neurogenous character may occur in isolation, complicate, cause or co-exist with upper limb neuropathy. For that reason such disorders should also be examined for. E.g. brachial plexopathy may complicate shoulder tendonitis; lateral epicondylitis or radio-humeral joint inflammation may harm the adjacent radial or posterior interosseous nerves; carpal tunnel syndrome may arise secondary to increased carpal pressure from inflamed flexor tendons at the volar wrist. Upper limb nerve afflictions are, however, more often seen in isolation without other demonstrable pathology [8,11].

Although testing of the presented nine muscles enables the examiner to diagnose or (with the additional examination of the mechanosensitivity of nerve trunks) to exclude an upper limb neuropathy with a high degree of certainty, the acknowledged weaknesses of this approach should be mentioned. In addition, the consequences of diagnosing peripheral upper limb nerve afflictions in terms of management and prevention shall be discussed.

3.1. Weaknesses of the method

Manual muscle testing (and other neurological assessment) is based on comparison between the two sides. For that reason it is more difficult (but still possible [7]) to assess patients with a symmetrical bilateral disorder. Weakness in a particular muscle (or an altered cutaneous sensitivity) should not be confused with paralysis (and analgesia/anesthesia, which, however, as well as cutaneous allodynia may occur). One should rather expect mild weaknesses, some of which may even become apparent only after the deliberate attempt to eventually create fatigue by testing a specific muscle several times. Sensory changes are also mostly modest only.

Moreover, patients are different. The internal and external topography and the innervation patterns of the peripheral nerves may vary considerably in between individual patients. The internal structure of the nerves may differ with the neurons innervating a specific muscle or with afferent function from a certain cutaneous area located superficially or more centrally in the nerve. This may be of importance because superficial fascicles are more vulnerable than those protected by a deeper location within the nerve trunk. In addition, anastomoses between nerves are quite frequent, and the clinician who does not recognize this is likely to be confused by non-expected findings. These circumstances may cause physical findings to diverge considerably from drawings in anatomy textbooks. Therefore, all physical findings should be interpreted humbly.

One can speculate whether the phenomenon that I term weakness in this chapter is actually synonymous with paresis. Paresis is a condition typified by partial loss of voluntary movement or by impaired movement, and neurologists use the term paresis to describe weakness. However, a weakness may occur with many disorders or even in an individual with a poor physical condition and without the occurrence of disease in neither nerve nor muscle.

Certain situations suggest that the identification of muscle weakness does reflect a paresis: Weakness in a muscle innervated by a nerve which is abnormally sore on palpation indicates that the weakness does represent an actual paresis. A pattern of weaknesses in several muscles in accordance with anatomic facts is another feature that suggests a relation to a focal nerve affliction and therefore represents a pattern of muscular pareses. Further support may derive from the identification of sensory alteration at appropriate locations, and e.g. differences of other neurological items in between the two sides.

3.2. Consequences of the diagnosis

The prognosis of the individual patient with peripheral nerve afflictions varies but relies on a correct diagnosis, a proper treatment, the severity of disease, predisposing conditions, complications, and patient cooperation. In addition to implications for prevention and treatment, the diagnosis is essential for optimizing the prognosis and therefore for the advice given to the patient with respect to the future life and work. To the experience of the author, the mere ability to coherently and understandably explain the background for the symptoms is important for the patient – even in cases where no effective treatment is available.

Some advice with regard to management such as avoiding the provocation of pain may be common to many upper limb disorders. To the experience of the author it is of particular importance for patients with upper limb neuropathic conditions that they should not provoke the pain so that it increases after use of the upper limbs. Otherwise, repetitive pain provocation may induce chronic pain due to factors such as sensitization and central nervous system plasticity.

This advice stands frequently in contrast to suggestions to many patients from the previously involved physicians and therapists. To my experience, well-intentioned advice, e.g. on universal working out to improve the upper limb muscle strength by machines in a gym, or by swimming, may have inadvertent and potentially harmful consequences. On the other hand, selective strengthening of weak antagonists to shortened muscles that should be stretched may be indicated, and this correction of an anomalous posture may be a prerequisite for the reestablishment of muscular balance and consequently for restoring nerve mobility. This type of treatment has been advocated by others [15]. It is, however, clear that for being efficient, any treatment whether surgical, physiotherapeutic, or pharmacologic should target the specific condition for which it is indicated. Similar considerations apply for preventive intervention, e.g. at worksites.

Patients with upper limb peripheral neuropathies may be treated by physiotherapy based on neurodynamic principles. This treatment, which is only mastered by a minority of physiotherapists, aims to mobilize nerves by resolving perineurial adhesions with manual techniques. The physiotherapeutic treatment is followed by instructions to the patient about carrying out stretching exercises specified to target the diagnosed nerve affliction(s) with its specific location(s). The effect of physiotherapy based on restoring muscular balance and neuromobilization has been sparsely documented [19]. It is, however, appreciated by most patients.

Surgery can lead to fine outcomes provided a precise previous location of nerve entrapment and the application of correct operative techniques. In cases of compression of the posterior interosseous nerve at the edge of the supinator muscle (radial tunnel syndrome) [20] and/or the median nerve at elbow level (pronator syndrome) [21], long-term follow-up studies have shown excellent results of surgery [18].

The pharmacological treatment of neuropathic pain is challenging and certainly differs from that of treatment of nociceptive pain. Although it is well known that antidepressants and antiepileptics are currently the drugs of choice for neuropathic pain, paracetamol, acetylic salicylic acid and non-steroid anti-inflammatory drugs are still used extensively in spite of being largely ineffective. The tendency to treat patients with opoids when milder analgesics fail is also worrying if prior treatment with drugs directed against neuropathic pain has not been tried.

Even with reduced pain and improved function following treatment, impairment may persist. Switching to a new job or vocational rehabilitation may be necessary. Thus, only two out of 21 patients with severe computer-related upper limb pain were able to resume graphical computer work [17]. This observation emphasizes the importance of early diagnosis and treatment, and in particular of preventive interventions at worksites in order to safeguard not only the patient but also colleague workers that are exposed to the same risk factors.

3.3. Causation and prevention

Painful upper limb neuropathic conditions are frequent consequences of trauma or adverse work-exposures such as prolonged static position such as with intensive PC work [17]. The condition seems to be further exacerbated by repetitive tasks or by the use of force as is prevalent in many manual occupations such as e.g. crafts, assembly work, food industry, and cleaning. Currently, the insufficient knowledge of causality with regard to work-related neuropathic upper limb conditions implies that evidence-based prevention is not feasible. However, certain work-exposures have been previously implicated with upper limb nerve afflictions with specific locations. Werner [22] and Hagert et al. [20] have reported on rotational load of the forearm causing radial tunnel syndrome rather than epicondylitis. Stål et al. has described pronator syndrome in a high proportion of female milkers [23]. Other researchers have also dealt with the work-relatedness of ulnar neuropathy [24], carpal tunnel syndrome [25,26], and brachial plexopathy, [13,27], of which the latter in particular was prevalent in our studies [8,10,11,17].

The limited evidence base with regard to causation complicates interventions aiming to prevent the development of upper limb neuropathic conditions at workplaces. Consequently, preventive interventions have to be mainly based on clinical experiences from exposure descriptions by patients and pathophysiological reasoning. General ergonomic principles may be applied with some effect. Pain exacerbation should not be provoked, and the patient should try to minimize the use of upper limb force and speed, to ensure task-variations to the maximal extent, and to predominantly use the upper limb close to the body. Preventive systematic stretching also seems of importance [28].

4. Conclusion

Manual muscle testing is an important part of the physical examination of upper limb patients. I have presented the rationale and methods for applying manual muscle testing as a key part of the physical neurological examination emphasizing a simple, rapid and valid assessment of the strength in nine upper limb muscles. To the experience of the author, the outcome of this screening can explain symptoms in a major proportion of patients with work-related upper limb disorders including those regarded as "non-specific".

This diagnostic contribution may represent a significant step towards a better understanding of these frequent conditions, which constitutes a major diagnostic challenge to clinicians. The patient will always favour of having the condition diagnosed but of equal importance is the demonstration of a positive impact on management or prevention of the application of the examination. The latter, however, demands further studies.

Colleagues are encouraged to routinely include the presented examination in their physical assessment of upper limb patients. For a precise diagnosis, subsequent complement with a more extensive neurological examination may be required.

Author details

Jørgen Riis Jepsen
Department of Occupational Medicine, Østergade 81-83, DK-6700 Esbjerg, Denmark
Centre of Maritime Health and Safety, Institute of Public Health, University of Southern Denmark, Niels Bohrs Vej 9-10, DK-6700 Esbjerg, Denmark

Acknowledgement

Professor Carl-Göran Hagert, Lund, Sweden has developed the method of the presented and validated manual examination of muscle strength and has kindly allowed me to use his hand-drawn figures in this chapter.

5. References

[1] Marx RG, Bombardier C, Wright JG (1999) What do we know about the reliability and validity of physical examination tests used to examine the upper extremity? J Hand Surg (Am); 24 (1): 185-93.

[2] Katz JN, Stock SR, Evanoff BA, Rempel D, Moore JS, Franzblau A, et al. (2000) Classification criteria and severity assessment in work-associated upper extremity disorders: Methods matter. Am J Ind Med; 38 : 369-72.

[3] Coggon D, Martyn C, Palmer KT, Evanoff B (2005) Assessing case definitions in the absence of a diagnostic gold standard. Int J Epidemiol; 34 (4): 949-52.

[4] Hagberg M (2005) Clinical assessment, prognosis and return to work with reference to work related neck and upper limb disorders. G Ital Med Lav Ergon; 27 (1): 51-7.

[5] Palmer K, Cooper C (2000) Repeated movement and repeated trauma affecting the musculoskeletal disorders of the upper limbs. In: Baxter P, Adams P, Aw T, Cockcroft A, Harrington J, editors. Hunter's Diseases of Occupations. 9 ed. London: Arnold. p. 453-75.

[6] Krarup C (1999) Pitfalls in electrodiagnosis. J Neurol; 246 (12): 1115-26.

[7] Jepsen J, Laursen L, Larsen A, Hagert CG (2004) Manual strength testing in 14 upper limb muscles. A study of the inter-rater reliability. Acta Orthop Scand; 75 (4): 442-8.
[8] Jepsen JR, Laursen LH, Hagert C-G, Kreiner S, Larsen AI (2006) Diagnostic accuracy of the neurological upper limb examination I. Inter-rater reproducibility of findings and patterns. BMC Neurology; 6 : 8.
[9] Miller TM, Johnston SC (2005) Should the Babinski sign be part of the routine neurologic examination? Neurology; 65 (8): 1165-8.
[10] Jepsen JR, Laursen LH, Hagert C-G, Kreiner S, Larsen AI (2006) Diagnostic accuracy of the neurological upper limb examination II. The relation to symptoms of patterns of findings. BMC Neurology; 6 : 10.
[11] Laursen LH, Sjogaard G, Hagert CG, Jepsen JR (2007) Diagnostic distribution of non-traumatic upper limb disorders: vibrotactile sense in the evaluation of structured examination for optimal diagnostic criteria. Med Lav; 98 (2): 127-44.
[12] Jepsen JR, Thomsen G (2006) A cross-sectional study of the relation between symptoms and physical findings in computer operators. BMC Neurology; 6 : 40.
[13] Pascarelli EF, Hsu YP (2001) Understanding work-related upper extremity disorders: clinical findings in 485 computer users, musicians, and others. J Occup Rehabil; 11 (1): 1-21.
[14] Novak CB (2003) Thoracic outlet syndrome. Clin Plast Surg; 30 (2): 175-88.
[15] Novak CB, Mackinnon SE (2002) Multilevel nerve compression and muscle imbalance in work-related neuromuscular disorders. Am J Ind Med; 41 (5): 343-52.
[16] Hagert C-G. Clinical assessment of the upper limb nerve tree. Scandinavian Society For Surgery Of The Hand, Autumn Meeting, Malmö , 50. 1993. Ref Type: Abstract
[17] Jepsen JR (2004) Upper limb neuropathy in computer operators? A clinical case study of 21 patients. BMC Musculoskeletal Disorders; 5 : 26.
[18] Hagert C-G, Hagert E (2008) Manual muscle testing - A clinical examination technique for diagnosing focal neuropathies in the upper extremity. In: Slutsky DJ, editor. Upper extremity nerve repair - Tips and techniques: A master skills publication. American Society for Surgery of the Hand, 6300, North River Rd. Suite 600, Rosemont, IL 60018-4256. p. 451-65.
[19] Ellis RF, Hing WA (2008) Neural mobilization: a systematic review of randomized controlled trials with an analysis of therapeutic efficacy. J Man Manip Ther; 16 (1): 8-22.
[20] Hagert C-G, Lundborg G, Hansen T (1977) Entrapment of the posterior interosseous nerve. Scand J Plast Reconstr Hand Surg; 11 : 205-12.
[21] Stål M, Hagert CG, Englund JE (2004) Pronator syndrome: a retrospective study of median nerve entrapment at the elbow in female machine milkers. J Agric Saf Health; 10 (4): 247-56.
[22] Werner CO (1979) Lateral elbow pain and posterior interosseus nerve entrapment. Acta Orthop Scand; Suppl.174 .
[23] Stål M, Hagert C-G, Moritz U (1998) Upper extremity nerve involvement in Swedish female machine milkers. Am J Ind Med; 33 : 551-9.

[24] Descatha A, Leclerc A, Chastang J-F, Roquelaure Y, The Study Group on Repetitive Work (2004) Incidence of ulnar nerve entrapment at the elbow in repetitive work. Scand J Work Environ Health; 30 (3): 234-40.

[25] Roquelaure Y, Ha C, Pelier-Cady MC, Nicolas G, Descatha A, Leclerc A, et al. (2008) Work increases the incidence of carpal tunnel syndrome in the general population. Muscle Nerve; 37 (4): 477-82.

[26] Roquelaure Y, Ha C, Nicolas G, Pelier-Cady MC, Mariot C, Descatha A, et al. (2008) Attributable risk of carpal tunnel syndrome according to industry and occupation in a general population. Arthritis Rheum; 59 (9): 1341-8.

[27] Mackinnon SE, Novak CB (2002) Thoracic outlet syndrome. Curr Probl Surg; 39 (11): 1070-145.

[28] Jepsen JR, Thomsen G (2008) Prevention of upper limb symptoms and signs of nerve afflictions in computer operators: The effect of intervention by stretching. J Occup Med Tox; 3 : 1.

Chapter 3

Autonomic Regulation in Musculoskeletal Pain

David M. Hallman and Eugene Lyskov

Additional information is available at the end of the chapter

http://dx.doi.org/10.5772/51086

1. Introduction

A large number of people suffer from musculoskeletal disorders (MSDs), including regional pain in the neck-shoulder region, lower back and the upper extremities, or more widespread pain, e.g., fibromyalgia (Lindell et al. 2000; Côté et al. 2009). The 12-month prevalence for neck pain typically ranges between 30% and 50% in the general population (Hogg-Johnson et al. 2009). Chronic pain is reported by 19% of the adult European population (Breivik et al. 2006), affecting more females than men.

Chronic MSDs are characterized by a localized, regional or widespread sensation of pain affecting muscles, joints, tendons or ligaments, accompanied by symptoms such as fatigue, tenderness at palpation and muscle stiffness. Diagnoses are often based on self-reported symptoms, as adequate objective markers are difficult to obtain at an individual level (Larsson et al. 2007). Many of these disorders are thus commonly referred to as non-specific myalgias, e.g., trapezius myalgia, tension neck, cervicalgia and cervico-brachial syndrome according to the international classification for diseases (ICD). Regional pain conditions, such as neck-shoulder pain, may be accompanied by diffuse symptoms that can progressively develop into more widespread pain, e.g., fibromyalgia (Sjörs et al. 2011; Larsson et al. 2012). Research indicates the involvement of both peripheral and central mechanisms in the pathogenesis of MSDs (Arendt-Nielsen and Graven-Nielsen 2003; Johansson et al. 2003). Furthering our understanding of core mechanisms could improve prevention, diagnostics and treatment of chronic MSDs.

2. Stress-related muscle pain

The aetiology of MSDs is multifactorial, involving the interactions of physiological, psychological, behavioural and external mechanical factors. During recent years, increased attention has been directed towards the impact of psychosocial factors on musculoskeletal health. Epidemiological studies have shown an association between MSDs and a wide range of stress-related exposures, including time pressure, lack of control and influence, low social support and high perceived stress (Torp et al. 2001; Bongers et al. 2006; Christensen and Knardahl 2011). It is well established that perceived stress can be manifested in various physiological disease indicators, such as increased heart rate, elevated blood pressure, and sustained muscle activity (Lundberg et al. 1994; Vrijkotte et al. 2000). Thus, exposures that induce perceived stress seem to play an important role in both the development and perpetuation of chronic muscle pain (Linton 2000; Keijsers et al. 2010). Recent data even suggest that cardiovascular disorders are risk factors for developing chronic musculoskeletal pain (Nolet et al. 2012).

Stress can been be defined as a state in which homeostasis (maintenance of balance in the internal milieu) is- , or is perceived to be, threatened (Chrousos 2009). These threats or challenges, also termed stressors, can be of different natures, e.g., psychological, physical, and physiological, but all can trigger adaptive physiological changes in order to actively preserve homeostasis (i.e., allostasis) (McEwen 2000). The adaptive physiological stress response is coordinated by the central nervous system, resulting in an orchestrated cascade of events in the periphery (Ulrich-Lai and Herman 2009).

On the other hand, chronic or frequently repeated stress without sufficient recovery can lead to an allostatic load, the price of adaptation resulting in disease (McEwen 1998). According to McEwen, there are four different scenarios that contribute to allostatic load. First, frequently repeated exposure to multiple stressors; second, lack of adaptation (e.g., when repeated stressors elicit similar response amplitudes); third, a prolonged response due to delayed shut-down of the stress systems; and fourth, an inadequate response that leads to compensatory hyperactivity of other mediators (McEwen 2007).

Thus, both over-activity or under-activity in physiological stress systems, such as the hypothalamic-pituitary-adrenal (HPA) axis or the autonomic nervous system (ANS), which are normally involved in adaptation to different challenges, may cause significant health problems (McEwen 1998). The ANS acts as a bridge between the central nervous system and the peripheral organs, and ANS activation in response to stressors is a key element in nociceptive and anti-nociceptive mechanisms (Schlereth and Birklein 2008). Pain itself is considered a powerful stressor, and intense, chronic pain may thus cause further adaptive or maladaptive changes in the ANS or other stress systems. Within this context, muscle pain can be viewed as a stress-related disorder.

In the following sections, we will analyse the possible link between ANS regulation and chronic muscle pain.

3. The autonomic nervous system

Physical (e.g., mechanical) or psychological stressors can facilitate chronic pain due to their effects on physiological stress systems (Kalezic et al. 2003). In particular, research has paid attention to the involvement of the ANS in the initiation and maintenance of chronic muscle pain. The ANS is a key stress response system in the body and helps to maintain internal balance via rapid activation during physical and mental load. ANS regulation involves a close and harmonious interplay between its two anatomically separated divisions: the sympathetic nervous system and the parasympathetic nervous system. The sympathetic system is generally considered an excitatory system associated with energy mobilization in situations requiring high physical or mental effort, while the parasympathetic system is activated during routine activities and rest, allowing for restoration of bodily resources.

ANS effects on different target organs

- **Sympathetic activation:** increases heart rate and blood pressure; generates peripheral vasoconstriction (muscle vasodilatation) and relaxation of bronchi; stimulates secretion of adrenaline and noradrenalin from the adrenal medulla.
- **Parasympathetic activation:** reduces heart rate; contracts bronchial muscles; stimulates digestive glands and the secretion of saliva.

Although some peripheral target organs (e.g., peripheral blood vessels, kidney, and liver) react mainly to one of these autonomic systems, many organs respond to both systems, often with each system eliciting opposite effects. For example, the sinus node of the heart is affected by both the sympathetic and parasympathetic (vagal) systems. Resting heart rate is under tonic parasympathetic inhibition, which reduces heart rate from its intrinsic value as driven by the sinus node. In different conditions, heart rate can increase instantaneously with reduced parasympathetic activation, with further increases above the intrinsic state resulting mainly from sympathetic activation. It is important to note that even in low heart rate conditions, autonomic regulation involves both sympathetic and parasympathetic components, and their complex interplay leads to continuous fluctuations in beat-to-beat heart rate. These variations are termed heart rate variability (HRV), and characterize a healthy autonomic state.

A predominance of sympathetic activity, either due reduced parasympathetic tone or excessive sympathetic activation, reduces the dynamic flexibility of the ANS and results in poor adaptation to altered internal or external demands. Thus, an autonomic imbalance or dysfunction may have detrimental consequences in terms of pathological conditions (Thayer et al. 2010).

Various structures at multiple levels of the central nervous system are involved in coordinating the stress responses, which affect the periphery. The ANS does not function independently, but rather constitutes an important part of a multi-stress system that is highly integrative and involves sophisticated co-activation and interaction between different homeostatic processes, and the immune and endocrine systems, including the HPA and the sympatho-adrenomedullary axis (Ulrich-Lai and Herman 2009). In this sense, an autonomic imbalance may also reflect altered regulation of the entire stress response system.

Further, basic physiological processes, for example, muscle circulation, muscle contractility, inflammatory processes, and sensory motor control, that have been linked to chronic MSDs are influenced by autonomic reflexes (Passatore and Roatta 2006; Visser and van Dieën 2006). Although autonomic nerves do not usually modulate nociceptor activation, this may change with chronic muscle pain (Martinez-Lavin 2007).

4. Autonomic regulation in acute and chronic pain

At the central level there is a strong connection between autonomic activation and nociception (Jänig 2003; Schlereth and Birklein 2008). Studies based on brain imaging techniques show a close anatomical and functional overlap between cortical and sub-cortical structures involved in pain processing and those controlling autonomic regulation. These include, but are not limited to, the periaqueductal grey matter and rostral ventrolateral medulla located in the brainstem, thalamus, hypothalamus, and insular, anterior cingulate, prefrontal and somatosensory cortices, and the amygdala (Critchley et al. 2000; Price 2000; Apkarian et al. 2005; Thunberg et al. 2005; Benarroch 2006) as illustrated in figure 1.

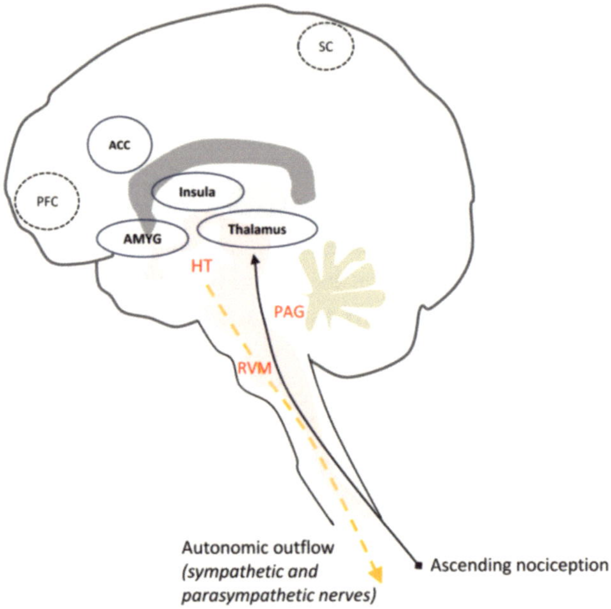

Figure 1. Simplified scheme of brain regions involved in pain processing and autonomic control, including brainstem: the periaqueductal grey matter (PAG) and rostral ventrolateral medulla (RVM), and cortical regions: thalamus, hypothalamus (HT), amygdala (AMYG) and the insular, anterior cingulate (ACC), prefrontal (PFC) and somatosensory (SC) cortices.

Studies indicate that autonomic responses to pain induced by electrical stimulation or heat are associated with brain activity in the cingulate and insular cortices (Dubé et al. 2009; Piché et al. 2010). Interestingly, higher brain activity in these brain regions has also been observed in patients with chronic pain, a condition previously assumed to be related to altered autonomic activity (Malinen et al. 2010).

Pain has a strong emotional component. This is manifested centrally via the involvement of the amygdala, which integrates polymodal information from different levels of the pain neuraxis, and attaches emotional significance to nociceptive stimuli. In turn, the amygdala projects to the hypothalamus, which is responsible for autonomic and neuroendocrine responses, and to the brainstem areas involved in endogenous pain modulation (Neugebauer et al. 2004; Rouwette et al. 2011).

The interactions between the ANS and pain are markedly different in acute and chronic pain conditions. In a healthy state, acute pain induces sympathetic arousal. Sympathetic arousal alleviates pain, which serves an adaptive stress response. The amplitude of pain-induced sympathetic reactivity depends on the intensity of the stimulus rather than on the state of wakefulness (sleep-wake) (Chouchou et al. 2011). Repeated painful stimulation over time may result in habituation with reduced perceived pain intensity and increased pain threshold (Bingel et al. 2007); the opposite may also occur. During acute physical or psychological stress, pain is normally suppressed via the activation of the descending anti-nociceptive pathways, involving opioid-dependent and noradrenalin-dependent mechanisms (Benarroch 2006; Schlereth and Birklein 2008).

With chronic musculoskeletal pain, and also with chronic stress, the interaction between the nociceptive and autonomic systems appears to become maladapted (Bruehl and Chung 2004; Schlereth and Birklein 2008). Chronic neck-shoulder pain is associated with increased local pain intensity, and reduced pain thresholds in response to sympathetic stimulation (Ge et al. 2006). Moreover, elevated blood pressure is normally associated with greater pain inhibition, but the opposite is observed in persons with chronic low back pain, and higher blood pressure is associated with increased sensitivity to pain (Bruehl and Chung 2004). The studies suggest that this inverse relationship results from altered function of the baro-receptors, which regulate blood pressure through changes in sympathetic outflow. Another study showed that elevated resting baroreflex sensitivity was associated with hypoalgesia in healthy normotensive subjects, but not in chronic low back pain patients (Chung et al 2008), and that an alfa-2 adrenergic blockade normalized the baroreceptor-pain association among the pain afflicted subjects. Additional studies supporting this model in chronic neck-shoulder pain are still lacking.

Under certain circumstances chronic pain may also be dependent on sympathetic neuronal activity, i.e., sympathetically maintained pain (Jänig 2003; Martinez-Lavin 2012). In such circumstances, sympathetic hyperactivity may activate nociceptive afferents, contributing to widespread pain, increased sensitivity to painful (hyperalgesia) and non-painful (allodynia) stimuli, and may be associated with additional symptoms, including fatigue and sleep disorders (Martinez-Lavin 2012). Different pain conditions may be affected in different ways, either directly (e.g., sympathetic-nociceptor activation) or indirectly (e.g., vasoconstriction-vasodilatation imbalance).

Taken together, it is possible that chronic muscle pain could be maintained and intensified due to pain-induced alterations in ANS regulation, particularly through the sympathetic branch of the ANS. In the next section, we will highlight some potential mechanisms for chronic neck-shoulder pain.

5. The sympathetic nervous system in musculoskeletal pain

Different explanatory models for MSDs have focused on ANS involvement in the pathogenesis of chronic pain. Autonomic activity, particularly of its sympathetic division, can modulate muscle function and pain via several mechanisms (see figure 2). These mechanisms are not considered mutually exclusive and may interact and play different roles depending on the time course and severity of the pain.

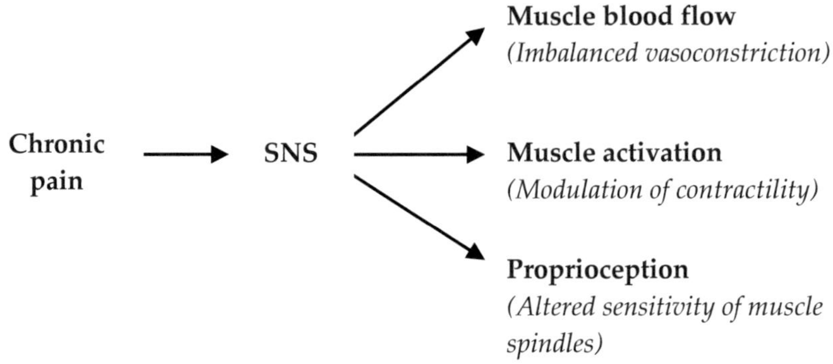

Figure 2. Local effects of sympathetic nervous system (SNS) activation induced by chronic pain

5.1. Sympathetic control of muscle blood flow

The neural control of blood flow in working muscles involves sympathetic and somatomotor interactions (Thomas and Segal 2004). Static contractions, often used in experimental protocols to assess systemic and local hemodynamics, induce sympathetic activation, which increases in proportion to the intensity and duration of muscular contractions (Saito et al. 1986). During exercise, sympathetic activation leads to vasoconstriction in skeletal muscles, and blood flow is re-directed to facilitate adequate oxygenation of working muscles. Somatomotor nerve activity leads to contraction of skeletal muscle, which generates the release of metabolites causing vasodilatation and functional hyperemia (Thomas and Segal 2004). Although other factors are also involved (e.g., central command, systemic blood pressure, and local factors), optimal regulation of muscle blood flow is highly dependent on these major components. Sympathetic reduction of blood flow in active and passive muscles has been demonstrated at different contraction intensities (Saito et al. 1986; Joyner et al. 1992; Buckwalter et al. 1997). Blood flow can also be influenced by mental stress via enhanced adrenaline secretion from the adrenal medulla into the circulating blood, resulting in β_2-adrenoreceptor mediated vasodilatation in contracting muscles (Larsson et al. 1995).

5.1.1. Insufficient blood flow regulation in chronic muscle pain

Impaired blood flow to the pain region has been observed in persons with both chronic regional and widespread pain during various provocations, e.g., cold water, needle stimulation by acupuncture, and static or dynamic contractions (Acero et al. 1999; Larsson et al. 1999; Sandberg et al. 2005; Elvin et al. 2006; Hallman et al. 2011); for comprehensive reviews on this topic see Passatore and Roatta (2006) and Vierck (2006).

In these pain conditions, it has been argued that enhanced sympathetic activity may contribute to impaired blood flow and nociceptive muscle pain due to an imbalance between vasoconstriction and vasodilatation (Passatore and Roatta 2006). When the oxygen demands are not adequately met, the muscles become ischemic and the local accumulation of metabolites may result in nociceptor activation, which, in turn, can enhance sympathetic outflow (Passatore and Roatta 2006; Vierck 2006). Hence, excessive sympathetic activation may play an important role in generation of muscle pain by mediating the response to various kinds of physical and psychological stressors. Once pain has become chronic, additional effects on ANS regulation can also be expected. First, amplification of afferent nociceptive signals may activate the sympathetic system through somato-sympathetic reflexes (Sato and Schmidt 1973); this occurs at a central level. This activation may result in further intensification of pain due to sensitization occurring at both the peripheral and central levels. Second, chronic pain is a strong psychological stressor that also activates the sympathetic system. As such, it seems possible that chronic pain can be maintained through a self-perpetuating (vicious) cycle.

Empirical support for this model is gained from studies examining widespread pain (fibromyalgia). Bengtsson and Bengtsson (1988) demonstrated that blocking the sympathetic stellate ganglions relieved pain in fibromyalgia patients, and they hypothesized that this was due to improved microcirculation. More recently, it was found, in a randomized controlled trial, that injections of norepinephrine (noradrenalin) evoked pain in fibromyalgia patients (Martinez-Lavin et al. 2002).

An alternative explanation for blunted blood flow response to stress in people with chronic muscle pain, proposed by Maekawa et al. (2002), is $ß_2$-receptor down regulation due to prolonged sympathetic activation . This would also explain a blunted blood flow response to stress, owing to a lack of vasodilatation. Further experimental and clinical studies are needed to elucidate the possible relationships between sympathetic function, impaired blood flow regulation and nociceptive sensitization in pathogenesis of chronic muscle pain.

5.2. Sustained muscle activity in chronic muscle pain

It is known that the sympathetic nervous system influences muscle contractility mechanisms (Roatta and Farina 2010). Sympathetic effects on muscle activity and motor-unit discharge rate have been observed in human experiments during fatiguing contractions and painful stimulation with cold water (Seals and Enoka 1989; Roatta et al. 2008). During acute stress exposure, skeletal muscles are activated to enable a `fight-or-flight' response involving extreme physical efforts or movements. Although this is a protective response, it may also result in sustained muscle activation or inadequate muscle relaxation, which plays an important role in the development of chronic MSDs

Studies on chronic neck pain have shown a different pattern of muscle activity as determined from electromyography (EMG) recordings, manifested in reduced muscle rest and increased activation of the neck-shoulder muscles in response to various functional tasks (Lundberg et al. 1999; Thorn et al. 2007; Johnston et al. 2008). We recently investigated autonomic and muscular responses, in subjects with chronic neck-shoulder pain and healthy controls, to sustained muscle contraction and a cold stimulation, known to provoke sympathetic activation (Hallman et al. 2011). We found that the pain group had significantly higher muscle activity during the rest period following the static contraction task, and during cold stimulation, than the control group did. The muscle activity increase in the cold condition was also correlated with pain intensity in the pain group. These findings suggest an augmented muscle response to sympathetic activation among those with chronic muscle pain. However, as we did not assess changes in muscle sympathetic nerve activity, the direct influence of sympathetic activation on muscle contractility could not be tested.

The neck-shoulder muscles are particularly susceptible to develop MSDs due to their high sensitivity to physical and mental stressors (Wang et al. 2011). For example, the trapezius muscle has been shown to be uniquely lacking in adaptation capacities to repeated stress exposures. In a recent study on healthy volunteers, the activity of different muscles was recorded by EMG during repeated exposure to mental stress (Stroop colour-word interference tests). All muscles showed lower reactivity during the second exposure except the trapezius muscles (Willmann and Bolmont 2012).

5.2.1. Stress induced muscle activity

Experimental studies have shown that mental stress can induce increased muscle activity that is unexplained by physical loads (Lundberg et al. 1994; Larsson et al. 1995). One hypothesis to explain such observations proposes that so-called low-threshold "Cinderella" motor units, which are recruited at all levels of contraction, may be especially affected by low-level mechanical loads and psychological stressors (Sjøgaard et al. 2000; Hägg 2003). In occupational settings with incorporated stress, this may result in increased low-level muscle activity and inadequate muscle relaxation, even in pauses between physical work bouts. In this way, these particular muscle fibres could become overused, and muscle fatigue and pain could develop.

Occupational tasks typically involve both physical and cognitive components. Research combining physical and mental tasks indicates a synergistic effect on trapezius muscle activity (Mehta and Agnew 2011). Further, Larsman et al. (2009) found that perceived work-related stress was positively associated with increased trapezius muscle activity and lower muscular rest during a combined mental stress and typing task. This relationship was more prominent among subjects with neck-shoulder pain (Larsman et al. 2009). However, not all studies have confirmed such effects. For instance, psychosocial exposures induced during breaks from computer keying work did not result in increased trapezius muscle activation (Blangsted et al. 2004). The interactions between physical (e.g., mechanical) and psychological exposures are complex and likely depend on many factors, including the type, duration and intensity of exposures, as well as the time pattern of alternation between work and rest. Muscle activity induced by mental or physical stress tests was also found to be correlated with cardiovascular indicators of sympathetic arousal (Lundberg et al. 1994; Krantz et al. 2004). These results may be interpreted as a `central effect´ that co-activates both the somatic and sympathetic nervous systems. In contrast, a peripheral sympathetic block did not affect pain and muscle activity in response to a stressful task (Nilsen et al. 2008).

5.3. Sympathetic nervous system involvement in sensory-motor control

Aberrant motor control has been identified as a potential factor in the continuation of chronic MSDs (Visser and van Dieën 2006). The transition from acute to chronic pain may be accompanied by alterations in motor variability. Chronic neck-shoulder pain was associated with reduced motor variability during a repetitive timing task (Madeleine et al. 2008). Chronic nociceptive stimuli may affect motor output via several mechanisms, including inhibition of motor neurons, reduced motor unit discharge rate, and compensatory activation of new motor units to maintain force production. In addition, increased sympathetic outflow induced by chronic pain, or psychological stress, can influence motor output, leading to reduced efficiency and precision of movements (Nijs et al. 2012). Studies also suggest that increased sympathetic tone may affect sensory-motor control through modulation of sensory receptors (i.e., muscle spindles) involved in afferent transmission of proprioceptive information (Johansson et al. 2003; Passatore and Roatta 2006; Nijs et al. 2012); this theory is, however, currently largely based on evidence from animal experiments.

In conclusion, an increase in sympathetic activity induced by chronic pain may contribute to pain sensitization at peripheral and central levels.

6. The parasympathetic nervous system in musculoskeletal pain

While research has mainly focused on the connection between the sympathetic nervous system and muscular pain, the involvement of the parasympathetic nervous system must also be considered. Studies have shown that parasympathetic withdrawal can facilitate sympathetic dominance of the ANS response and thus contribute to inadequate stress responses and cardiovascular adjustments during recovery following exercise, or during sleep (Gockel et al. 1995; Kingsley et al. 2009; Lerma et al. 2011).

It is known that conditions of psychological stress or pain can result in reduced parasympathetic (vagal) activity, a state that is associated with increased morbidity and all-cause mortality (Thayer et al. 2010). For instance, reduced heart rate variability (HRV) reflected diminished parasympathetic (vagal) activity in workers who reported high levels of perceived stress (Vrijkotte et al. 2000) and in people afflicted with chronic muscle pain (Martinez-Lavin 2007).

6.1. Inflammation

Studies show that inflammatory processes are modulated by the parasympathetic nervous system (Tracey 2002). During acute stress, activation of sympathetic and vagal nerves provides local and systemic anti-inflammatory effects without affecting the heart. The cholinergic anti-inflammatory pathway consists of the efferent vagus nerve and the secretion of acetylcholine. The afferent vagus provides information about the state of peripheral inflammation to the brain, resulting in compensatory vagal activation to attenuate pro-inflammatory cytokine production by the release of acetylcholine (Rosas-Ballina and Tracey 2009). Such anti-inflammatory effects have been demonstrated in response to electrical stimulation of the vagus nerve (Borovikova et al. 2000). In contrast, acute systemic inflammation may temporarily alter parasympathetic function in healthy subjects (Jae et al. 2010). In injury, or excessive overload, local inflammation may play a significant role in development of MSDs, especially in early stages (Barbe and Barr 2006). However, the possible role of the ANS as a mediator of this relationship is still unknown.

6.2. Sleep

Night time sleep is generally considered highly restorative when it is adequate. Not surprisingly, insufficient (non-restorative) sleep negatively impacts physical and mental health. Studies examining self-reports and objective measures by polysomnography report disturbed sleep as a common symptom in chronic muscle pain (Spaeth et al. 2011); this would partly explain why these individuals may experience general fatigue and tiredness (Fishbain et al. 2004). Even occasional nights with poor sleep may affect pain perception in the following days (Edwards et al. 2008). The mechanisms responsible for sleep disturbances in chronic MSDs, however, are not fully understood, and may in part be related to co-morbidity of psychological stress, depression or a reduction in physical activity. Pain is also a possible factor for sleep alterations in MSDs due to its effects on cortical and autonomic arousals (Chouchou et al. 2011).

Diurnal variations or 24-hour day-night patterns in cardiovascular autonomic regulation show higher sympathetic day-time activation, and reduced activity during sleep (non-rapid eye movement). The enhancement of parasympathetic (vagal) activation during sleep is dependent on a variety of factors, for example changes in physical activity and light, circadian biological rhythms, and coupling between sleep mechanisms and cardiovascular regulation (Trinder et al. 2012). The relationship between sleep and autonomic activity is bi-directional. During normal sleep, the cardiovascular system can exhibit brief periods of distinct activation, i.e., arousals, reflecting changes in autonomic regulation. However, poor sleep may result in a higher frequency and amplitude of nocturnal arousals, and *vice versa,* and in such circumstances, altered autonomic balance can be expected (Trinder et al. 2012).

7. Autonomic aberrations in chronic neck-shoulder pain: recent findings

Findings from clinical and applied studies show that chronic muscle pain is associated with peripheral ANS aberrations at both systemic and local levels. ANS dysfunctions have been extensively studied in patients with widespread chronic pain (Martínez-Lavín et al. 1998; Haley et al. 2004; Martinez-Lavin 2007; Reyes del Paso et al. 2010; Lerma et al. 2011) often by using ECG-based methods, e.g., heart rate variability (HRV) analyses. In general, at a group level these patients show autonomic imbalance in terms of high sympathetic activation and low parasympathetic tone at rest and blunted sympathetic response to various types of stressors (Martinez-Lavin 2007).

Our research group has recently shown similar findings among persons with regional chronic pain, as compared to symptom-free controls. In subjects with chronic low back pain, assessment of ANS regulation during a rest condition revealed higher heart rate, electrodermal activity and low frequency HRV in the pain group, indicating increased basal sympathetic activity (Kalezic et al. 2007). Individuals with whiplash-associated disorders had increased heart rate and arterial blood pressure in response to a chewing test, as compared to healthy controls (Kalezic et al. 2010).

We recently investigated autonomic responses to a battery of functional tests in persons with chronic trapezius myalgia and in healthy controls. After a 15 minute resting condition subjects performed a hand grip test, a cold pressor test and a deep breathing test, interspaced by 5 minute rest periods. Autonomic regulation was assessed using HRV, arterial blood pressure, local trapezius muscle blood (photoplethysmography) and muscle activity (electromyography). During the initial rest condition, persons with chronic pain showed reduced HRV in comparison with controls. In response to the static contraction, blunted trapezius blood flow and arterial blood pressure with simultaneous increased HRV were observed in the pain group compared with the controls (Hallman et al. 2011), reflecting aberrations in ANS regulation at both systemic and local levels. Similar results were obtained from 24-hour ambulatory monitoring of ECG in persons with chronic neck-shoulder pain and in healthy controls. Increased heart rate and diminished HRV were found during sleep, which indicated increased sympathetic and reduced parasympathetic activity among the pain afflicted individuals, in comparison with controls (Hallman and Lyskov 2010). Overall, these results indicate that regional chronic muscle pain is associated with ANS imbalance at rest, and with altered sympathetic nervous system response to laboratory stressors.

These findings were in line with an earlier observation of altered sympathetic function in persons with regional neck-shoulder symptoms, as observed from cardiovascular variables (Gockel et al. 1995). However, contradictory findings have also been reported. For example, altered cardiovascular responses to low-grade mental stress were found in fibromyalgia patients, whereas a group of subjects with neck-shoulder pain did not react significantly differently than healthy controls (Nilsen et al. 2007). More recently, a study of individuals with trapezius myalgia showed an elevated heart rate at rest but no differences in stress responses compared with controls (Sjörs et al. 2009).

Our results on local muscle blood flow were in concert with previous findings, which generally reflected insufficient muscle circulation in people with chronic neck-shoulder pain. In a series of studies, Larsson and colleagues investigated local microcirculation using laser Doppler flowmetry in patients with chronic neck pain. During static contractions, reduced microcirculation was observed in painful muscles among patients (Larsson et al. 1994). In addition, a greater reduction in blood flow was associated with a higher pain intensity and mitochondrial changes in patients (Larsson et al. 1990). Similar findings were later observed using noninvasive techniques. Acero et al. (1999) used near-infrared spectroscopy (NIRS) to assess blood volume during a cold pressor test, known to induce pain and sympathetic activation, in persons with chronic neck pain. During cold stimulation, blood volume was found to be lower in the pain group; this was interpreted as a lack of vasodilatation, possibly induced by chronic stress. In a recent study in trapezius myalgia, NIRS recordings on patients reflected reduced oxygenation of relaxed trapezius muscle in response to cycling (Andersen et al. 2010). Similar results have been shown by photoplethysmography recordings of changes in local blood flow during acupuncture (Sandberg et al. 2005). Although muscular contractions at lower intensities induced normal, or slightly aberrant, responses in subjects with neck-shoulder pain, trapezius blood flow remained increased in these patients after simulated office work (Strøm et al. 2009) and repetitive low-force exercise (Rosendal et al. 2004). Hence, a different mechanism may be involved when the physical work induces distinct sympathetic activation, which possibly did not occur in the latter studies applying low-intensity mechanical loads.

Doppler ultrasound has been used to assess vascular responses to muscular work in patients with diffuse forearm pain. Vasoconstriction of the radial artery and lack of a vasodilatory response to exercise were found in patients (Pritchard et al. 1999). Further, changes in skin temperature determined by thermography (i.e., far infrared images) showed reduced temperature in the afflicted region among patients with forearm pain, possibly reflecting sympathetic dysfunction (Sharma et al. 1997; Gold et al. 2009).

Although aberrations in autonomic regulation are relatively small and have not always been seen at the individual level, the cross-sectional findings outlined above provide convincing support for autonomic involvement at both the systemic and local levels in chronic neck-shoulder pain. Given the lack of prospective studies to date, the causal relations still remain unclear.

7.1. Difficulties in interpreting stress reactivity

Studies generally show a wide spectrum of physiological reactions to laboratory stressors, which are not easily interpreted in terms of ANS hypo- or hyper-reactivity. There are, however, several explenations that may account for this. First, there could be methodological issues related to discrepancies in application of stress stimuli (e.g., different types, intensities and durations of stressors) and varied diagnosis or exclusion criteria for patient groups. Furthermore, it is possible that there exist sub-groups of pain patients with different aetiologies and underlying mechanisms. Also, co-morbidity factors (including depression, chronic fatigue, and posttraumatic stress syndromes, frequent usage of medication) affecting autonomic function may also play significant roles in ANS reactions as similar signs of cardiovascular system aberrations are observed across a variety of stress-related disorders (Cohen et al. 2000; Newton et al. 2011; Kemp et al. 2012). Alternatively, physiological variables could be insensitive and unspecific regarding discrimination between pain and control groups, consequently masking group differences.

A second explanation for the heterogeneous results to date is the inconsistency in symptom duration, severity, and anatomical spread in pain-group participants. It has been suggested that regional chronic pain may represent an earlier stage of widespread pain (Riva et al. 2012). This may account for observations of cardiovascular hypo-reactivity in patients with fibromyalgia, and the less consistent observations among persons with chronic neck-shoulder pain. This theory is in line with the allostatic load model of chronic stress (McEwen

1998), where a hyper-reactive stress system, i.e., regional neck-shoulder pain, might progress into hypo-reactivity, i.e., widespread chronic pain, due to beta receptor down regulation (Martinez-Lavin 2007). Although this is an intriguing idea, it still needs to be verified by prospective studies.

7.2. Predictive value of heart rate variability

Measures of HRV, especially when derived from 24-h ambulatory recordings including night time sleep, are valuable predictors of mortality from cardiovascular diseases (Kleiger et al. 2005). Also, individual differences in HRV seem to be associated with pain variables (Campbell et al. 2003).

In a recent animal study (Oliveira et al. 2012), chronic widespread pain was induced in rats by two injections of acidic saline, administered five days apart. One day after the second injection, HRV spectral power had shifted towards lower frequency ranges indicating a change in cardiac autonomic regulation in terms of increased sympathetic predominance. These findings support the theory that chronic pain may alter autonomic balance. In a study on patients with chronic regional pain or fibromyalgia, it was found, across both pain conditions, that age, gender, pain sensation, pain anxiety and physical functioning could all predict resting HRV (Mostoufi et al. 2012). In an ambulatory study, nocturnal HRV was similarly shown to be a strong predictor of widespread pain (Lerma et al. 2011). Further, increased baroreflex sensitivity was associated with higher pain tolerance and lower pain intensity in patients with widespread pain (Reyes del Paso et al. 2011). Thus, a bi-directional relationship likely exists with chronic pain affecting ANS regulation and *vice versa*. Studies on regional pain conditions have shown contradictory results. For instance, a study on chronic low back pain (Gockel et al. 2008) found no association between perceived pain intensity and autonomic function assessed by HRV among patients, while functional disability was associated with impaired autonomic function in the same sample.

It is not yet clear whether lower HRV among persons with chronic regional muscle pain is specific to pain or whether it reflects poor health in general. Physical activity is another recognized factor that may influence HRV, and because altered activity patterns have been found in chronic muscle pain (Griffin et al. 2012), this possible relationship should be taken into account in forthcoming studies.

8. A hypothetical model of ANS involvement in chronic muscle pain

In the present hypothetical model of possible ANS involvement in chronic pain, it is assumed that the causal relations look different depending on the progression of symptoms, i.e., development or maintenance of pain (see figure 3). The current model is centred on:

- the acute response to external exposures, which may become maladaptive and lead to initiation of muscle pain if it is extended for a long period of time or frequently repeated without recovery

- the prolonged response induced by chronic pain, which is characterized by a basal state of ANS imbalance and by altered reactivity to stressors, which may eventually lead to worsening of symptoms.

It is hypothesized that long-term exposure to mechanical (e.g., low-level repetitive work) and/or psychological (e.g., time pressure) stressors may give rise to an unfavourable physiological response, including sustained muscle activity and lack of muscle rest, inadequate circulation, and altered sensory-motor control, via activation of the sympathetic nervous system, resulting in local accumulation of noxious substances that activate afferent nociceptors, producing local or regional pain. The latter may result in further sympathetic activation that acts back to the periphery. In chronic pain, alterations between (anti)nociceptive mechanisms and ANS regulation may contribute to maintenance of pain, and sensitization, via a self-perpetuating (vicious) cycle, which adds an additional loading on the allostatic stress systems via involvement of positive feedback loops. ANS imbalance, resulting from pain, in terms of sympathetic hyperactivity and diminished parasympathetic tone, may eventually lead to sympathoadrenal hyporeactivity (beta-receptor down regulation) to stressors. This may also be expressed in additional subjective symptoms, including sleep disorders, fatigue, and psychological stress, as well as reduced physical activity.

A variety of individual predisposing factors, such as age, gender, anthropometrics, and genetics/epigenetics, should also be taken into account in attempts to understand individual differences in susceptibility to chronic pain. Among other factors, perceived stress is assumed to play a mediating role at different levels of the model, both in the initiation and continuation of pain, by inducing inadequate ANS reactions. In chronic pain states, accumulated symptoms, which may be accompanied by perceived stress, fatigue and physical inactivity (reduced cardio-respiratory fitness), may all worsen the state of allostatic load (see figure 3).

9. Complexity in assessment of autonomic regulation of MSDs

Various methods exist for assessing ANS regulation; these, however, are individually suitable for experimental application depending on the specific circumstances. Here, relevant methods and tests for characterizing different aspects of ANS activity will be briefly summarized. We will focus on relevant physiological measures and tests applicable to patients with chronic MSDs.

9.1. Measures of autonomic regulation at systemic and local levels

Heart rate variability (HRV) analysis has emerged as a reliable instrument for assessment of autonomic regulation. Heart rhythm is inconstant and varies in a complex and seemingly chaotic way due to efferent sympathetic and parasympathetic modulation of the sinus node of the heart; in general, increased variability reflects healthy ANS regulation. Time series of beat-to-beat RR intervals can be derived from continuous ECG recordings, and variability assessed.

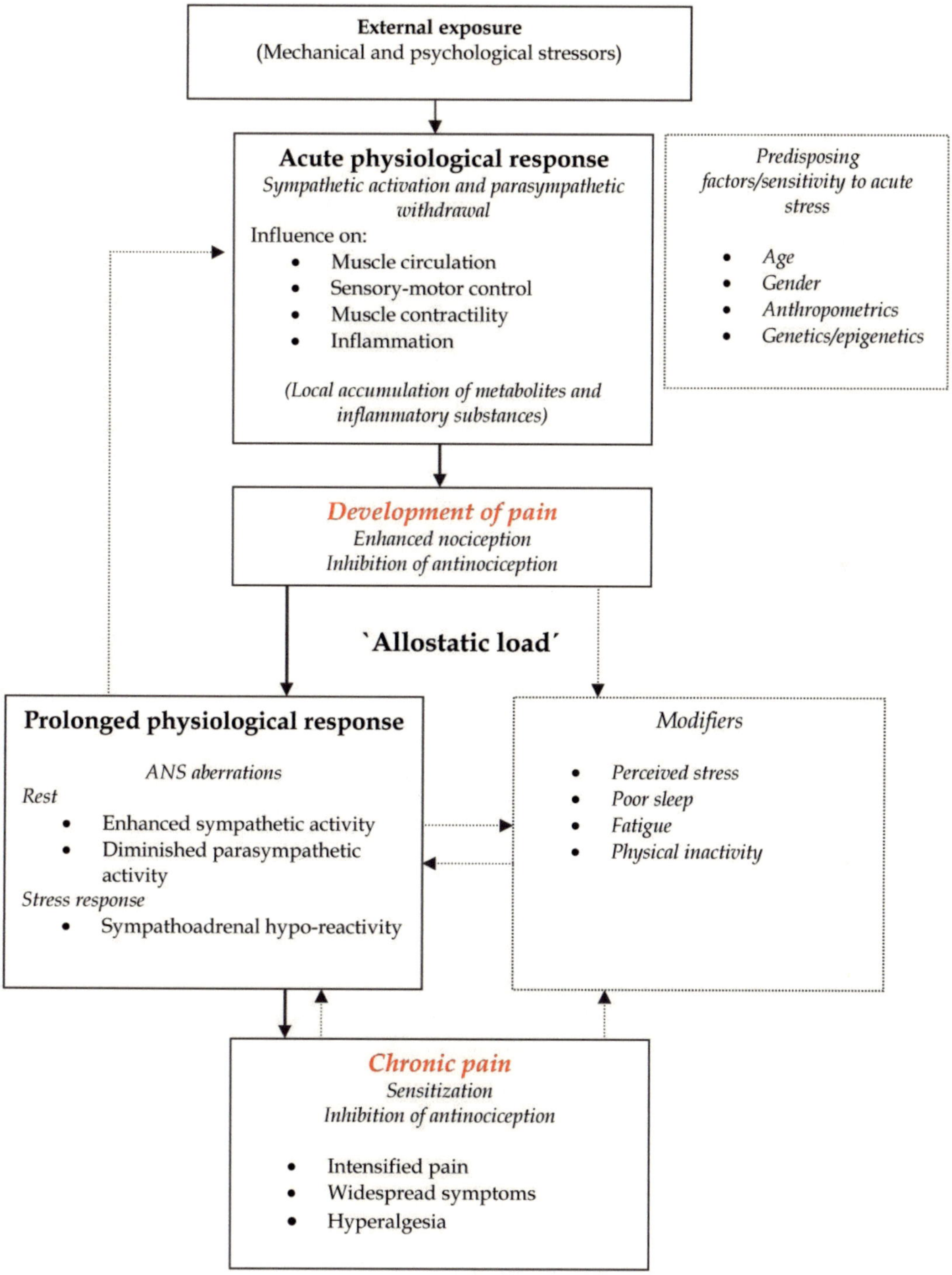

Figure 3. The autonomic nervous system (ANS) involvement in the pathogenesis of chronic musculoskeletal pain

Based on time series of RR intervals, HRV can be analysed in the time domain in units of milliseconds. The standard deviation of all RR-intervals is a measure of ANS regulation, while other measures of short-term variability, for example the root mean square of successive differences between adjacent pairs of RR intervals, are closely related to parasympathetic (vagal) activity as mediated through breathing mechanisms (i.e., respiratory sinus arrhythmia). Frequency domain measures of HRV, via analysis of spectral power density in various frequency ranges, can be informative regarding both the sympathetic and parasympathetic contributions to ANS regulation and balance. The RR interval power spectra contains a low frequency peak between 0.04-0.15 Hz, reflecting baroreceptor modulation with a combination of sympathetic and parasympathetic influences, and a high frequency peak (0.15-0.4 Hz), which predominantly reflects parasympathetic influences, according to Task force standards (1996). Short-term HRV, usually derived over 5 minute ECG segments, is suitable for laboratory experiments, and can be analysed under rest conditions or in response to different sympathetic or parasympathetic manoeuvres. Long-term 24-hour recordings may provide useful information about circadian rhythms (Bilan et al. 2005) and autonomic balance during sleep (Hallman and Lyskov 2010).

Arterial blood pressure is another important cardiovascular characteristic of ANS regulation, which can be easily monitored continuously by non-invasive techniques. Also assessment of sudomotor parameters (e.g., skin conductance and sweat) and temperature changes are common indicators of sympathetic arousal. These variables seem to be rather far removed from local muscle processes, although they may provide relevant information regarding the autonomic state at rest or in response to laboratory, or real-life, stressors in individuals with musculoskeletal pain.

Moreover, indicators of local circulation (blood flow, blood volume, and oxygenation) are relevant measures of sympathetic influences on vasoconstriction, and they can be used reliably in experimental assessment of regional MSDs, such as neck-shoulder pain, or widespread pain conditions, without acting disturbing. Changes in muscle blood flow or blood volume can be derived from different non-invasive methods, including NIRS, photoplethysmography, and doppler ultrasound.

Muscle sympathetic nerve activity, although an invasive method, can be directly recorded from human peripheral nerves using microneurography. Quantification of spontaneous sympathetic bursts gives information regarding efferent sympathetic neural activity to skeletal muscle, and its effects on muscle circulation.

Muscle activity, assessed using surface EMG, has been widely used in exposure assessment as an adequate indicator of muscle fatigue. EMG characteristics may also add information about individual differences in stress reactivity, with a relatively clear connection to ANS function (Lundberg et al. 1994).

In conclusion, ANS testing in chronic MSDs may include a combination of these measures, as well as other methods not mentioned here, for adequate assessment of autonomic reactions. Some methods are preferably used in the laboratory setting, while others can be used in both lab and field studies.

9.2. Laboratory tests and ambulatory monitoring

Laboratory tests assessing systemic and local cardiovascular reactions are valuable tools for characterizing ANS function at the group level for persons afflicted with chronic MSDs, although they are more often applied in evaluation of autonomic neuropathies, and risk assessment for cardiovascular disease. Autonomic provocations should preferably be standardized, non-invasive and target specific reflex pathways. In preparation, it is important to avoid substances that may affect ANS regulation, such as beta blocker drugs, and to be fully recovered from any acute illnesses. Furthermore, subjects should avoid caffeine, nicotine, large meals, and extensive physical activity at the day of testing (Weimer 2010). Commonly used tests include: sustained hand grip, cold pressor, deep breathing, orthostatic, and mental stress tests.

The sustained (static) hand grip test can be used to assess sympathetic nervous function, so long as the subject is able to perform a proper calibration contraction close to their maximal voluntary effort. The static test consists of pressing a dynamometer with the hand at 30% of maximal voluntary contraction for duration of approximately 3 minutes. The hand grip test activates mechanical and chemically sensitive muscle receptors that tend to give rise to a distinct cardiovascular response due to an initial reduction of parasympathetic (vagal) activity followed by an increase in sympathetic tone, i.e., the exercise pressor reflex (Khurana and Setty 1996; Smith et al. 2006). Static contractions have been applied in several studies to differentiate between chronic MSDs and healthy subject groups (Gockel et al. 1995; Hallman et al. 2011).

The cold pressor test is also frequently used to test autonomic function, and is based on submersion of the hand or foot in cold water (between 1 and 5 degrees Celsius). This test activates nociceptive afferents, which in turn activate the efferent sympathetic nervous system, and inhibit vagal modulation of the heart, which is associated with increases in heart rate, arterial blood pressure and muscle sympathetic nerve activity (Victor et al. 1987). Previous studies have demonstrated its applicability in cases of chronic MSDs (Vaeroy et al. 1989; Acero et al. 1999). Due to pain intolerance, a maximum of 3 minute test duration can be recommended for assessment of this population.

Orthostatic stressors are widely excepted tests for reliable assessment of sympathetic (adrenergic) function by recording blood pressure and heart rate changes in response to head-upright tilt (i.e., passive orthostatic test) or standing up from a supine position (i.e., active orthostatic test). These procedures induce a sequence of cardiovascular reflexes controlled by the sympathetic nervous system, mainly characterized by increases in heart rate and diastolic blood pressure, to maintain adequate perfusion to the brain (Weimer 2010). Signs of orthostatic intolerance have been found among fibromyalgia patients, with reduced blood pressure during upright standing indicating impaired sympathetic function (Bou-Holaigah et al. 1997; Furlan et al. 2005; El-Sawy et al. In press)

A multitude of mental stressors, such as the colour-word interference test, mental arithmetic, public speech, and the social trial stress test have been used in experiments for assessment of sympathetic reactions at local and systemic levels. The physiological responses induced by mental stressors may vary to greatly axross individuals, as well as between different types of tasks (Fechir et al. 2008), and are largely dependent on cognitive and behavioural processes. Increased sympathetic reactivity to mental stress is correlated with subjective stress ratings, and is associated with a wide range of pathological conditions, including chronic MSDs (Lundberg 2006).

Deep breathing by following a paced stimulus (e.g., 5 breaths per minute) is a strong parasympathetic provocation, and it induces large oscillations in beat-to-beat heart rate. This test can thus be used for assessment of parasympathetic cardiac regulation, as derived by computing the mean difference between the shortest RR interval at inhalation and the longest RR interval at exhalation.

To ensure the quality of the results obtained using any of the above tests, it is essential to control for possible confounding factors, that is, factors that influence both the independent variable and the outcome variable. For example, if the purpose is to investigate the effect of gender on resting blood pressure, a possible confounder is psychological stress. Stress may be more prevalent in females than males, and may thus result in elevated female blood pressure. One advantage of performing tests in a laboratory setting is that it is possible to control for many potential confounders that can have a direct influence on ANS regulation, including temperature, noise, body position, prior food and medication intake. However, it is also important to account for other behavioural (physical activity, sleep), psychological (depression, anxiety, stress) and physiological (various diseases, circadian rhythms) factors, which may influence autonomic regulation, leading to erroneous results.

One must also consider, however, whether the results obtained under experimental conditions can be generalized to real life conditions. How well do laboratory stressors used in the lab match those occurring in a real working environment with regard to type, intensity and duration? Ambulatory monitoring can, therefore, be used as an effective complement to laboratory testing, as it allows assessment of many physiological variables under real-life conditions. Due to the fast development of ambulatory devices and their accompanying signal processing software, ambulatory monitoring is mainly non-invasive, and relatively easy to wear under periods of several days. Thus, such methods can be used in research, by clinicians, and for coaching (e.g., in sports and exercise).

10. ANS involvement in chronic MSDs, implications for treatment

The above studies suggest that deviations in ANS regulation constitute an important element of the pathogenesis of chronic muscle pain. Chronic MSDs are considered to be a state of allostatic load, including continuation of pain due to maladaptive ANS regulation of anti-nociceptive and nociceptive processes. It is thus hypothesized that treatment of chronic MSDs will benefit from restoring ANS balance.

How do individuals recover from this complex vicious cycle? Although the external exposures, such as those mechanical and psychological strains people may encounter at work, could be partly avoided by staying at home or by changing to another occupation, it is not possible to just switch off the internal exposure: increased sympathetic activity due to nociception.

It does not seem to be a coincidence that effective treatments of chronic MSDs are also beneficial for ANS balance, particularly for improving cardiovascular control. A variety of forms of physical activity and exercise are established strategies for treatment of muscle strength and function, perceived pain reduction , and for improving cardiovascular fitness and general health (Ylinen et al. 2003; Andersen et al. 2008). Physical activity may also reduce perceived stress and acts preventing against various chronic diseases (Warburton et al. 2006). Although increased physical activity is strongly associated with long-term effects on autonomic regulation, surprisingly little is known about this relationship regarding chronic MSDs. Considering the proposed model of ANS involvement in chronic musculoskeletal pain at local and systemic levels, we would expect that improvement of pain by increasing or adjusting the level of physical activity may be accompanied by restoration of ANS regulation. Relaxation techniques, for example by using individually based slow breathing (Hallman et al. 2011), or psychological treatments aiming at reducing perceived stress, may also be considered for improving ANS balance in people with musculoskeletal pain. Thus, combined strategies, including both adjustments of physical activity levels and psychological stress, may prove to be effective for prevention and treatment of chronic MSDs.

11. Conclusion

Studies indicate that the involvement of the ANS at both the systemic and local levels is an important element of the pathogenesis of chronic musculoskeletal pain. It is hypothesized that treatment of chronic MSDs will benefit from improving ANS balance. Future studies on chronic MSDs should look closer at the possible causal relations between the ANS and pain. There is also a need to consider many other factors that could affect this relationship.

Author details

David M Hallman and Eugene Lyskov
University of Gävle, Centre for Musculoskeletal Research, Sweden

12. References

Acero, C. O., Kuboki, T., Maekawa, K., Yamashita, A. and Clark, G. T. (1999). Haemodynamic responses in chronically painful, human trapezius muscle to cold pressor stimulation. *Archives of Oral Biology* 44(10): 805-812.

Andersen, L., Blangsted, A., Nielsen, P., Hansen, L., Vedsted, P., Sjøgaard, G., et al. (2010). Effect of cycling on oxygenation of relaxed neck/shoulder muscles in women with and without chronic pain. *European Journal of Applied Physiology* 110(2): 389-394.

Andersen, L. L., Jørgensen, M. B., Blangsted, A. K., Pedersen, M. T., Hansen, E. A. and Sjøgaard, G. (2008). A Randomized Controlled Intervention Trial to Relieve and Prevent

Neck/Shoulder Pain. *Medicine & Science in Sports & Exercise* 40(6): 983-990 910.1249/MSS.1240b1013e3181676640.

Apkarian, A. V., Bushnell, M. C., Treede, R.-D. and Zubieta, J.-K. (2005). Human brain mechanisms of pain perception and regulation in health and disease. *European Journal of Pain* 9(4): 463-463.

Arendt-Nielsen, L. and Graven-Nielsen, T. (2003). Central sensitization in fibromyalgia and other musculoskeletal disorders. *Current Pain and Headache Reports* 7(5): 355-361.

Barbe, M. F. and Barr, A. E. (2006). Inflammation and the pathophysiology of work-related musculoskeletal disorders. *Brain, Behavior, and Immunity* 20(5): 423-429.

Benarroch, E. (2006). Pain-autonomic interactions. *Neurological Sciences* 27(0): s130-s133.

Bilan, A., Witczak, A., Palusinski, R., Myslinski, W. and Hanzlik, J. (2005). Circadian rhythm of spectral indices of heart rate variability in healthy subjects. *Journal of Electrocardiology* 38(3): 239-243.

Bingel, U., Schoell, E., Herken, W., Büchel, C. and May, A. (2007). Habituation to painful stimulation involves the antinociceptive system. *Pain* 131(1–2): 21-30.

Blangsted, A., Søgaard, K., Christensen, H. and Sjøgaard, G. (2004). The effect of physical and psychosocial loads on the trapezius muscle activity during computer keying tasks and rest periods. *European Journal of Applied Physiology* 91(2): 253-258.

Bongers, P., Ijmker, S., van den Heuvel, S. and Blatter, B. (2006). Epidemiology of work related neck and upper limb problems: Psychosocial and personal risk factors (Part I) and effective interventions from a bio behavioural perspective (Part II). *Journal of Occupational Rehabilitation* 16(3): 272-295.

Borovikova, L. V., Ivanova, S., Zhang, M., Yang, H., Botchkina, G. I., Watkins, L. R., et al. (2000). Vagus nerve stimulation attenuates the systemic inflammatory response to endotoxin. *Nature* 405(6785): 458-462.

Bou-Holaigah, I., Calkins, H., Flynn, J. A., Tunin, C., Chang, H. C., Kan, J. S., et al. (1997). Provocation of hypotension and pain during upright tilt table testing in adults with fibromyalgia. *Clinical and experimental rheumatology* 15(3): 239-246.

Breivik, H., Collett, B., Ventafridda, V., Cohen, R. and Gallacher, D. (2006). Survey of chronic pain in Europe: Prevalence, impact on daily life, and treatment. *European Journal of Pain* 10(4): 287-333.

Bruehl, S. and Chung, O. Y. (2004). Interactions between the cardiovascular and pain regulatory systems: an updated review of mechanisms and possible alterations in chronic pain. *Neuroscience & Biobehavioral Reviews* 28(4): 395-414.

Buckwalter, J. B., Mueller, P. J. and Clifford, P. S. (1997). Sympathetic vasoconstriction in active skeletal muscles during dynamic exercise. *J Appl Physiol* 83(5): 1575-1580.

Campbell, T. S., Ditto, B., Séguin, J. R., Sinray, S. and Tremblay, R. E. (2003). Adolescent Pain Sensitivity Is Associated With Cardiac Autonomic Function and Blood Pressure Over 8 Years. *Hypertension* 41(6): 1228-1233.

Chouchou, F., Pichot, V., Perchet, C., Legrain, V., Garcia-Larrea, L., Roche, F., et al. (2011). Autonomic pain responses during sleep: A study of heart rate variability. *European Journal of Pain* 15(6): 554-560.

Christensen, J. O. and Knardahl, S. (2011). Work and neck pain: A prospective study of psychological, social, and mechanical risk factors. *Pain* 151(1): 162-173.

Chrousos, G. P. (2009). Stress and disorders of the stress system. *Nature Reviews Endocrinology* 5(7): 374-381.

Cohen, H., Benjamin, J., Geva, A. B., Matar, M. A., Kaplan, Z. and Kotler, M. (2000). Autonomic dysregulation in panic disorder and in post-traumatic stress disorder: application of power spectrum analysis of heart rate variability at rest and in response to recollection of trauma or panic attacks. *Psychiatry Research* 96(1): 1-13.

Côté, P., van der Velde, G., Cassidy, J. D., Carroll, L. J., Hogg-Johnson, S., Holm, L. W., et al. (2009). The Burden and Determinants of Neck Pain in Workers: Results of the Bone and Joint Decade 2000-2010 Task Force on Neck Pain and Its Associated Disorders. *Journal of Manipulative and Physiological Therapeutics* 32(2, Supplement 1): S70-S86.

Critchley, H. D., Corfield, D. R., Chandler, M. P., Mathias, C. J. and Dolan, R. J. (2000). Cerebral correlates of autonomic cardiovascular arousal: a functional neuroimaging investigation in humans. *The Journal of Physiology* 523(1): 259-270.

Dubé, A.-A., Duquette, M., Roy, M., Lepore, F., Duncan, G. and Rainville, P. (2009). Brain activity associated with the electrodermal reactivity to acute heat pain. *NeuroImage* 45(1): 169-180.

Edwards, R. R., Almeida, D. M., Klick, B., Haythornthwaite, J. A. and Smith, M. T. (2008). Duration of sleep contributes to next-day pain report in the general population. *Pain* 137(1): 202-207.

El-Sawy, N., El-Tantawi, G., Achmawi, G. A. H., Sultan, H. and Younis, S. (In press). Autonomic changes in fibromyalgia: Clinical and electrophysiological study. *Alexandria Journal of Medicine.*

Elvin, A., Siösteen, A.-K., Nilsson, A. and Kosek, E. (2006). Decreased muscle blood flow in fibromyalgia patients during standardised muscle exercise: A contrast media enhanced colour doppler study. *European Journal of Pain* 10(2): 137-144.

Fechir, M., Schlereth, T., Purat, T., Kritzmann, S., Geber, C., Eberle, T., et al. (2008). Patterns of sympathetic responses induced by different stress tasks. *Open Neurobiology Journal* 2: 25-31.

Fishbain, D. A., Cutler, R. B., Cole, B., Lewis, J., Smets, E., Rosomoff, H. L., et al. (2004). Are Patients with Chronic Low Back Pain or Chronic Neck Pain Fatigued? 5: 187-195.

Furlan, R., Colombo, S., Perego, F., Atzeni, F., Diana, A., Barbic, F., et al. (2005). Abnormalities of cardiovascular neural control and reduced orthostatic tolerance in patients with primary fibromyalgia. *The Journal of Rheumatology* 32(9): 1787-1793.

Ge, H.-Y., Fernández-de-las-Peñas, C. and Arendt-Nielsen, L. (2006). Sympathetic facilitation of hyperalgesia evoked from myofascial tender and trigger points in patients with unilateral shoulder pain. *Clinical Neurophysiology* 117(7): 1545-1550.

Gockel, M., Lindholm, H., Alaranta, H., Viljanen, A., Lindquist, A. and Lindholm, T. (1995). Cardiovascular functional disorder and stress among patients having neck-shoulder symptoms. *Annals of the Rheumatic Diseases* 54(6): 494-497.

Gockel, M., Lindholm, H., Niemist, L. and Hurri, H. (2008). Perceived Disability but Not Pain is Connected with Autonomic Nervous Function Among Patients with Chronic Low Back Pain. *Journal of Rehabilitation Medicine* 40: 355-358.

Gold, J., Cherniack, M., Hanlon, A., Dennerlein, J. and Dropkin, J. (2009). Skin temperature in the dorsal hand of office workers and severity of upper extremity musculoskeletal disorders. *International Archives of Occupational and Environmental Health* 82(10): 1281-1292.

Griffin, D. W., Harmon, D. C. and Kennedy, N. M. (2012). Do patients with chronic low back pain have an altered level and/or pattern of physical activity compared to healthy individuals? A systematic review of the literature. *Physiotherapy* 98(1): 13-23.

Haley, R. W., Vongpatanasin, W., Wolfe, G. I., Bryan, W. W., Armitage, R., Hoffmann, R. F., et al. (2004). Blunted circadian variation in autonomic regulation of sinus node function in veterans with Gulf War syndrome. *The American Journal of Medicine* 117(7): 469-478.

Hallman, D., Lindberg, L.-G., Arnetz, B. and Lyskov, E. (2011). Effects of static contraction and cold stimulation on cardiovascular autonomic indices, trapezius blood flow and muscle activity in chronic neck–shoulder pain. *European Journal of Applied Physiology* 111(8): 1725-1735.

Hallman, D. and Lyskov, E. (2010). Monitoring of heart rate variability, physical activity and percieved stress and energy in daily life among persons suffering from neck-shoulder pain. Nordic Conference Odense, Danmark, University of Southern Danmark: 57.

Hallman, D., Olsson, E., von Schéele, B., Melin, L. and Lyskov, E. (2011). Effects of Heart Rate Variability Biofeedback in Subjects with Stress-Related Chronic Neck Pain: A Pilot Study. *Applied Psychophysiology and Biofeedback* 36(2): 71-80.

Hogg-Johnson, S., van der Velde, G., Carroll, L. J., Holm, L. W., Cassidy, J. D., Guzman, J., et al. (2009). The Burden and Determinants of Neck Pain in the General Population: Results of the Bone and Joint Decade 2000-2010 Task Force on Neck Pain and Its Associated Disorders. *Journal of Manipulative and Physiological Therapeutics* 32(2, Supplement 1): S46-S60.

Hägg, G. M. (2003). The Cinderella hypothesis. 127-132.

Jae, S., Heffernan, K., Park, S.-H., Jung, S.-H., Yoon, E., Kim, E., et al. (2010). Does an acute inflammatory response temporarily attenuate parasympathetic reactivation? *Clinical Autonomic Research* 20(4): 229-233.

Johansson, H., Windhorst, U., Djupsjöbacka, M. and Passatore, M., Eds. (2003). *Chronic Work-Related Myalgia. Neuromuscular Mechanisms behind Work-Related Chronic Muscle Pain Syndromes*. Gävle, Gävle University Press.

Johnston, V., Jull, G., Darnell, R., Jimmieson, N. and Souvlis, T. (2008). Alterations in cervical muscle activity in functional and stressful tasks in female office workers with neck pain. *European Journal of Applied Physiology* 103(3): 253-264.

Joyner, M. J., Nauss, L. A., Warner, M. A. and Warner, D. O. (1992). Sympathetic modulation of blood flow and O2 uptake in rhythmically contracting human forearm muscles. *American Journal of Physiology - Heart and Circulatory Physiology* 263(4): H1078-H1083.

Jänig, W. (2003). Relationship Between Pain and Autonomic Phenomena in Headache and Other Pain Conditions. *Cephalalgia* 23(1 suppl): 43-48.

Kalezic, N., Noborisaka, Y., Nakata, M., Crenshaw, A. G., Karlsson, S., Lyskov, E., et al. (2010). Cardiovascular and muscle activity during chewing in whiplash-associated disorders (WAD). *Archives of Oral Biology* 55(6): 447-453.

Kalezic, N., Roatta, S., Lyskov, E. and Johansson, H. (2003). Stress - An Introductory Overview. *Chronic Work-related Myalgia. Neuromuscular Mechanisms behind Work-related Chronic Muscle pain Syndromes*. H. Johansson, U. Windhorst, M. Djupsjöbacka and M. Passatore. Gävle, Gävle University press: 57-71.

Kalezic, N., Åsell, M., Kerschbaumer, H. and Lyskov, E. (2007). Physiological Reactivity to Functional Tests in Patients with Chronic Low Back Pain. *Journal Of Musculoskeletal Pain* 15(1): 29 - 40.

Keijsers, E., Feleus, A., Miedema, H. S., Koes, B. W. and Bierma-Zeinstra, S. M. A. (2010). Psychosocial factors predicted nonrecovery in both specific and nonspecific diagnoses at arm, neck, and shoulder. *Journal of Clinical Epidemiology* 63(12): 1370-1379.

Kemp, A. H., Quintana, D. S., Felmingham, K. L., Matthews, S. and Jelinek, H. F. (2012). Depression, Comorbid Anxiety Disorders, and Heart Rate Variability in Physically Healthy, Unmedicated Patients: Implications for Cardiovascular Risk. *PLoS ONE* 7(2): e30777.

Khurana, R. and Setty, A. (1996). The value of the isometric hand-grip test-studies in various autonomic disorders. *Clinical Autonomic Research* 6(4): 211-218.

Kingsley, J. D., Panton, L. B., McMillan, V. and Figueroa, A. (2009). Cardiovascular Autonomic Modulation After Acute Resistance Exercise in Women With Fibromyalgia. *Archives of Physical Medicine and Rehabilitation* 90(9): 1628-1634.

Kleiger, R. E., Stein, P. K. and Bigger, J. T. (2005). Heart Rate Variability: Measurement and Clinical Utility. *The Annals of Noninvasive Electrocardiology* 10(1): 88-101.

Krantz, G., Forsman, M. and Lundberg, U. (2004). Consistency in physiological stress responses and electromyographic activity during induced stress exposure in women and men. *Integrative Physiological and Behavioral Science* 39(2): 105-118.

Larsman, P., Thorn, S., Søgaard, K., Sandsjö, L., Sjøgaard, G. and Kadefors, R. (2009). Work related perceived stress and muscle activity during standardized computer work among female computer users. *Work: A Journal of Prevention, Assessment and Rehabilitation* 32(2): 189-199.

Larsson, B., Björk, J., Börsbo, B. and Gerdle, B. (2012). A systematic review of risk factors associated with transitioning from regional musculoskeletal pain to chronic widespread pain. *European Journal of Pain*: n/a-n/a. (In press).

Larsson, B., Søgaard, K. and Rosendal, L. (2007). Work related neck-shoulder pain: a review on magnitude, risk factors, biochemical characteristics, clinical picture and preventive interventions. *Best Practice & Research Clinical Rheumatology* 21(3): 447-463.

Larsson, R., Öberg, P. A. and Larsson, S. E. (1999). Changes of trapezius muscle blood flow and electromyography in chronic neck pain due to trapezius myalgia. *Pain* 79: 45-50.

Larsson, S. E., Bodegård, L., Henriksson, K. G. and Öberg, P. Å. (1990). Chronic trapezius myalgia. Morphology and blood flow studied in 17 patients. *Acta Orthopaedica Scandinavica* 61: 394-398.

Larsson, S. E., Larsson, R., Zhang, Q., Cai, H. and Öberg, P. Å. (1995). Effects of psychophysiological stress on trapezius muscles blood flow and electromyography during static load. *European Journal of Applied Physiology and Occupational Physiology* 71: 493-498.

Larsson, S. E., Ålund, M., Cai, H. and Öberg, P. Å. (1994). Chronic pain after soft-tissue injury of the cervical spine: trapezius muscle blood flow and electromyography at static loads and fatigue. *Pain*. 57: 173-180.

Lerma, C., Martinez, A., Ruiz, N., Vargas, A., Infante, O. and Martinez-Lavin, M. (2011). Nocturnal heart rate variability parameters as potential fibromyalgia biomarker: correlation with symptoms severity. *Arthritis Research & Therapy* 13(6): R185.

Lindell, L., Bergman, S., Petersson, I. F., Jacobsson, L. T. H. and Herrström, P. (2000). Prevalence of fibromyalgia and chronic widespread pain. *Scandinavian Journal of Primary Health Care* 18(3): 149-153.

Linton, S. J. (2000). A Review of Psychological Risk Factors in Back and Neck Pain. *Spine* 25(9): 1148-1156.

Lundberg, U. (2006). Stress, subjective and objective health. *International Journal of Social Welfare* 15: S41-S48.

Lundberg, U., Elfsberg Dohns, I., Melin, B., Sandsjö, L., Palmerud, G., Kadefors, R., et al. (1999). Psychophysiological stress responses, muscle tension, and neck and shoulder pain among supermarket cashiers. *Journal of Occupational Health Psychology* 4(3): 245-255.

Lundberg, U., Kadefors, R., Melin, B., Palmerud, G., Hassmén, P., Engström, M., et al. (1994). Psychophysiological stress and emg activity of the trapezius muscle. *International Journal of Behavioral Medicine* 1(4): 354-370.

Madeleine, P., Mathiassen, S. and Arendt-Nielsen, L. (2008). Changes in the degree of motor variability associated with experimental and chronic neck–shoulder pain during a standardised repetitive arm movement. *Experimental Brain Research* 185(4): 689-698.

Maekawa, K., Clark, G. T. and Kuboki, T. (2002). Intramuscular hypoperfusion, adrenergic receptors, and chronic muscle pain. *The Journal of Pain* 3(4): 251-260.

Malik, M. (1996). Task force of the European Society of Cardiology and The North American Society of Pacing and Electrophysiology. Heart Rate Variability : Standards of Measurement, Physiological Interpretation, and Clinical Use. *European Heart Journal* 93(5): 1043-1065.

Malinen, S., Vartiainen, N., Hlushchuk, Y., Koskinen, M., Ramkumar, P., Forss, N., et al. (2010). Aberrant temporal and spatial brain activity during rest in patients with chronic pain. *Proceedings of the National Academy of Sciences* 107(14): 6493-6497.

Martinez-Lavin, M. (2007). Biology and therapy of fibromyalgia. Stress, the stress response system, and fibromyalgia. *Arthritis Research & Therapy* 9(4): 216.

Martinez-Lavin, M. (2012). Fibromyalgia: When Distress Becomes (Un)sympathetic Pain. *Pain Research and Treatment* 2012.

Martínez-Lavín, M., Hermosillo, A. G., Rosas, M. and Soto, M. E. (1998). Circadian studies of autonomic nervous balance in patients with fibromyalgia: A heart rate variability analysis. *Arthritis & Rheumatism* 41(11): 1966-1971.

Martinez-Lavin, M., Vidal, M., Barbosa, R.-E., Pineda, C., Casanova, J.-M. and Nava, A. (2002). Norepinephrine-evoked pain in fibromyalgia. A randomized pilot study [ISRCTN70707830]. *BMC Musculoskeletal Disorders* 3(1): 2.

McEwen, B. S. (1998). Stress, Adaptation, and Disease: Allostasis and Allostatic Load. *Annals of the New York Academy of Sciences* 840(1): 33-44.

McEwen, B. S. (2000). The neurobiology of stress: from serendipity to clinical relevance. *Brain Research* 886(1-2): 172-189.

McEwen, B. S. (2007). Physiology and Neurobiology of Stress and Adaptation: Central Role of the Brain. *Physiological Reviews* 87(3): 873-904.

Mehta, R. K. and Agnew, M. J. (2011). Effects of concurrent physical and mental demands for a short duration static task. *International Journal of Industrial Ergonomics* 41(5): 488-493.

Mostoufi, S. M., Afari, N., Ahumada, S. M., Reis, V. and Wetherell, J. L. (2012). Health and distress predictors of heart rate variability in fibromyalgia and other forms of chronic pain. *Journal of Psychosomatic Research* 72(1): 39-44.

Neugebauer, V., Li, W., Bird, G. C. and Han, J. S. (2004). The Amygdala and Persistent Pain. *The Neuroscientist* 10(3): 221-234.

Newton, J. L., Pairman, J., Hallsworth, K., Moore, S., Plotz, T. and Trenell, M. I. (2011). Physical activity intensity but not sedentary activity is reduced in chronic fatigue syndrome and is associated with autonomic regulation. *QJM*. vol, issue, pages: 104(8):681-687

Nijs, J., Daenen, L., Cras, P., Struyf, F., Roussel, N. and Oostendorp, R. A. B. (2012). Nociception Affects Motor Output: A Review on Sensory-motor Interaction With Focus on Clinical Implications. *The Clinical Journal of Pain* 28(2): 175-181 110.1097/AJP.1090b1013e318225daf318223.

Nilsen, K. B., Sand, T., Borchgrevink, P., Leistad, R. B., Rø, M. and Westgaard, R. H. (2008). A unilateral sympathetic blockade does not affect stress-related pain and muscle activity in patients with chronic musculoskeletal pain. *Scandinavian Journal of Rheumatology* 37(1): 53-61.

Nilsen, K. B., Sand, T., Westgaard, R. H., Stovner, L. J., White, L. R., Bang Leistad, R., et al. (2007). Autonomic activation and pain in response to low-grade mental stress in fibromyalgia and shoulder/neck pain patients. *European Journal of Pain* 11(7): 743-755.

Nolet, P. S., Côté, P., Cassidy, J. D. and Carroll, L. J. (2012). The Association Between Self-Reported Cardiovascular Disorders and Troublesome Neck Pain: A Population-Based Cohort Study. *Journal of Manipulative and Physiological Therapeutics* 35(3):176-183.

Oliveira, L. R., de Melo, V. U., Macedo, F. N., Barreto, A. S., Badaue-Passos Jr, D., Viana dos Santos, M. R., et al. (2012). Induction of chronic non-inflammatory widespread pain increases cardiac sympathetic modulation in rats. *Autonomic Neuroscience* 167(1): 45-49.

Passatore, M. and Roatta, S. (2006). Influence of sympathetic nervous system on sensorimotor function: whiplash associated disorders (WAD) as a model. *European Journal of Applied Physiology* 98(5): 423-449.

Piché, M., Arsenault, M. and Rainville, P. (2010). Dissection of perceptual, motor and autonomic components of brain activity evoked by noxious stimulation. *Pain* 149(3): 453-462.

Price, D. D. (2000). Psychological and Neural Mechanisms of the Affective Dimension of Pain. *Science* 288(5472): 1769-1772.

Pritchard, M., Pugh, N., Wright, I. and Brownlee, M. (1999). A vascular basis for repetitive strain injury. *Rheumatology* 38(7): 636-639.

Reyes del Paso, G. A., Garrido, S., Pulgar, Á. and Duschek, S. (2011). Autonomic cardiovascular control and responses to experimental pain stimulation in fibromyalgia syndrome. *Journal of Psychosomatic Research* 70: 125-134.

Reyes del Paso, G. A., Garrido, S., Pulgar, Á., Martín-Vázquez, M. and Duschek, S. (2010). Aberrances in Autonomic Cardiovascular Regulation in Fibromyalgia Syndrome and Their Relevance for Clinical Pain Reports. *Psychosomatic Medicine* 72(5): 462-470.

Riva, R., Mork, P. J., Westgaard, R. H. and Lundberg, U. (2012). Comparison of the cortisol awakening response in women with shoulder and neck pain and women with fibromyalgia. *Psychoneuroendocrinology* 37(2): 299-306.

Roatta, S., Arendt-Nielsen, L. and Farina, D. (2008). Sympathetic-induced changes in discharge rate and spike-triggered average twitch torque of low-threshold motor units in humans. *The Journal of Physiology* 586(22): 5561-5574.

Roatta, S. and Farina, D. (2010). Sympathetic actions on the skeletal muscle. *Exerc Sport Sci Rev* 38(1): 31-35.

Rosas-Ballina, M. and Tracey, K. J. (2009). Cholinergic control of inflammation. *Journal of Internal Medicine* 265(6): 663-679.

Rosendal, L., Larsson, B., Kristiansen, J., Peolsson, M., Søgaard, K., Kjær, M., et al. (2004). Increase in muscle nociceptive substances and anaerobic metabolism in patients with trapezius myalgia: microdialysis in rest and during exercise. *Pain* 112(3): 324-334.

Rouwette, T., Vanelderen, P., Roubos, E. W., Kozicz, T. and Vissers, K. (2011). The amygdala, a relay station for switching on and off pain. *European Journal of Pain*: 16(6):782-792.

Saito, M., Mano, T., Abe, H. and Iwase, S. (1986). Responses in muscle sympathetic nerve activity to sustained hand-grips of different tensions in humans. *European Journal of Applied Physiology and Occupational Physiology* 55(5): 493-498.

Sandberg, M., Larsson, B., Lindberg, L.-G. and Gerdle, B. (2005). Different patterns of blood flow response in the trapezius muscle following needle stimulation (acupuncture) between healthy subjects and patients with fibromyalgia and work-related trapezius myalgia. *European Journal of Pain* 9(5): 497-510.

Sato, A. and Schmidt, R. F. (1973). Somatosympathetic Reflexes: Afferent Fibers, Central Pathways, Discharge Characteristics. *Physiological Reviews* 53(4): 916-947.

Schlereth, T. and Birklein, F. (2008). The Sympathetic Nervous System and Pain. *NeuroMolecular Medicine* 10(3): 141-147.

Seals, D. R. and Enoka, R. M. (1989). Sympathetic activation is associated with increases in EMG during fatiguing exercise. *Journal of Applied Physiology* 66(1): 88-95.

Sharma, S. D., Smith, E. M., Hazleman, B. L. and Jenner, J. R. (1997). Thermographic changes in keyboard operators with chronic forearm pain. *BMJ* 314(7074): 118-.

Sjøgaard, G., Lundberg, U. and Kadefors, R. (2000). The role of muscle activity and mental load in the development of pain and degenerative processes at the muscle cell level during computer work. *European Journal of Applied Physiology* 83(2): 99-105.

Sjörs, A., Larsson, B., Dahlman, J., Falkmer, T. and Gerdle, B. (2009). Physiological responses to low-force work and psychosocial stress in women with chronic trapezius myalgia. *BMC Musculoskeletal Disorders* 10(1): 63.

Sjörs, A., Larsson, B., Persson, A. and Gerdle, B. (2011). An increased response to experimental muscle pain is related to psychological status in women with chronic non-traumatic neck-shoulder pain. *BMC Musculoskeletal Disorders* 12(1): 230.

Smith, S. A., Mitchell, J. H. and Garry, M. G. (2006). The mammalian exercise pressor reflex in health and disease. *Experimental Physiology* 91(1): 89-102.

Spaeth, M., Rizzi, M. and Sarzi-Puttini, P. (2011). Fibromyalgia and Sleep. *Best Practice & Research Clinical Rheumatology* 25(2): 227-239.

Strøm, V., Røe, C. and Knardahl, S. (2009). Work-induced pain, trapezius blood flux, and muscle activity in workers with chronic shoulder and neck pain. *Pain* 144(1-2): 147-155.

Thayer, J. F., Yamamoto, S. S. and Brosschot, J. F. (2010). The relationship of autonomic imbalance, heart rate variability and cardiovascular disease risk factors. *International Journal of Cardiology* 141(2): 122-131.

Thomas, G. D. and Segal, S. S. (2004). Neural control of muscle blood flow during exercise. *J Appl Physiol* 97(2): 731-738.

Thorn, S., Søgaard, K., Kallenberg, L. A. C., Sandsjö, L., Sjøgaard, G., Hermens, H. J., et al. (2007). Trapezius muscle rest time during standardised computer work – A comparison of female computer users with and without self-reported neck/shoulder complaints. *Journal of Electromyography and Kinesiology* 17(4): 420-427.

Thunberg, J., Lyskov, E., Korotkov, A., Ljubisavljevic, M., Pakhomov, S., Katayeva, G., et al. (2005). Brain processing of tonic muscle pain induced by infusion of hypertonic saline. *European Journal of Pain* 9(2): 185-194.

Torp, S., Riise, T. and Moen, B. E. (2001). The Impact of Psychosocial Work Factors on Musculoskeletal Pain: A Prospective Study. *Journal of Occupational and Environmental Medicine* 43(2): 120-126.

Tracey, K. J. (2002). The inflammatory reflex. *Nature* 420(6917): 853-859.

Trinder, J., Waloszek, J., Woods, M. and Jordan, A. (2012). Sleep and cardiovascular regulation. *Pflügers Archiv European Journal of Physiology* 463(1): 161-168.

Ulrich-Lai, Y. M. and Herman, J. P. (2009). Neural regulation of endocrine and autonomic stress responses. *Nat Rev Neurosci* 10(6): 397-409.

Vaeroy, H., Qiao, Z. G., Morkrid, L. and Forre, O. (1989). Altered sympathetic nervous system response in patients with fibromyalgia (fibrositis syndrome). *The Journal of rheumatology* 16(11): 1460-1465.

Wang, Y., Szeto, G. and Chan, C. (2011). Effects of physical and mental task demands on cervical and upper limb muscle activity and physiological responses during computer tasks and recovery periods. *European Journal of Applied Physiology* 111(11): 2791-2803.

Warburton, D. E. R., Nicol, C. W. and Bredin, S. S. D. (2006). Health benefits of physical activity: the evidence. *CMAJ* 174(6): 801-809.

Weimer, L. H. (2010). Autonomic Testing: Common Techniques and Clinical Applications. *The Neurologist* 16(4): 215-222

Victor, R., Leimbach, W., Seals, D., Wallin, B. and Mark, A. (1987). Effects of the cold pressor test on muscle sympathetic nerve activity in humans. *Hypertension* 9(5): 429-436.

Vierck, J. C. J. (2006). Mechanisms underlying development of spatially distributed chronic pain (fibromyalgia). *Pain* 124(3): 242-263.

Willmann, M. and Bolmont, B. (2012). The trapezius muscle uniquely lacks adaptive process in response to a repeated moderate cognitive stressor. *Neuroscience Letters* 506(1): 166-169.

Visser, B. and van Dieën, J. H. (2006). Pathophysiology of upper extremity muscle disorders. *Journal of Electromyography and Kinesiology* 16(1): 1-16.

Vrijkotte, T. G. M., van Doornen, L. J. P. and de Geus, E. J. C. (2000). Effects of Work Stress on Ambulatory Blood Pressure, Heart Rate, and Heart Rate Variability. *Hypertension* 35(4): 880-886.

Ylinen, J., Takala, E.-P., Nykänen, M., Häkkinen, A., Mälkiä, E., Pohjolainen, T., et al. (2003). Active Neck Muscle Training in the Treatment of Chronic Neck Pain in Women. *JAMA: The Journal of the American Medical Association* 289(19): 2509-2516.

Chapter 4

Work Related Musculoskeletal Pain and It's Management

David McBride and Helen Harcombe

Additional information is available at the end of the chapter

http://dx.doi.org/10.5772/51706

1. Introduction

This chapter reviews current best evidence in the identification and management of work related factors causing musculoskeletal pain and discomfort.

Work related MSDs of the low back and upper extremity are an important cause of morbidity and have a high economic cost to society, which in 2001 was estimated to cost the United States $54 billion per annum[1]. The cause of the morbidity is pain and discomfort caused by a mis-match between the physical and physiological factors of tissue load and tissue tolerance which causes a combination of structural damage and metabolic waste accumulation. Some of these strains and sprains are acute overexertion, where there may be direct damage to the muscle fibres, the tendons or the ligaments, with either micro-tears or more gross structural damage. This in turn leads to activation of peripheral nociceptors (type II and IV pain fibres) by direct mechanical or chemical action. This may, in turn, result in central sensitization.

A subacute mechanism may also occur whereby there is a gradual onset of tissue damage over time. Chronic MSDs are also associated with pain syndromes or the 'overuse' syndromes. The combination of peripheral and central sensitization has led to investigation into how psychosocial factors modify the experience of pain. There are social and cultural associations with these chronic pain syndromes which have resulted in 'epidemics' of non-specific musculoskeletal symptoms, for example repetition strain injury (RSI) in Australia[2]. Patients may lie at the extremes of this spectrum of disorder, some have acute pathology readily amenable to intervention while others are disabled by 'chronic pain syndromes.' Many do however lie between these extremes and there is now more general agreement that work related MSDs have a multifactorial aetiology.

When attempting to manage any of these conditions it is therefore essential to recognize when work related factors are part of the aetiology because there is a greater likelihood of successful treatment and rehabilitation if these are successfully identified and dealt with. The important work related factors which must be assessed include force, posture and repetition, factors which have an important bearing on muscle loading and the ability to recover. Once an MSD has occurred, early identification and reporting will ensure that interventions can be applied and in planning these there are work related and organizational factors which must be understood. Chief amongst these is the ability to modify the work to avoid or reduce the effect of precipitating factors. Organisational factors encompass the availability of medical resources, but also include the environment in which recovery takes place. The psychosocial climate of the workplace, for example whether co-workers and management are perceived as being supportive or not, is acknowledged to be important[1,3].

It is essential in dealing with workplaces and employees that the doctor recognizes their role. If they are acting for a third party such as an employer or an insurance organization (the 'double agent' scenario)[4] there is a fundamental change in the nature of the clinical relationship. It may not be a traditional 'doctor patient' relationship but may become a 'doctor client' relationship. The role of the doctor is to be impartial and honest with all of the agents and it is essential to be explicit about this point with the client. This may be perceived as running contrary to the Hippocratic principle of 'do no harm' because the consultation may not always achieve outcomes perceived by the 'patient' as being in their best interest, for example cessation of a benefit and returning to work with low back pain. The philosophical framework within which we make our judgments is in fact complex[5], and an area of practice well worthy of further study. The ethical implications of our work become clearer with experience. For this reason the practitioner is urged to reflect on the effects of the decisions that they make. Opening up an ethical dialogue with the client will help in this matter

2. The epidemiology of work related MSDs

There are significant difficulties in implementing studies which examine the relationships between work related factors and MSD outcomes. Prospective studies are best suited to clarifying causal issues, but the dynamic nature of MSDs, with a tendency towards recurrence, causes difficulties in identifying incident cases. Case identification is usually based on measures of frequency, duration, severity or disability. If meaningful comparisons are to be made between studies consistent case definitions are required, which is often not the case. This means that the results do not lend themselves to inclusion in meta-analysis, thus losing opportunities for more powerful estimation of the magnitude of the risks. Many studies also rely on self-reported symptoms as an outcome measure, without the additional benefit of clinical examination or investigation. The exposures, for example work related physical factors, have the multiple domains of force, posture and repetition. All are subject to misclassification errors, as is the classification into exposure groups. Lastly, there are the complicating factors of the epidemiological confounders, not least of which are psychological factors. Despite these problems, many studies on occupational MSDs have been carried out and the relationships with work are becoming clearer.

3. MSD classification

A convenient classification of work related MSDs is into the 'axial' anatomical areas of the neck, neck/shoulder and back and the 'peripheral' areas of the shoulder, elbow and hand-wrist. Both low back pain (LBP) and neck pain (NP) are amongst the commonest MSDs, with over 80% of individuals experiencing some degree of discomfort in the area over a life-time: over 80% in the low back[6] and 67% in the neck[7]. It has been suggested that the most important causes of LBP are genetic, this influence causing a tendency towards spinal degeneration[8]. The reality is however more complex because the normal biological pain experience is modulated by psychological and social factors, the biopsychosocial model providing a heuristic framework for understanding the pain process[9]. There is evidence that occupational factors play a significant role within this model. As the most prevalent MSDs, LBP and NP provide a useful framework for understanding the other MSDs: the aetiological factors have the same nature and the investigation and management follow similar principles.

4. Axial pain: Acute low back pain

If LBP is of acute or subacute onset, of less than three months duration and has neither radiation suggestive of radicular involvement nor 'red flags' (features of cauda equina syndrome; severe worsening pain, especially at night or when lying down; significant trauma; weight loss; history of cancer; fever; use of intravenous drugs or steroids and patients over 50 years old) suggesting other pathology it can be considered 'non specific' or mechanical in nature.

There are many risk factors that have been associated with LBP and they have opportunities to act at various points during the complex 'natural history' of the disorder, affecting incidence, prevalence, recurrence, the chronic pain state, the transition to a chronic pain state, sickness absence and disability. The risk factors themselves can be classified into work related factors, being the physical nature of the work and the psychosocial work climate, along with the personal factors of physical and psychological attributes.

4.1. Work related physical factors in LBP

There have been many epidemiological studies of the relationship between the physical attributes of work and MSDs in general. Well designed studies are necessary to understand exactly how these attributes, including the main occupational factors of force, posture and repetition, contribute to the development of musculoskeletal pain and ill health. The quality of some epidemiological studies has been criticized[10], the problems already having been mentioned.

One of first major reviews of the physical causes of MSDs, including LBP, was carried out by the National Institute of Occupational Safety and Health (NIOSH)[3]. The factors that the review team looked at were force, leading to muscular stress; repetition, which increases the cumulative loading; awkward postures which put the tissues at a mechanical disadvantage and vibration which causes adverse effects on blood vessels and nerves. The conditions for which the review panel found 'strong evidence' for an association with physical workplace factors were neck pain with posture; a combination of force, posture and repetition with elbow tendonitis, carpal tunnel syndrome and hand/wrist tendonitis and lifting/forceful movement with LBP. The factors where reviewers considered that there was 'evidence' of an association were neck pain with repetition and force; shoulder with posture and repetition; elbow with force; hand/wrist with repetition, force and vibration; tendinitis with repetition, force and posture and back pain with heavy physical work and awkward posture.

A more recent look at the evidence mandated by NIOSH and the National Institutes of Health emphasised the complex interrelationships involved in the causation of MSDs. The panel on musculoskeletal disorders and the workplace[1] (panel on MSDs), approached the problem (p.2) "..from a whole-person perspective, that is, from a point of view that does not isolate disorders of the low back and upper extremities from physical and psychosocial factors in the workplace, from the context of the overall texture of the worker's life, including social support systems and physical and psychosocial stresses outside the workplace, or from personal responses to pain and individual coping mechanisms." Their synthesis of the evidence was that the pattern of evidence for both the low back and upper extremity (p.7) "supports an important role for physical factors".

Systematic reviews provide important contributions to understanding occupational MSDs. Important points about these reviews is that they follow strict rules by providing explicit information about the quality classification of studies that they include in the first place. They then use similarly explicit criteria to assess the quality of the evidence, for example the number of studies showing a positive association, the consistency of the results and the strengths of the associations. There are then many methods for presenting the evidence base, for example support for the relationship between exposure and outcome is usually expressed qualitatively as, for example, 'strong; limited; insufficient or no evidence' or 'strong, moderate or insufficient' evidence.

An alternative approach, the 'narrative review', an expert consensus which follows fewer rules but sometimes gives a broader perspective, can give evidence which differs from that given by systematic reviews. This contrast is illustrated by the differences between the panel review support for a relationship between physical factors and MSDs and a more recent systematic review which found 'conflicting' evidence about the relationship between force, in terms of heavy or physically demanding work, and the incidence of LBP[11]. It also illustrates some of the pitfalls because this review group were criticized for the way in which they categorised the evidence. They were taken to task by their definition of 'conflicting' as "inconsistent evidence in the available studies" by Takala (p.E282)[12] and also (p.E1011) for "mechanistic interpretation of statistical testing", the latter further elaborated by Olsen[13] (pE576) as "counting and comparing the number of statistically significant and nonsignificant associations". These commentaries suggest that the 'conflicting' classification is misleading. The 'mechanistic' criticism implies that some systematic reviews are prone to the effects of rather arbitrary choices between 'numbers of counts' in deciding when a relationship is significant or not. Systematic reviews do involve qualitative (in the research sense) decisions. Such decisions have in fact been common practice in occupational epidemiology as the decision to choose a 'cut point' between exposure categories can also be somewhat arbitrary. Meta-analyses avoid this particular problem.

One should not of course ignore the results of individual good quality studies, for example well powered prospective cohort studies. A good example is a large Danish cohort study[14] which concluded (p.1) that "Uncomfortable working positions, lifting or carrying loads, and pushing or pulling loads increased the risk of onset of long term sickness absence".

As regards posture, there is little evidence that sitting is a risk factor, and strong evidence that standing and walking has no association[11].

Whole body vibration (WBV) is a prevalent exposure for workers who drive or operate plant and machinery. Vibration acceleration is measured in three standard axes, X, fore and aft; Y, lateral; and Z, vertical. Acceleration acting in the Z axis is likely to place significant dynamic compressive loads on the spine. Exposure, like noise, is rarely steady and there are two main acceleration exposure indices, the 'equal energy' root mean square (r.m.s.) acceleration measured in ms^{-2}, or a measure of vibration dose, the vibration dose value (VDV) measured in $ms^{-1.75}$. The latter gives more weighting to 'shock' vibration, a quality which will have been apparent to those who have travelled 'cross country' in an all terrain vehicle or '4 wheel drive'.

There are standards for such exposure[15], probably the most useful values to remember being the European 'exposure action value' of 0.5 ms^{-2} which requires employers to activate a programme to reduce the exposures and a value of 1.5 ms^{-2} as the 'exposure limit value' above which workers should not be exposed.

The panel for MSDs[1] was of the opinion that WBV was an important factor for LBP, with (p.99) 16 out of 17 studies reporting a positive association, risk factors lying between 1.3 and 9.0. This is an example of when systematic reviews give a different perspective. Taking the quality of studies into account Bakker et al.[11] were able to include only 6 studies in a review, reporting (p.E284) "conflicting evidence for whole-body vibration as a risk factor for LBP". Although it is always difficult to interpret how epidemiological studies text should influence clinical decision making when dealing with individual cases, the European (or other) limits should be borne in mind when managing LBP in those who may be subject to WBV.

4.2. The psychosocial work climate in LBP

The psychosocial work climate has been difficult to characterize and therefore to study, but three systematic reviews summarise the evidence[1618]. Hartvigsen et al.[16], in a review of prospective studies, provided a useful categorisation of work related factors: perceptions of work (e.g. job satisfaction, feelings toward work); organisational aspects of work (job security, job demands); social support at work (recognition and respect, social support) and stress at work (stress, job strain). This review considered both LBP and the consequences of LBP, but after assessing 40 prospective studies (p.3) "no clear picture of the relation between work related psychosocial factors and LBP emerges". Hoogendorn et al.[17], assessing cohort and case-control studies, said that (p.2122) "comparing the results of this and other reviews on psychosocial factors showed that although there was evidence for the effect of some psychosocial work characteristics in all reviews, the results were rather heterogenous". Linton[19], in his review of prospective studies, did find significant associations. These were 'strong' for job satisfaction; monotonous work; work relations and perceived demands/load, 'moderate' for job control and pace and 'insufficient' for job content. The apparent disparity in these findings once again reflects the quality criteria applied in selection of the studies and how the evaluation of strength of association was carried out.

4.3. Individual demographic factors in LBP

Examining basic demographic factors and the association with low back pain highlights the heterogeneity of MSD outcomes of interest. Age has been shown to have a strong association with duration of sick leave[20]; an association with poor recovery[21]; an inconsistent relationship with work disability[22]; and no relation with either to return to work[23] or chronic disability[24]. The review showing a strong association with age and duration of sick leave[20] looked specifically at factors predicting duration of sick leave in workers in the early stages of an LBP related sick leave episode. On the other hand that showing no association between age and sickness absence[23] was specifically aimed at patients with non-specific low back pain and distinguishing predictors for either reporting sick (absence threshold) or to returning to work (return to work threshold). The concepts of absence threshold and return to work threshold are part of a sickness absence model first described by Steers and Rhodes[25] but adapted by Allegro and Veerman[26], which is, as usual, multifactorial. The model has a number of complex decision points for the patient with multiple opportunities for the psychosocial environment to exert an influence on their choices. The environment includes the economic and socio-political environment with factors such as the availability of alternative employment, sick leave and ill health retirement. These factors are all plausible reasons for the differences between studies.

4.4. Individual psychological factors

In 2002 Pincus et al.[27] carried out a review of psychological factors and their relationship with chronicity and disability in relation to low back and neck pain. The authors acknowledged the epidemiological uncertainties introduced by the characteristics of the specific populations in question and the measurement tools applied. The measurement tools, to be specific using questionnaires designed to measure psychological attributes in psychiatric patients (in contrast to MSD patients), proved to be a limiting factor. Because of the shortcomings in psychological instruments this review group could not differentiate between psychological distress, depressive symptoms and depressive mood, so grouped them together as 'distress'. They did however find that distress was a significant predictor and, acknowledging the importance of the population from which the sample is drawn, that this was especially so in the primary care setting. Linton[19], in examining low back and neck pain, also reported a 'clear link' between distress, as well as anxiety; stress; mood and emotions; cognitive functioning and pain behaviours. Cognitive variables such as fear avoidance beliefs have been associated as (Linton, p.1152) "a stable factor" for both LBP and neck pain, as have expectations of recovery. Linton also gives a particular mention as to how the person experiencing the pain perceives that the problem will develop, saying that (p.1152) "This anticipated outcome may be of special importance in assessing risk factors given the simplicity in obtaining such information".

4.5. Clinical assessment

The history should include aspects surrounding the onset of the pain and whether there is any history of radiation or neurological disturbance. It is also important to ask about previous episodes and any disability that resulted, as well as current limitations. In the absence of red flags as discussed in section 4, page 3, further investigation, at least in the first 6 weeks, is not indicated.

In the clinical assessment of LBP, as in all occupational MSDs, a thorough occupational history must be elicited. The history of the events preceding the acute episode is important, but many episodes occur spontaneously.

Occupationally, it is important to identify activities that may have caused the pain, or may be associated with limitations. This part of the history should include a review of the job in question in terms of occupational tasks and activities, best described from start to finish of each task or activity, working through them in a temporal or other logical sequence. Each task will require a description of the relevant work place physical factors of force, posture and repetition. As regards force and LBP there is no absolute 'cut-off' in magnitude of weight that it is safe or unsafe to lift, but carried close to the body, with arms flexed at the elbow and shoulders not extended, 16 kg for females and 25kg for males is a recommended maximum[28]. Postural factors modify this, reducing acceptable force to less than half if there is a mechanical disadvantage, for example with shoulders or elbows extended (figure 1). Twisting moments are thought to place additional biomechanical strain on the spine.

In terms of repetition there are no strict definitions, but a cycle of tasks occurring more frequently every 30 seconds should be classified as high.

There is no substitute for observing the person at work, actually performing the job tasks, however regular workplace visits may not be logistically practicable for many practitioners. If dealing with referrals from a workplace on a routine basis, it is however well worthwhile to carry out a workplace familiarisation visit during which relevant ergonomic factors can be assessed.

Any sporting activities in which the patient participates should also be assessed in much the same way as the occupational assessment, along with activities of daily living.

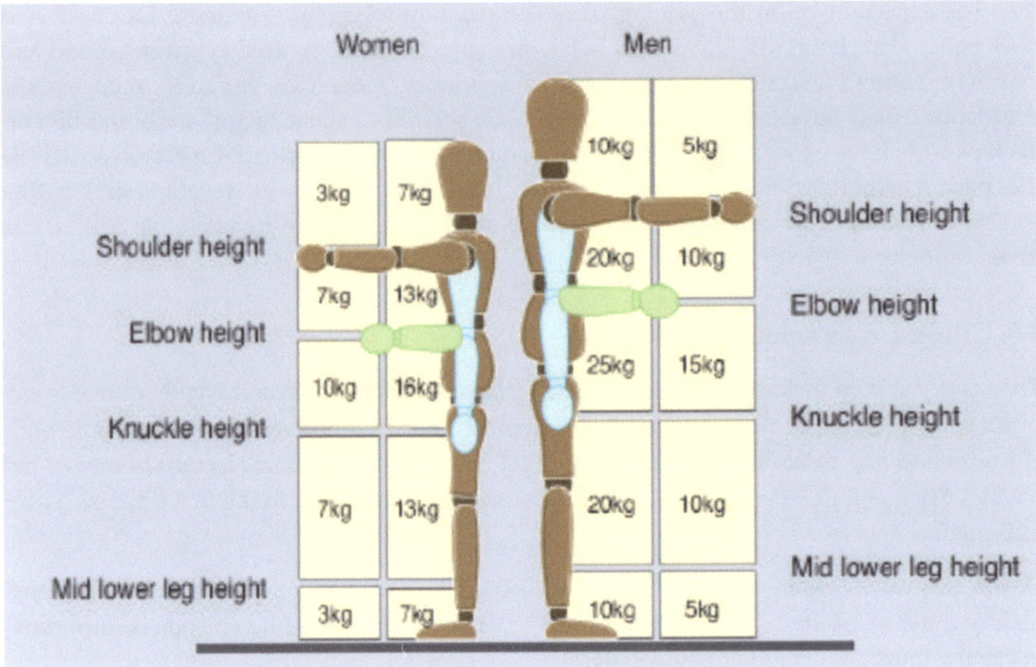

Source: HSE Leflet, Getting to Grips with Manual Handling

Figure 1.

There are a number of detailed assessment tools which are available to help in the assessment of the risk of MSDs. The Rapid Upper Limb Assessment (RULA) is an example, giving algorithms which may be used in the workplace setting[29].

4.6. Management of LBP

The management of LBP has been the subject of many reviews and much debate. In common with many areas of medical treatment, a sound evidence base, in the form of high quality randomised controlled trials (RCTs) is often lacking. The Cochrane Back Review Group[30] is instructive in the matter of treatment for LBP.

Adequate analgesia is necessary, paracetamol being a good initial choice. Non steroidal anti inflammatory drugs (NSAIDs) are also effective in acute and chronic LBP without sciatica, however a Cochrane review group found that effect sizes were small, that NSAIDs had more potential for adverse effects and that no one NSAID was more effective than another[31].

'Physiotherapy' includes many modalities of treatment including exercise therapy, but spinal manipulative therapy (SMT) and mobilisation (MOB) are common techniques. Other healthcare providers such as osteopaths and chiropractors also carry out these techniques.

A review of the evidence for their effectiveness[32], reported that, for acute LBP, (p.339) "There is moderate evidence that SMT has better short-term efficacy than spinal mobilization and detuned diathermy. There is limited evidence that SMT has better short-term efficacy than a combination of diathermy, exercise and ergonomic instruction."

When there was a mix of acute and chronic LBP[32], as is commonly the case, SMT/MOB provided (p.332) "either similar or better pain outcomes in the short and long term when compared with placebo and with other treatments, such as McKenzie therapy, medical care, management by physical therapists, soft tissue treatment and back school."

For chronic LBP, Bronfort et al.[32] reported that SMT/MOB was effective compared with a placebo, general practitioner care or other physical therapy and similarly effective as NSAIDs. However, a later review of SMT (which in this case included both manipulation and mobilisation techniques)[33], reported that (p.3) "SMT appears to be as effective as other common therapies prescribed for chronic low back pain such as exercise therapy, standard medical care or physical therapy."

4.7. Intervention strategies

Good quality interventions can only be designed on the basis of RCTs, which have proved a challenge to implement, follow up being difficult in the modern more dynamic workforce. In keeping with the multifactorial aetiology of MSDs, and knowledge about injury reduction interventions, it is becoming clear that single faceted approaches to primary and secondary prevention are not effective[34]. An example of a single faceted approach is an ergonomic intervention in which work-stations are physically changed. A multi faceted approach would include additional educational programmes and training.

As noted by Boocock et al.[35], Westgaard and Winkel[36] provided a useful construct for understanding ergonomic or 'mechanical' exposures and how the 'confounders' of other physical and psychosocial factors can be influenced by intervention strategies. They identified three main groups of intervention: mechanical exposure, production systems/organisational culture and modifier interventions. The first two are designed to change job exposures. Mechanical exposure interventions are aimed at improving the design of the work to reduce mechanical stresses. Production systems interventions change the exposure by changing the systems and culture of a company with focus on how the work is done and participation, for example using teams instead of individuals, influencing product flow and work technique training. Modifier interventions are not designed to change the exposure but to put the worker in a better position to deal with demands such as providing micro-breaks and pauses in work. These intervention strategies are considered further in section 6.2.

4.8. Rehabilitation

A fundamental tenet of occupational rehabilitation for all MSDs is that the patient should stay at work if possible, as physical activity will benefit most patients and protect against the adoption of a 'sick role'. There is evidence that if a worker is on sick leave for 4-12 weeks they have a 10-40% risk of still being off work at one year[37].

This tenet must however be tempered with the knowledge gained from a review of the job, and will require that the demands of the job are balanced with the abilities of the individual. Functional capacity of the individual client can be assessed, on a pragmatic basis, by asking them which tasks are giving difficulty, if (and with what degree of difficulty) they can be carried out, for how long, if there are any alternative tasks in the workplace that they could manage and if, in their opinion, the job or tasks could be modified. In general, task modification can be by means of hardware or software. Hardware in this context refers to the interface between the person and the work. A regards prevention of LBP loads should be presented to the worker so that they can perform manual handling in as 'near neutral' a posture as possible. Transfer points, for example the ends of conveyors, should therefore be adjustable to avoid trunk flexion. Software interventions include administrative arrangements which facilitate job rotation. This can shorten intensive job cycles and bring into play different muscle groups. Another strategy to reduce musculoskeletal stress is to provide adequate pauses and breaks.

This is a good point at which to consider the ethical implications of any recommendations. A return to work is undoubtedly good therapy for those who have an MSD, but the work context must be taken into account. One should consider whether the work, for example whole body shock vibration in a bulldozer driver, will cause excessive discomfort. The effect on the work should also be assessed, another good illustration being the effect of discomfort on cognitive performance in safety critical jobs.

The knowledge gained from this overall assessment should form the basis of a return to work contract between patient and treating practitioner. This must be communicated to the workplace in as specific and detailed a manner as possible in terms of the tasks that can be carried out, along with any limitations such as restrictions in the force or weight that can be borne, tasks that cannot be undertaken or that require modification and restrictions in 'duty cycle' (the frequency and or duration of tasks) that may be necessary. Objective assessment and agreement between practitioner and patient is essential, in particular the time frames that can be expected for a return to normal work, for which there are guidelines: the normal expectation should be of recovery from LBP within two to four weeks. The process from here will be a matter of adjustment and matching between the physical capabilities of the individual and the demands of the workplace.

4.9. Barriers to adjustment and return to work

A number of psychological factors have been associated with the prevalence of MSDs, their chronicity and poorer outcomes. These have been described as 'yellow flags'[38]. They will not be present in every patient, but barriers should be suspected if recovery is delayed beyond the usual 2-4 weeks. These can be broadly classified into personal and work related factors. The point at which they act, either in aggravation of the experience of acute pain or in the transition from acute to chronic pain cannot be identified with any certainty. They do however need to be identified and are discussed in the next section on chronic LBP. The New Zealand Guidelines Group provide a practical guide to assessing 'yellow flags', in the form of a screening questionnaire and clinical guide-line[39].

5. Chronic low back pain

Chronic low back pain can be classified by the frequency, duration, and intensity of the pain that is experienced, by the degree of disability that results, by the amount of sick leave that is taken or a combination of these indicators. All may be variously defined, which does give rise to some difficulty in making comparisons.

A number of variables seem to be important in the transition between acute and chronic LBP, these include biological, cognitive, affective and behavioural elements. It is very important to bear in mind that research into these factors has been conducted in many settings, be it presenting for treatment in primary care, in a workplace, a specialist referral centre or for disability benefit assessment. The setting will influence how the risk factor influences both the prevalence and strength of association. When identifying the significance of risk factors one must therefore examine carefully the population from which the study is drawn. With psychological variables it must be clear what instruments were used to measure the psychological constructs and how outcome measures, in terms of 'unfavourable outcomes', were defined.

It has been suggested that cognitive and behavioural factors might play a part in the transition from acute to chronic LBP. A review by Ramond et al.[40] looked at the problem prospectively in the primary care setting. Coping strategies were evaluated in four studies and fear-avoidance beliefs in seven, with statistical associations in about half of these. The authors specifically mention high pain related fear as being a powerful predictor in a Dutch study[41].

Presence of a belief about future harm from, or being disabled by, LBP has been shown to result in adverse outcomes in a number of studies. It is relatively simple to gain information in this respect[19], so it is an area where reassurance may be helpful.

In people with both non-chronic[42, 43] and chronic LBP[23] more positive expectations of recovery have been associated with better sick leave related outcomes.

6. Axial pain: Neck pain

Shoulder/neck disorders are an important 'cross-over' region. There is debate about 'specific' shoulder pain, discussed below, and 'non specific' shoulder pain in the cervico-thoracic area. The latter seems to have few occupational risk factors and thus seemingly spontaneous onset, for example 'tension neck syndrome'. A considerable range of clinical conditions is therefore represented. Epidemiologically, this can give rise to classification problems, many studies using self reported neck pain as an outcome rather than the result of a clinical assessment.

There is no doubt that neck pain is common, The annual prevalence for neck pain has been reported to range between 16.7% to 75.1%, with a mean of 37.2%, similar figures to LBP[44].

Diagnostically, there is a great deal of variation in the terminology used to describe neck pain and the clinical diagnostic protocols involved. Larsson et al.[45] make a good point in saying that (p.455) "The basis for the diagnostic criteria of neck and shoulder myalgia is relatively vague, and the diagnostic terminology and methods for assessment of neck and upper-limb musculoskeletal disorders are variable." They introduce a standardized clinical examination protocol as a diagnostic aide for neck and upper extremity disorders, which includes standardised questions on pain, tiredness and stiffness on the day of examination, with physical tests including range of motion and 'tightness' of muscles, pain threshold and sensitivity, muscle strength, and palpation of tender points, to which should be added tests of sensation.

A broad and functional diagnostic classification would distinguish between muscular and vertebral dysfunction. Acute muscular dysfunction is recognisable as torticollis, with acute or subacute onset and severe muscle spasm and limitation of movement. It is usually idiopathic however if there has been a motor vehicle crash or other incident involving sudden neck acceleration it may be classified as a 'whiplash' injury. Vertebral dysfunction arises because of facet joint, intervertebral disc or spondolytic problems. Nerve root problems will be suggested by the presence of cervical nerve root symptoms including dermatomal radiation but especially if sensorimotor symptoms are present. Cervical outlet syndrome will be suggested by symptoms and signs in the ulnar nerve distribution.

Non-specific neck pain, a diagnosis of exclusion, lies in a continuum. It may only involve the neck muscles, but may also spread beyond that boundary, seldom strictly classified but would include the middle and lower fibres of the trapezius. If tender points are palpable in the trapezius area, some would advocate a diagnosis of 'trapezius myalgia', which may occur at the more chronic limit of the spectrum.

As with LBP, it is essential to rule out 'red flag' disorders.

Of the risk factors, sex does appear to play a significant role in neck pain, females having a higher prevalence than males [44]. There is no ready explanation for this.

6.1. Interventions in neck and upper extremity pain

As for LBP, adequate analgesia is necessary in the acute phase, along with an explanation that the discomfort will settle.

Conservative treatments, including physiotherapy, have played a major role in treatment and intervention in these conditions, however there is not a good evidence base for the efficacy of such treatment, partly because there have been fewer high quality intervention studies. A Cochrane review was carried out by Verhagen et al. in 2006[46]. Although subsequently withdrawn for reasons of being 'out of date' (the new protocol is however available[47]) it summarised the evidence available at the time. The reviewers examined the role of physiotherapy and workplace ergonomic interventions for adults suffering from 'complaints of the arm, neck and/or shoulder' or CANS. The results, in terms of quality of the studies, was disappointing. From 126 references selected for full text retrieval only 21 trials were included in the review. The reviewers concluded that (p.4) "…there is limited evidence about the positive effectiveness of exercises when compared to massage; adding breaks during computer work; massage as add-on treatment on manual therapy, manual therapy as add-on treatment on exercises; and some keyboards in people with carpal tunnel syndrome when compared to placebo. There is conflicting evidence concerning the efficacy of exercises over no treatment or as an add-on treatment, and no differences between various kinds of exercises can be found yet. At the moment there is also conflicting evidence about the effectiveness of ergonomic programs over no treatment."

6.2. Workplace interventions in neck pain

Boocock and colleagues[35] carried out a review specifically based on the classification of Westgaard and Winkel[36]. Once again, although 451 studies were suitable for review, only 31 were selected for full assessment. Of these 31 (p.293) "Ten were classified as mechanical exposure interventions, two as production systems/organisational culture interventions and 19 as modifier interventions." Of the 10 mechanical exposure interventions, four looked at work environment/workstation adjustments. These showed some evidence of positive health effects. Three studies looked at changes to workstation equipment (keyboards and mouse design) in visual display unit workers with upper extremity symptoms and there was moderate evidence to support this intervention. Two of three studies examining the introduction of ergonomic equipment concerned vibration reduction, and although reporting positive health outcomes, were of low quality and gave insufficient evidence of benefit. Two low quality studies did not find improvements after organisational and work-task design changes in office workers and manufacturing assembly workers therefore there was not sufficient evidence to support these interventions.

Nineteen studies focussed on modifier interventions. Three medium-quality studies, including one randomised controlled trial, in workers with neck/upper extremity conditions (not including fibromyalgia) investigated exercise such as strengthening, flexibility and coordination and provided some evidence of the effectiveness of this type of intervention.

Another four studies looked at the benefits of this type of intervention in fibromyalgia sufferers, with some evidence in support of exercise regimes.

The effects of multiple modifier interventions including exercise were examined in eight studies, four that excluded fibromyalgia and four that included the condition. These also gave some evidence that such regimes were beneficial.

Lastly, one RCT examined multiple modifier interventions excluding exercise but including cognitive behavioural training and education from which non fibromyalgia patients showed positive benefits. However, there was insufficient evidence to support this approach in patients with fibromyalgia.

Boocock et al. specifically compare their results with that of Verhagen et al.[46] who carried out the Cochrane review. The results for the mechanical intervention group were similar, bearing in mind that the 'limited evidence' category of the earlier review compares with the 'some evidence' category of the latter. Both reviews agreed that production systems interventions showed little benefit. However, one significant difference was that the Boocock et al. review showed that there was some evidence that modifier intervention would provide benefit.

As regards overall recommendations, there does seem to be benefit in introducing mechanical interventions. The majority of the studies in this category in the Boocock et al. review were of office workers using computers and either involved either work environment change (primarily lighting) and/or adjustment to office layout or equipment or looked at new keyboards and introduction of adjustable equipment. Fewer studies focussed on manufacturing, where force and repetition would be most prevalent and where one would expect most benefit in terms of mechanical interventions to reduce demand. Two studies did however look at hand-arm vibration reduction in a manufacturing setting again showing showing some benefit.

7. Peripheral pain

The acronyms associated with MSDs have already been introduced. The term RSI has been used as a broad term to describe conditions of the upper limb that have an association with force, posture and repetition, also known as cumulative trauma disorder in the US, with the term occupational overuse syndrome used in Australia and New Zealand emphasising the occupational associations.

There is good epidemiological evidence that peripheral MSDs have specific occupational associations. There is a much greater level of evidence than is the case with LBP and NP that the physical factors of force, posture and repetition play a significant role in these conditions, for example the postural factor of working above head height is associated with shoulder disorders[3]. As a general rule if a combination of these factors is present they should be considered significant.

An example of a population based study supporting the role of work comes from Roquelaire et al.[48] who carried out a population based cross sectional study over 3 years, taking a random sample from workers undergoing mandatory health screening by 83 occupational physicians. All the patients underwent a standardised clinical examination. Occupational risk factors were assessed by questionnaire. From the total of 3,710 workers a total of 472 had at least one MSD. Rotator cuff syndrome was, with 274 cases (7.4%) the most prevalent condition, followed by 113 cases (3.1%) CTS; 90 (2.6%) lateral epicondylitis; 45 (1.2%) De Quervain's disease; 30 (2.6%) ulnar tunnel syndrome and 29 (0.8%) wrist tendinitis. The risk of an MSD increased with age, those aged 50-54 having a higher risk (in comparison to those aged less than 30, an Odds Ratio (OR) of 4.9, 95% confidence interval (CI) 2.7-8.6 for men and an OR of 5.0, 95% CI 2.7-9.3 for women. A final multivariate logistic model showed an increased risk with age (all age groups compared to those less than 30 years; obesity (OR 1.6, 95%CI 1.1-2.4) and a prior history of upper extremity MSD (OR 3.3, 95% CI 2.6-4.2);

The associated physical factors were high repetitiveness (OR 1.6, 95% CI 1.2-2.0); arms at or above shoulder level (OR 1.5, 95% CI 1.1-2.0) and wrist bending in extreme postures (OR 1.5, 95% CI 1.2-2.0). The only work-related psychosocial factor remaining in the final model was low supervisor support (OR 1.3, 95% CI 1.1-1.7).

7.1. Shoulder pain

Occupational shoulder pain does have specific workplace associations with forceful repetitive work especially when the work is carried out above shoulder height[3]. Such work provides a biomechanically plausible mechanism for many of these injuries, but especially for rotator cuff syndrome (supraspinatus, infraspinatus, or bicipital tendinitis) where increased pressure may impair the microcirculation and cause microtrauma.

Rotator cuff syndrome is a common condition, and the most common source of shoulder pain in those over the age of 35, the prevalence rising with age. In those over the age of 70, tears may be found in more than 50% of those presenting with shoulder pain[39].

The pathological changes in rotator cuff are becoming clearer with time, but involve either tendinosis or a tendon tear, either full or part thickness. Tendinosis may occur due to the changes outlined above with microtrauma, but degenerative changes also occur due to age and there is an association with systemic conditions including diabetes. Tears occur with more forceful activity or where tendons are weakened due to degenerative changes. These may be classified as partial, full thickness or massive (involving more than one rotator cuff tendon).

The history should include the mode of onset of the pain, the location (typically at the point of the shoulder), whether the onset was acute or chronic and whether night pain is present. A detailed occupational history should include the factors of force, posture and repetition, and a sporting and recreational history is essential. The occupations which involve work at or above shoulder height include automotive engineers, builders, electricians and assembly line workers.

There is no single clinical finding that is pathognomonic of the condition, but a 'painful arc' is highly suggestive, and weakness in shoulder abduction may indicate the presence of a tear.

If a tear is suspected, diagnostic ultrasound of the shoulder should be carried out: this is a valid test for full thickness tears but the validity for detecting tendinosis or in differentiating other causes of painful shoulder has not been demonstrated[39].

Differential diagnoses include subacromial bursitis and acromioclavicular joint problems. The clinical findings (location of the pain and aggravating movements) may be sufficient to distinguish between them. Plain X-ray of the shoulder may exclude osteoarthritis in the older patient.

7.1.1. Interventions in shoulder pain

Treatment is aimed at pain relief and restoration of function.

The initial approach should include an adequate dose of NSAIDs. The occupational review should identify the activities giving rise to discomfort, and if these are causing significant pain the particular task or activity should be avoided or modified.

Corticosteroid injections are quite often used as an adjunct treatment for tendinopathy if NSAIDs have been given an adequate trial. For rotator cuff syndrome, the injection may be given either sub-acromially or intra-articularly. A Cochrane review of sub-acromial injections showed that they had a small benefit over placebo in some trials with generally short term benefit. Only 3 trials comparing steroid to NSAIDs were available for comparison, and there were however no significant benefit of injection.[49]

Physiotherapy is commonly used for shoulder conditions and Green et al.[50] (p.2) say that "There is some evidence from methodologically weak trials to indicate that some physiotherapy interventions are effective for some specific shoulder disorders. For example, the review group found that mobilisation plus exercise was better than exercise alone in people with rotator cuff disease.

Surgery has been advocated for rotator cuff syndrome, particularly in young and active patients. A variety of open and arthrosopic techniques has been developed, including subacromial decompression, debridement and repair of tendons, with multiple techniques often being used. A Cochrane review[51] summarised the evidence. Only two trials of rotator cuff tear repair met the inclusion criteria and neither had advantageous outcomes. The review group concluded that (p.9) "Based upon our review of 14 trials, all highly susceptible to bias, we cannot draw firm conclusions about the efficacy or safety of surgery for rotator cuff disease".

7.2. Elbow

The classical forms of elbow tendinitis are tennis (lateral) and golfers (medial) epicondylitis. These are, apart from the sporting connotations, well recognised occupational entities.

Lateral epicondylitis is caused by injury to the extensor tendons of the forearm caused by repeated resisted contraction of the extensor muscles, the force coming classically from resistance to the action in the backhand swing in tennis or the more prevalent action of carrying heavy shopping or suitcases. The pathology is thought to be small tears or granulation tissue occurring at the attachment of the common extensor origin at the lateral side of the elbow. The pain originates here and may radiate to the forearm or wrist.

Occupationally the pain is caused by repetitive wrist extension and supination against resistance.

Medial epicondylitis is much less common and is caused by wrist flexion and pronation, or the forces acting against this motion, classically a golf swing.

There is strong evidence that a combination of the risk factors of force, posture and repetition are associated with both of these conditions. The occupational history should include the nature of the tasks undertaken, and observation, as always, is useful. Workers involved in assembly or construction work using screwdrivers are at particular risk, as are those using air or electrically driven screwdrivers or torque wrenches especially if the torque is not controlled adequately as tightening occurs. Hammering, and the repetitive motions of meat packing may also be causative. If a tool is being used, the grip should be of the right size- neither too large nor small.

The history should also include any sporting activities that are undertaken.

On examination in lateral epicondylitis, pain will be present distal to the insertion of the extensor carpi radialis brevis tendon at the elbow, and increased by wrist extension, especially with a pronated, radially deviated wrist in elbow extension. Classically, an introductory hand shake with the patient will exacerbate the discomfort.

In medial epicondylitis, the pain occurs with resisted wrist flexion and resisted forearm pronation.

The main differential diagnosis in the occupational setting will be non-specific forearm pain. This is more likely if the pain is diffuse, there is no clear history of force, posture or repetition in the job, no clear precipitating factors and the pain is atypical with a burning or other dysaesthetic quality.

Investigations are seldom needed in the presence of a typical history.

Treatment is by the avoidance of the provoking activities and maintenance and improvement of strength and range of motion by exercises which can be provided by a physiotherapist. It may be difficult to achieve the desired degree of rest in the occupations which give rise to epicondylitis, as they are often truly forceful and repetitive. If the treating physician is not familiar with the workplace, a task analysis will be necessary. This can often be carried out by an occupational therapist or physiotherapist who has training in, and experience of, workplace assessment. There may be ways in which the work can be changed, for example job rotation, to reduce cumulative loading on the individual. Individual technique and the design of any tools used also requires assessment. Bissett et al.[52] comment upon interventions for tennis elbow with outcomes including pain relief, functional improvement and 'global improvement', the latter including return to work, or normal activities, or both. Corticosteroid injections seemed more effective than placebo or no intervention at increasing global improvement at 6 weeks, but not at one year. The authors comment that corticosteroid injection may however increase the recurrence rate. Autologous blood injection is a relatively new technique, with the benefits unknown at present, but case series have reported significant improvements[53]. Compared with placebo, it seems that topical NSAIDs reduce pain at 4 weeks but may not give functional improvement[52].

7.3. Hand/wrist pain

The classical hand-wrist occupational disorder is carpal tunnel syndrome, entrapment of the median nerve at the wrist. Ulnar neuropathy at the elbow is less common.

De Quervains tendonitis and wrist tendonitis also have occupational associations.

The occupations involved will generally be those involving significant forces or effort in performing the job, for example those carrying in assembly work, for example in the automotive industries, and those involved in meat processing, for example butchering or packing.

7.4. Carpal tunnel syndrome (CTS)

CTS is a condition which results from pressure on the median nerve at the wrist where it passes under the transverse carpal ligament. The pressure in this space may arise due to either tendinopathy or by enlargement of the other wrist structures. The symptoms are sensory changes, tingling and pain, in the distribution of the median nerve at the wrist. The motor branches may also be affected, with wasting of the thenar eminence. The prevalence in the general population[54] depends on the depth of screening, with 354 individuals (14.4%) of 2466 responders in a general population survey reporting symptoms, 94 (3.8%) confirmed 'clinically certain', 168 (6.8%) 'clinically uncertain' and 120 (4.9%) from both groups having neurophysiological tests reported as positive.

CTS is associated with endocrine disorders (diabetes and thyroid disorders) and pregnancy and there seems to be a familial tendency[55].

The diagnosis is primarily by the history of tingling and numbness, with loss of manual dexterity supporting the diagnosis. The pain is classically present at night, waking the patient, and may radiate either proximally or distally.

The symptoms typically localise to the palmar aspect of the first (thumb) to fourth (ring) fingers and the distal palm, being the sensory innervation of the median nerve at the wrist.

Numbness predominantly in the fifth finger or extending to the thenar eminence or dorsum of the hand should suggest other diagnoses. The pain may be atypical with more generalised radiation. This may indicate autonomic fibre involvement and does not exclude CTS from the diagnosis. There may also be a loss of motor function: the median nerve also supplies motor fibres to the thenar muscles and the lateral two lumbricals. Apart from the 'hands falling asleep' the deficit in motor function may cause loss of dexterity and grip strength. The functional loss may cause the patient to drop things.

Investigations should include inflammatory indices and thyroid function.

Nerve conduction studies (NCS) are often advocated in the diagnosis of CTS. Using the results of such diagnostic tests in diagnostic algorithms does however require insight as to the properties of such a screening test. One must firstly bear in mind that there are many modalities of NCS and that a specific prescription for the test is required. A New Zealand review[56] looked at (p.59) "intra-individual comparative tests of the measurable conduction of the median nerve over equally long nerve segments in the hand" The specificity (a low number of false positives, the likelihood of correctly identifying those who do not have the disorder) was reported as lying between 83 and 100%. The sensitivity (a low number of false positives, so likely to identify those who do have the disorder) was reported as being in the order of 70-80%. Relying on the results of NCS requires the application of rules. NCS is therefore good at "ruling in"[57]: if it is negative then a patient is unlikely to have the condition. It is not however good at "ruling out" because a positive test does not necessarily means that the patient has the condition. CTS is therefore a very good example of a condition which has a complex diagnostic algorithm.

Ultrasound and MRI scanning can also demonstrate compression, but are not superior to NCS[56].

Bearing in mind the prevalence of CTS, the occupational associations have been questioned. A review by Palmer et al.[58] found reasonable evidence that regular and prolonged use of hand-held vibratory tools increased the risk of CTS by a factor of 2 (a prevalence Odds Ratio of 2 or more) and also "found substantial evidence for similar or even higher risks from prolonged and highly repetitious flexion and extension of the wrist, especially when allied with a forceful grip" (p.57). The studies reviewed did have limitations, many being cross sectional in nature, but the clinical advice given in this paper is sound. The authors comment that highly repetitive gripping should be avoided by ergonomic design of tasks and tools, and by scheduling appropriate rest breaks. They defined repetitive wrist movements as flexion/extension every 30 seconds or more often. A detailed job assessment should be carried out in all cases of suspected occupational CTS.

Treatment is, in the first instance, expectant. A wrist splint, worn especially at night (as with De Quervains tenosynovitis, may improve the nocturnal symptoms and local corticosteroid injection may also be helpful in the short term. Definitive treatment is by surgical division of the retinaculum, which can be performed endoscopically.

7.5. Ulnar neuropathy

Ulnar neuropathy at the elbow (UNE) is, after CTS, the second most common upper limb compression neuropathy. The nerve is in a superficial position at the medial epicondyle of the elbow and this, along with the arrangement of the muscular septae in this area, means that it is prone to ischaemia and traction injuries. Compression also occurs in the Guyon canal at the wrist. It has proved difficult to estimate incidence and prevalence, but between 1995 and 2000 Juratli et al.[59]. reported that 2,863 cases were diagnosed by the Washington State workers compensation system. It seems that the condition is expensive: this group reported (abstract) that of 250 surgical cases selected at random "The mean wage replacement and medical benefits paid per case were $19,100 and $15,200, respectively."

The diagnosis is suggested by pain and dysaesthesiae in the ring and little fingers of the hand. As in CTS this may be noticed at night and there may also be discomfort at the elbows. The sensory changes usually precede any motor loss, which involves the ulnar innervated small muscles of the hand. It is possible to have concurrent CTS and UNE in which case the clinical picture can be complex. Ulnar nerve conduction studies can be performed to help confirm the diagnosis, but there is little information on the validity of such testing. X-ray of the elbow and wrist may also be indicated if there are anatomical abnormalities or a history of trauma.

The work relatedness of the condition appears not to have been widely studied. Descatha and colleagues[60] describe a longitudinal study in which they were able to follow 598 workers with 15 incident cases. The variables most strongly associated with UNE were (p.237) "holding a tool in position"; BMI and another work related MSD. This does suggest that occupational activities may be important, the most likely suspects being those that are associated with epicondylitis and CTS. Direct pressure on the elbow (as in driving or leaning on the elbows at a work bench) and trauma around the elbow are also associated with UNE.

Treatment guidelines e.g. those of the Washington State Department of Labor and Industries[61], suggest that conservative treatment should be tried for 6 weeks. Surgery is usually reserved for cases that limit activities (i.e. with motor involvement). A Cochrane review group[62] could not recommend a single best treatment or when to treat a patient conservatively or surgically, Of the two main surgical options, decompression or transposition, both seemed equally effective.

7.6. De Quervains tenosynovitis

De Quervains tenosynovitis is caused by entrapment of the tendons of the abductor pollicis longus (APL) and the extensor pollicis brevis (EPB) tendons where the extensor retinaculum binds the tendon sheaths at the radial styloid process. The pathophysiological process is thought to be the same as with rotator cuff syndrome, with repetitive microtrauma giving rise to impaired circulation and granulation tissue.

Clinically the condition is characterised by wrist pain at the anatomical snuffbox that may radiate proximally or distally. There may also be localized swelling and crepitus on thumb and wrist movement.

There will be localized pain on palpation over the APL and EPB tendons, and discomfort on resisted abduction or extension of the thumb.

The original NIOSH panel was of the opinion that there was 'strong' evidence that a combination of force, posture and repetition (in other words highly repetitious, forceful hand/wrist exertion) was associated with hand wrist tendinitis[3], which includes De Quervains. The populations studied have included meat workers and assembly line workers, the wrist motions involved being complex in nature, but involving a strong grip.

The treatment involves avoiding the provoking activities, and wrist splinting (at least in daytime) for a period of two to six weeks may be helpful. Splinting should be applied in wrist extension of 10° and first carpo-metacarpal and metacarpo-phalangeal joints also both splinted in slight extension. If there is no improvement in four to six weeks, corticosteroid injection may be tried, as may adjunct NSAIDs. The evidence of effectiveness of the latter two, as in other MSDs, is uncertain.

7.7. Wrist tendonitis

Tenosynovitis of the wrist is a disorder of the tendon sheaths at the wrist, localised to the involved tendons, with symptoms on wrist movement. The prevalence in the general population is thought to be about 1% in men and 2% in women[63]. It is higher in working populations. A study of 5,338 workers in the Henan province of China[64] found the prevalence of self reported wrist discomfort to be 33.5% and associated with physical job characteristics: prolonged wrist bending or twisting; exerting great forces with arms or hands and using vibrating tools. In a study of garment workers[65], 146 out of 520 individuals (35.6%) reported hand/wrist pain for at least two days in the past month. Fifteen of the 374 who were pain free had one or more physical signs at the wrist and only 21 of the 146 reporting pain had one or more sign on examination. Tendinopathy examination findings were recorded as flexor carpi radialis (2.5%) or flexor carpi ulnaris (1.1%) tendinopathies; digital flexor tendonitis (0.9%) and extensor tendonitis (2.7%). Only about half of those diagnosed with signs reported symptoms. With the wrist stabilised, pain should be exacerbated by resisted movement of the affected tendon.

Conservative treatments include rest, NSAIDs physiotherapy and workplace interventions [66]. A review of conservative treatments[67] did however identify that there was no evidence to support or refute these strategies.

A systematic review of the efficacy of corticosteroid and other injections for the management of tendinopathies[68] concluding (p.1762) that "We have shown strong evidence that corticosteroid injection is beneficial in the short term for treatment of tendinopathy, but is worse than are other treatment options in the intermediate and long terms."

7.8. Hand arm vibration syndrome (HAVS)

HAVS is characterised by disorders of the intrinsic muscles, nerves, bone, joints and circulatory systems and is caused by vibration being transmitted to the hands by a vibrating tool or a work piece. Vibration White Finger (VWF) is the most common syndrome in the

UK and in other countries with similar climates, but the vascular changes are not so prevalent in more temperate climates.

This condition occurs following exposure to hand vibration, the first symptom being vascular, manifest as blanching of the fingers. The attacks usually occur on exposure to cold (and not directly after the vibration exposure): touching a cold surface, being exposed to a cold damp environment, or immersing the hands in cold water (cold water provocation, one of the diagnostic tests) will precipitate the blanching sign. Attacks are therefore more common in the winter.

There is a gradual progression of symptoms: the finger tips are first to be affected, but with increasing vibration dose the middle and proximal digits are affected. This blanching lasts for a period of minutes to hours, and ends with a reactive hyperaemia with pins and needles or frank discomfort or pain.

VWF also has a neurological component, noticed as tingling, numbness and a loss of manual dexterity. At first this is most noticeable after the vibration exposure stops and it recovers after exposure, but it may get worse with continued exposure and become permanent.

The two main mechanisms, vascular and neurological, have separate mechanisms. The vascular component is caused by ischaemia, and interest has focused on direct damage to the vessel walls and also the sympathetic neural network which regulates the arterioles. Neural changes seem to progress independently of the vascular damage, and result in the loss of sensation and motor function.

Other possible changes seen in the musculoskeletal system of the hand, wrist and arm in vibration exposed workers have been muscle fatigue, callus formation in palms and digits, enlargement of metacarpophalangeal joints, bone changes and alteration in grip force, but these have been difficult to quantify.

It is also difficult to differentiate between these effects caused by vibration and the effects of heavy physical work on the hand. Repetitive flexion and extension of the wrist, which action is also prevalent in some of these occupations, may lead to CTS and this may complicate the clinical picture.

7.9. Diagnosis

The clinical assessment is based on the extent of involvement according to the vascular and neurological components separately according to the 'Stockholm classification' (table 1) [69].

It is more usual for the vascular signs and symptoms to occur first, in other words the vibration white finger. The 1987 Stockholm classification of the vascular component mentioned above gives some guidance as to the onset. It is more usual for the blanching to affect the tips only of one or more fingers. The vibration exposure itself does not usually cause white finger, it is exposure to cold and wet conditions that trigger the vascular spasm, which is most commonly followed by hyperaemia.

<table>
<tr><th colspan="3">Vascular component</th></tr>
<tr><td>Stage</td><td>Grade</td><td>Description</td></tr>
<tr><td>1</td><td>Mild</td><td>Occasional blanching attacks affecting tips of one or more fingers</td></tr>
<tr><td>2</td><td>Moderate</td><td>Occasional attacks affecting distal and middle phalanges of one or more fingers</td></tr>
<tr><td>3</td><td>Severe</td><td>Frequent attacks affecting all phalanges of most fingers</td></tr>
<tr><td>4</td><td>Very severe</td><td>As in 3, with trophic skin changes (tips)</td></tr>
<tr><th colspan="3">Neurological component</th></tr>
<tr><td>Stage</td><td colspan="2">Description</td></tr>
<tr><td>0SN</td><td colspan="2">no symptoms</td></tr>
<tr><td>1SN</td><td colspan="2">Intermittent or persistent numbness with or without tingling</td></tr>
<tr><td>2SN</td><td colspan="2">As in 1SN with reduced sensory perception</td></tr>
<tr><td>3SN</td><td colspan="2">As in 2SN with reduced tactile discrimination and manipulative dexteritv</td></tr>
</table>

Table 1. Stockholm Classification (1987)

The onset is usually gradually progressive with cumulative exposure, spreading to more fingers and farther down the fingers.

There are many occupations which involve exposure to vibration. Some of the highest exposures are to be found in the silviculture, construction and metalworking industries.

Primary and secondary Raynauds phenomenon must be ruled out.

Secondary Raynauds phenomenon (including vibration) may complicate other conditions, the most frequent of these being connective tissue disorders. Blood indices and inflammatory markers are required. A cervical rib will be excluded radiologically.

Routine laboratory investigations should therefore include rheumatoid factor, antinuclear serum antibodies, possibly cryoglobulins and serum protein electrophoresis. Scleroderma must be excluded.

There are a number of objective tests described to assess HAVS: vascular (cold provocation), the neurological component includes tactile, vibrotactile, and thermal threshold impairment (detected by aesthesiometry and altered vibration perception threshold). Musculoskeletal testing is sometimes carried out (dynamometry, pinch test and pick-up test), but not all clinicians agree on what should be present in the test battery. Single tests such as the Allen test are of very limited validity.

Primary prevention of HAVs should be aimed at reducing exposures to a 'safe' level. The exposure action value[1] is an r.m.s acceleration value of 2.5 ms^{-2}, and the exposure limit value 5 ms^{-2}[15]. Exposure at 2.5 ms^{-2} will result in HAVS in 10% of persons after 12 years of exposure, and at 5 ms^{-2} after 5.8 years. Many vibrating tools, for example chainsaws and construction equipment, frequently exceed this value.

There is no specific treatment for HAVS, but with cessation of exposure the condition should remain static.

8. Summary

There is no clinical hallmark with which to distinguish occupational MSDs from those due to any other agency apart from the evidence gained from the occupational history. The astute clinician will always ask about the occupation of the patient during a consultation, knowing that important opportunities for disease prevention and treatment will otherwise be missed. In the clinical interpretation of epidemiological data it is as well to bear in mind that there are many methodological pitfalls in the study of MSDs. Not least of these is the dynamic nature of these disorders in that they tend towards recurrence. It can be therefore be difficult to distinguish between 'new' incident cases and those which are in fact recurrent or persistent. This misclassification of outcome will distort the relationship with risk factors. There are also problems with case definition either in terms of the self reported outcome measures of frequency, duration and severity or on the other hand clinical case identification. Exposure assessment and classification is also difficult, particularly assessing the elements of force, posture and repetition. There are also many important psychosocial confounders in the personal and work domains, the importance of which are becoming clearer. It can therefore be difficult to demonstrate a causal relationship when studying MSDs, for example the temporal relationship is often uncertain; the strength of the relationship can be diluted by confounding or misclassification and, as it is technically very demanding to measure physical exposures, dose response information is often lacking. Although the work-relatedness of some MSDs has been questioned, it is nevertheless of vital importance to understand the role of the work place in both causation and rehabilitation. The authors cannot do better than quote the words of Ramazzini, the 'father of occupational medicine', whose advice given to the profession was[70] (page 13) "There are many things that a doctor, on his first visit to a patient, ought to find out from the patient or from those present. For so runs the oracle of our inspired teacher: "when you come to a patients house, you should ask him what sort of pains he has, what caused them, how many days he has been ill whether the bowels are working and what sort of food he eats" So says Hippocrates in his work *Affections*. I may venture to add one more question: what occupation does he follow?"

---

[1] For definitions see section 4.1 (page 65)

Author details

David McBride and Helen Harcombe
University of Otago, Dunedin, New Zealand

9. References

[1] Panel on Musculoskeletal Disorders and the Workplace, National Research Council and Institute of Medicine and Commission on Behavioral and Social Sciences and Education. (2001). Musculoskeletal disorders and the workplace: low back and upper extremities. Washington, DC, National Academy Press. Available http://www.nap.edu/openbook.php?isbn=0309072840 Accessed 2012 19 July.
[2] Dodwell P (2003). OOS or MUD? Time for a cleanup. NZ Med J. 116: 1-6.
[3] National Institute of Occupational Safety and Health. (1997). Musculoskeletal disorders and workplace factors, a critical review of the epidemiological evidence for work-related musculoskeletal disorders of the neck, upper extremity, and low back. Cincinnati, National Institute of Occupational Safety and Health. Available http://www.cdc.gov/niosh/docs/97-141/ Accessed 2012 19 July.
[4] McCunney R J and Brandt-Rauf P (1991). Ethical conflict in the private practice of occupational medicine. Journal of Occupational Medicine. 33: 80-82.
[5] Brandt-Rauf P W, Brandt-Rauf S I and Fallon Jr L F (1989). Management of ethical issues in the practice of occupational medicine. Occup Med (Philadelphia). 4: 171-176.
[6] Walker B F (2000). The prevalence of low back pain: A systematic review of the literature from 1966 to 1998. J Spinal Disord. 13: 205-217.
[7] Cote P, Cassidy J D and Carroll L (1998). The Saskatchewan health and back pain survey: The prevalence of neck pain and related disability in Saskatchewan adults. Spine. 23: 1689-1698.
[8] Battie M C, Videman T, Gibbons L E, et al. (1995). Determinants of lumbar disc degeneration: A study relating lifetime exposures and magnetic resonance imaging findings in identical twins. Spine. 20: 2601-2612.
[9] Gatchel R J, Peng Y B, Peters M L, et al. (2007). The Biopsychosocial Approach to Chronic Pain: Scientific Advances and Future Directions. Psychol Bull. 133: 581-624.
[10] Punnett L and Wegman D H (2004). Work-related musculoskeletal disorders: The epidemiologic evidence and the debate. J Electromyogr Kinesiol. 14 13-23.
[11] Bakker E, Verhagen A, Trijffel E V, et al. (2009). Spinal mechanical load as a risk factor for low back pain: a systematic review of prospective cohort studies. Spine. 34: E281.
[12] Takala E P, Andersen J H, Burdorf A, et al. (2010). Re: Bakker EW, Verhagen AP, van Trijffel E, et al. Spinal mechanical load as a risk factor for low back pain: a systematic review of prospective cohort studies. Spine 2009; 34:E281-93. Spine. 35: E1011-1012.
[13] Olsen O (2010). Re: Bakker EW, Verhagen AP, van Trijffel E, et al. Spinal mechanical load as a risk factor for low back pain: A systematic review of prospective cohort studies. Spine. 35: E576.

[14] Lund T, Labriola M, Christensen K B, et al. (2006). Physical work environment risk factors for long term sickness absence: prospective findings among a cohort of 5357 employees in Denmark. BMJ. 332: 449-452.

[15] Griffin M J (2004). Minimum health and safety requirements for workers exposed to hand-transmitted vibration and whole-body vibration in the European Union; a review. Occup Environ Med. 61: 387-397.

[16] Hartvigsen J, Lings S, Leboeuf-Yde C, et al. (2004). Psychosocial factors at work in relation to low back pain and consequences of low back pain; a systematic, critical review of prospective cohort studies. Occup Environ Med. 61: e2.

[17] Hoogendoorn W E, vanPoppel M N, Bongers P M, et al. (2000). Systematic Review of Psychosocial Factors at Work and Private Life as Risk Factors for Back Pain. Spine. 25: 2114-2125.

[18] Linton S J (2001). Occupational psychological factors increase the risk for back pain: a systematic review. J Occup Rehabil. 11: 53-66.

[19] Linton S (2000). A Review of Psychological Risk Factors in Back and Neck Pain. Spine. 25: 1148-1156.

[20] Steenstra I A, Verbeek J H, Heymans M W, et al. (2005). Prognostic factors for duration of sick leave in patients sick listed with acute low back pain: A systematic review of the literature. Occup Environ Med. 62: 851-860.

[21] Kent P M and Keating J L (2008). Can we predict poor recovery from recent-onset nonspecific low back pain? A systematic review. Man Ther. 13: 12-28.

[22] Shaw W S, Pransky G and Fitzgerald T E (2001). Early prognosis for low back disability: intervention strategies for health care providers. Disabil Rehabil. 23: 815-828.

[23] Kuijer W, Groothoff J, Brouwer S, et al. (2006). Prediction of Sickness Absence in Patients with Chronic Low Back Pain: A Systematic Review. J Occup Rehabil. 16: 439-467.

[24] Truchon M and Fillion L (2000). Biopsychosocial determinants of chronic disability and low-back pain: A review. J Occup Rehabil. 10: 117-142.

[25] Steers R M and Rhodes S R (1978). Major influences on employee attendance: A process model. J Appl Psychol. 63: 391-407.

[26] Allegro J and Veerman T (1998). Sickness absence. Handbook of work and organisational psychology. Drenth JD, Thierry H and de Wolff CJ. East Sussex, Psychology Press: 121-144.

[27] Pincus T, Burton a K, Vogel S, et al. (2002). A systematic review of psychological factors as predictors of chronicity/disability in prospective cohorts of low back pain. Spine. 27: E109-120.

[28] Health and Safety Executive. (2011). Getting to grips with manual handling. Bootle, Health and Safety Executive. Available http://www.hse.gov.uk/pubns/indg143.pdf Accessed 2012 16 July.

[29] McAtamney L and Corlett E N (1993). RULA: a survey method for the investigation of work-related upper limb disorders. Appl Ergon. 24: 91-99.

[30] Cochrane Back Review Group. (2012). Available http://back.cochrane.org/ Accessed 2012 19 June.

[31] Roelofs P D, Deyo R A, Koes B W, et al. (2008). Non-steroidal anti-inflammatory drugs for low back pain. Cochrane database of systematic reviews (Online). Available http://onlinelibrary.wiley.com/doi/10.1002/14651858.CD000396.pub3/abstract Accessed 2012 19 July.

[32] Bronfort G, Haas M, Evans R L, et al. (2004). Efficacy of spinal manipulation and mobilization for low back pain and neck pain: A systematic review and best evidence synthesis. Spine Journal. 4 (3): 335-356.

[33] Rubinstein S M, van Middelkoop M, Assendelft W J, et al. (2011). Spinal manipulative therapy for chronic low-back pain. Cochrane database of systematic reviews (Online). Available http://onlinelibrary.wiley.com/doi/10.1002/14651858.CD008112.pub2/abstract Accessed 2012 19 July.

[34] Lilley R, Cryer C, Lovelock K, et al. (2009). Effective Occupational Health Interventions in Agriculture - An International Literature Review of Primary Intervention Designed to Reduce Injury & Disease in Agriculture. Dunedin, Injury Prevention Research Unit, University of Otago. Available http://ipru3.otago.ac.nz/ipru/ReportsPDFs/OR075.pdf Accessed 2012 25 July

[35] Boocock MG, McNair PJ, Larmer PJ, et al. (2007). Interventions for the prevention and management of neck/upper extremity musculoskeletal conditions: a systematic review. Occup Environ Med. 64: 291-303.

[36] Westgaard R H (1997). Ergonomic intervention research for improved musculoskeletal health: A critical review. International Journal of Industrial Ergonomics. 20: 463-500.

[37] Waddell G and Burton A K (2001). Occupational health guidelines for the management of low back pain at work: Evidence review. Occup Med (London). 51 (2): 124-135.

[38] Samanta J, Kendall J and Samanta A (2003). 10-Minute consultation: Chronic low back pain. BMJ. 326 (7388): 535.

[39] New Zealand Guidelines Group. (2004). The diagnosis and management of soft tissue shoulder injuries and related disorders: best practice guideline Wellington, ACC. Available http://www.acc.co.nz/about-acc/research-sponsorship-and-projects/research-and-development/evidence-based-healthcare-reports/WPC096922 Accessed 2012 16 July.

[40] Ramond A, Bouton C, Richard I, et al. (2011). Psychosocial risk factors for chronic low back pain in primary care-a systematic review. Fam Pract. 28: 12-21.

[41] Swinkels-Meewisse I E J, Roelofs J, Schouten E G W, et al. (2006). Fear of movement/(re)injury predicting chronic disabling low back pain: A prospective inception cohort study. Spine. 31: 658-664.

[42] Shaw S, Pransky G and William T E (2001). Early Disability Risk Factors for Low Back Pain Assessed at Outpatient Occupational Health Clinics. Spine. 30: 572-580.

[43] Iles R Systematic Review of the Ability of Recovery Expectations to Predict Outcomes in Non-Chronic Non-Specific Low Back Pain. J Occup Rehabil. 19: 25-40.

[44] Fejer R, Ohm-Kyvik K and Hartvigsen J (2006). The prevalence of neck pain in the world population: a systematic critical review of the literature. Eur Spine J. 15: 834-848.

[45] Larsson B, Søgaard K and Rosendal L (2007). Work related neck–shoulder pain: a review on magnitude, risk factors, biochemical characteristics, clinical picture and preventive interventions. Best Pract Res Clin Rheumatol. 21: 447-463.

[46] Verhagen AP, Karels CC, Bierma-Zeinstra SMA, et al. (2006). Ergonomic and physiotherapeutic interventions for treating work-related complaints of the arm, neck or shoulder in adults. Cochrane database of systematic reviews (Online). Available http://onlinelibrary.wiley.com/doi/10.1002/14651858.CD003471.pub4/abstract Accessed 2012 19 July.

[47] Verhagen AP, Karels CC, Bierma-Zeinstra SMA, et al. (2010). Ergonomic and physiotherapeutic interventions for treating work-related complaints of the arm, neck or shoulder in adults (Protocol). Cochrane database of systematic reviews (Online). Available http://onlinelibrary.wiley.com/doi/10.1002/14651858.CD008742/abstract Accessed 2012 19 July.

[48] Roquelaure Y, Ha C, Rouillon C, et al. (2009). Risk factors for upper-extremity musculoskeletal disorders in the working population. Arthritis Care and Research. 61 (10): 1425-1434.

[49] Buchbinder R, Green S and Youd J M. (2003). Corticosteroid injections for shoulder pain. Cochrane database of systematic reviews (Online). Available http://onlinelibrary.wiley.com/doi/10.1002/14651858.CD004016/abstract Accessed 2012 19 July.

[50] Green S, Buchbinder R and Hetrick S. (2003). Physiotherapy interventions for shoulder pain. Cochrane database of systematic reviews (Online). Available http://onlinelibrary.wiley.com/doi/10.1002/14651858.CD004258/abstract Accessed 2012 19 July.

[51] Coghlan J A, Buchbinder R, Green S, et al. (2008). Surgery for rotator cuff disease. Cochrane database of systematic reviews (Online). Available http://onlinelibrary.wiley.com/doi/10.1002/14651858.CD005619.pub2/abstract Accessed 2012 19 July.

[52] Bissett L, Coombes B and Vicenzino B. (2011). Tennis elbow. Clin Evid (Online). Available http://clinicalevidence.bmj.com/x/systematic-review/1117/credits.html Accessed 2012 16 July.

[53] Rabago D, Best T M, Zgierska A E, et al. (2009). A systematic review of four injection therapies for lateral epicondylosis: Prolotherapy, polidocanol, whole blood and platelet-rich plasma. Br J Sports Med. 43 (7): 471-481.

[54] Atroshi I, Gummesson C, Johnsson R, et al. (1999). Prevalence of carpal tunnel syndrome in a general population. JAMA. 282 (2): 153-158.

[55] Nordstrom D L, Vierkant R A, DeStefano F, et al. (1997). Risk factors for carpal tunnel syndrome in a general population. Occup Environ Med. 54 (10): 734-740.

[56] Accident Compensation Corporation. (2009). Distal Upper Limb: Guidelines for Management of Some Common Musculoskeletal Disorders. Wellington, Accident Compensation Corporation. Available http://www.acc.co.nz/about-acc/research-sponsorship-and-projects/research-and-development/evidence-based-healthcare-reports/WPC096922 Accessed 2012 16 July.

[57] MacDermid J C and Doherty T (2004). Clinical and electrodiagnostic testing of Carpal Tunnel Syndrome. A narrative review. J Orthop Sports Phys Ther. 34 (10): 565-588.

[58] Palmer K T, Harris E C and Coggon D (2007). Carpal tunnel syndrome and its relation to occupation: a systematic literature review. Occup Med (London). 57: 57-66.

[59] Juratli S M, Nayan M, Fulton-Kehoe D, et al. (2010). A population-based study of ulnar neuropathy at the elbow in Washington State workers' compensation. Am J Ind Med. 53: 1242-1251.

[60] Descatha A, Leclerc A, Chastang J F, et al. (2004). Incidence of ulnar nerve entrapment at the elbow in repetitive work. Scand J Work Environ Health. 30: 234-240.

[61] Washington State Department of Labor and Industries. (2010). Work-Related Ulnar Neuropathy at the Elbow (UNE) Diagnosis and Treatment. Seattle, Washington State Department of Labor and Industries. Available http://www.lni.wa.gov/ClaimsIns/Files/OMD/MedTreat/UlnarNerve.pdf Accessed 2012 16 July.

[62] Caliandro P, La Torre G, Padua R, et al. (2011). Treatment for ulnar neuropathy at the elbow. Cochrane database of systematic reviews (Online). 2: CD006839.

[63] Walker-Bone K, Palmer K T, Reading I, et al. (2004). Prevalence and impact of musculoskeletal disorders of the upper limb in the general population. Arthritis Care and Research. 51 (4): 642-651.

[64] Yu S, Lu M L, Gu G, et al. (2012). Musculoskeletal symptoms and associated risk factors in a large sample of Chinese workers in Henan Province of China. Am J Ind Med. 55: 281-293.

[65] Wang P C, Rempel D M, Hurwitz E L, et al. (2009). Self-reported pain and physical signs for musculoskeletal disorders in the upper body region among Los Angeles garment workers. Work. 34: 79-87.

[66] Andreu J L, Oton T, Silva-Fernandez L, et al. (2011). Hand pain other than carpal tunnel syndrome (CTS): The role of occupational factors. Best Prac Res Clin Rheumatol. 25: 31-42.

[67] Crawford J O and Laiou E (2007). Conservative treatment of work-related upper limb disorders - A review. Occup Med (London). 57: 4-17.

[68] Coombes B K, Bisset L and Vicenzino B (2010). Efficacy and safety of corticosteroid injections and other injections for management of tendinopathy: A systematic review of randomised controlled trials. Lancet. 376 (9754): 1751-1767.

[69] Brammer AJ, Taylor W and Lundborg G (1987). Sensorineural stages of the hand-arm vibration syndrome. Scand J Work Environ Health. 13: 279-283.

[70] Ramazzini B (1940). De morbis artificum: Diseases of workers Trans. Wilmer Cave Wright. Chicago, The University of Chicago Press.

Chapter 5

Management of Chronic Musculoskeletal Pain in the Elderly: Dilemmas and Remedies

Ayse Ozcan Edeer and Hulya Tuna

Additional information is available at the end of the chapter

http://dx.doi.org/10.5772/50780

1. Introduction

Aging is perhaps better understood as a process of gradual change from birth to death, since there is no universally accepted definition of old age. Projections show dramatic increases in older population; approximately by 2030 there will be an estimated 8 million people who are 85 years or older [1-3]. Moreover, 25% of the population in USA will be age 65 years or older in 2050. The percentage over the age of 85 is expected to triple [4-7]. Europe has experienced the similar transition to an older population profile over the last century which reflects a world-wide demographic trend towards an ageing population. Department of Health reports that in Britain, the number of people aged over 65 years has doubled in the last 70 years and the number of people over 90 years is expected to double in the next 25 years [8]. Similarly D'Astolfo et al state that older adults aged 65 plus, are the fastest growing segment of the Canadian population [9].

The European Union has identified the provision of health and social care for this population as a crucial challenge for the 21st century. In a shift away from merely extending life, ways of reducing morbidity and coping with disability, preventing incapacity, extending the quality of life and enhancing the functional independence of older people will be an important component of service provision [10,11]. Recent efforts have begun to concentrate on the predictors of successful aging, but age-based comparisons of the pain experience remain challenging due to the complexity and non-uniformity of the aging process [12]. Therefore, there is an urgent and growing need for interventions that are effective in decreasing pain, suffering, and pain-related disability in this group.

2. Prevalence of pain in older adults

Although chronic pain is a highly prevalent and often disabling condition among older adults, the prevalence in the elderly is not properly defined. Some studies suggest that fifty percent of community dwelling adults aged 60 years or above have been found to experience pain and this number increases to 45–80% in the nursing home population with analgesics being used in 40% to 50% of residents [1,13-19]. Brown et al report higher percentage and state that more than 90% of the elderly living in the community experienced pain within the past month [6]. Given the prevalence of chronic pain, its impact on health, and its costs, which approach $100 billion annually, chronic pain represents a major public health issue [20].

While the existence of acute pain remains approximately the same across the adult life span, there is an age-related increase in the prevalence of chronic pain at least until the seventh decade of life [13,15]. Approximately 57% of older adults report experiencing pain for 1 or more years compared with less than 45% of younger people. Furthermore, long-term care data indicate that over 40% of patients, who were known to have pain at an initial assessment, had worsening or severe pain at the time of the second assessment 2–6 months later [21].

3. Chronic musculoskeletal pain

Chronic musculoskeletal pain (CMP) is the most common, non-malignant disabling condition that affects at least one in four older people [22,23]. The most musculoskeletal pain in the joints of the upper and lower extremities, especially hips, knees, and hands, is associated with the degenerative changes of osteoarthritis. Older adults may also develop tendonitis and bursitis, as well as inflammatory joint and muscle disease [24]. The most common painful musculoskeletal conditions among older adults are osteoarthritis, low back pain, fibromyalgia, chronic shoulder pain, knee pain, myofascial pain syndrome and previous fracture sites [7,23,25].

It is reported that the most common causes of pain identified in nursing home patients included arthritis and previous fractures. Arthritis alone affects well over 20 million Americans with an increase to 40 million expected by 2020. Twenty-nine percent of Medicare patients in nursing homes with a fracture in the prior 6 months suffer with daily pain [13]. Also surgical procedures are more frequently performed on older people. In the Medicare population in the United States for example, rates of total joint replacement surgery for patients with severe hip or knee osteoarthritis are more than doubled between 1988 and 1997. Over the same time period, rates of spine surgery in Medicare patients increased by 57% [23]. Chronic low back pain (CLBP) is one of the most common, poorly understood, and potentially disabling chronic pain conditions in older adults [26]. Many older adults remain quite functional despite CLBP, and because age-related co-morbidities often exist independently of pain, the unique impact of CLBP is unknown [27]. The Framingham Study (1992-1993) reported 63% of women pain in one or more regions, compared to 52% of men. Widespread CMP was more prevalent among women than men (15 versus 5%, respectively) [28].

Finding that CMP is linked with the subsequent development of severe mobility disability may have important public health implications for the rapidly aging population [29]. Among 898 nondisabled community-dwelling older adults, it was found that the risk of disability increases with the number of areas reported with CMP [30]. The results of the another study indicated that more than 90% of the elderly living in the community experienced pain within the past month, with 41% reporting discomforting, distressing, unbearable, or severe pain. CMP was found to be the most predominant pain, and inactivity was the most effective strategy used to lessen pain [6]. D'Astolfo et al emphasized that CMP is a significant burden on the Canadian health care system. It is considered the third most expensive disorder in terms of spent health care dollars, surpassed only by cancer and heart disease [9].

4. Consequences of chronic musculoskeletal pain

The impact of CMP is a cycle of disuse and inactivity. This cycle in turn leads to a further reduction in function, accompanying psychological effects and decreased quality of life [7,31]. Interrelated problems caused by the inadequate treatment of pain in older adults have been highlighted by several authors. Consequences of poorly managed CMP in this population may include fear of movement, decreased ambulation, functional decline, functional dependence, disability, impaired posture, risk of pressure sores, muscle atrophy, increased subsequent exacerbation of frailty. Older adults may also have impaired appetite, malnutrition, impairment of excretory functions (bowel and bladder) and impaired memory, the impairment of enjoyable recreational activities, impaired dressing and grooming, sleep disturbance, behavioral problems, social isolation, depression, anxiety and even suicidal thoughts [7,10,14-16]. Furthermore, depression, behavioral changes, and cognitive impairment can complicate therapy and make assessment more difficult. Pain-induced decline in mobility and activity may further lead to increase the risk of trauma, particularly caused from falls [14].

Falls are one of the major causes of death among older adults and the most important cause of hospitalization and increased healthcare utilization and costs in this population [9]. CMP measured according to number of locations, severity, or pain interference with daily activities is associated with greater risk of falls in older adults [32-35]. Leveille et al conducted the population-based study. At baseline, 40% of participants reported polyarticular chronic pain, and another 24% reported chronic pain in only one joint area. A total of 1,029 falls were reported during 18 months of follow-up. The researchers found that patients who had chronic pain had higher rates of falls during follow-up than those who were pain-free [33]. In the another population based study, total of 605 participants aged 75 years and older, CMP was reported by 48% of the participants, of whom majority had moderate to severe pain in lower extremities or back. The participants with moderate to severe pain had more than twice (odds ratio 2.33, 95% confidence interval 1.44-3.76) the risk for impaired balance compared with those without pain. The researchers came up with a conclusion that there was a direct relationship between the moderate to severe CMP and impaired postural balance [36].

5. Ineffective management of chronic musculoskeletal pain in older adults

In spite of high prevalence and consequences of CMP among older adults, there have been relatively few studies in older populations with pain. Studies have indicated that less than

1% of the thousands of papers published on pain focus on the aging society [13,17]. Therefore, health care professionals remain ineffective in assessing and treating pain. Improving the health care professionals' knowledge and skills related to pain assessment in older adults and adopting aggressive approaches to comprehensive pain assessment are crucial to improve older adult's quality of life [15,37]. The study conducted recently reported that although CLBP was a common and debilitating problem in older adults, primary care physicians did not feel "very confident" in their ability to diagnose any of the contributors of CLBP listed (most items <40%). The results point to a need for more primary care physician education about CLBP in older adults [38].

Older people may not report pain, and nurses or caregivers may not enquire about it. Both older people and their caregivers can hold age related attitudes regarding pain and view pain as an expected consequence of the ageing process. Older adults may not report pain because they do not want to be a burden for their families and caregivers. It results mostly in lack of information by healthcare professionals about pain control of older people. Furthermore, extensive documentation requirement may deter health-care professionals from appropriately prescribing effective treatments [39,40]. Other factors such as inadequate reimbursement and financial incentives for pain management efforts, negative reinforcement in training programs for attending to pain while being rewarded for less important and more detailed interventions, lack of training for pain management skills, lack of recognition and interaction among various medical disciplines (and even among different pain groups), limited access to diagnostic or therapeutic facilities or experts, inadequate pharmacy services, insufficient staffing for proper pain assessment and interventions, inflexible access to medications based on formulary selections, and other restrictive policies may also contribute to failure in treatment of pain [4,40].

6. Management of chronic musculoskeletal pain in older adults

Treatments for CMP are focused at decreasing pain, making it more tolerable and improving patients function. Considering the needs of individual older patients can better explain what their expectations are regarding pain treatment outcomes. Treating pain should be done individually as well as following some general principles. Multidisciplinary pain programs that combine several modes of pharmacological and non-pharmacological treatment have demonstrated efficacy for the management of chronic pain in older adults. However, those programs appear to be not being used effectively, because older patients are less likely to be offered this treatment in pain management clinics, and receive fewer treatment options when attending such clinics due to inadequate representation [12,41].

Pharmacological therapy for chronic musculoskeletal pain is the most effective when combined with non-pharmacological approaches: physical therapy (e.g., exercise program, TENS, application of heat or cold), psychological methods (e.g., relaxation, biofeedback, hypnosis, cognitive-behavioral therapy), educational programs, social interventions and complementary therapies (e.g., acupuncture) [14,16,37,41,]. In an older population, where the risk of adverse events is higher, the non-pharmacologic options will usually cost less and cause fewer side effects.

7. Pharmacological therapy

Although the high risk for adverse drug reactions in the older adults, pharmacologic interventions remain the primary modality for treating CMP in the geriatric population [20]. The management of CMP in older patients mostly consists of opioids, non-opioids and adjuvant analgesics.

Drug distribution usually is different in older patients as compared to younger patients because of changes in blood flow to organs, protein binding, and body composition that occur with aging [3]. In addition, many older adults continue to report substantial pain despite the regular use of analgesic medications. Polypharmacy, as well as inappropriate prescribing, for the older patients is a major problem and a challenge that contributes to costs, adverse drug events, confusion, compliance issues, and errors in management. [42-44] It is reported that CMP is one of the most common geriatric consultation and admission the hospital. Geriatric consultations increase the total number of medications and the cost of medications used by elderly patients. These restrictions have led to a need for effective non-pharmacological interventions to manage CMP [42].

7.1. Nonopioids

According to American Geriatric Society (AGS) nonopioids are generally the first line of therapy for mild to moderate or "tolerable" CMP [16,23,43]. Acetaminophen (APAP) and nonsteroidal anti-inflammatory drugs (NSAIDs) are among the most common analgesics used to. APAP is usually the first choice because it is relatively safe for older people. It was reported that APAP treatment reduced pain behaviors associated with musculoskeletal pain in persons with dementia in community-dwelling [45,46]. Dosing of APAP should be limited to avoid liver toxicity, and topical analgesics are preferred for focal pain. The long-term use of NSAIDs should be avoided when possible because of their high frequency of adverse effects; e.g., risks of gastrointestinal bleeding and renal dysfunction which are significantly higher in older adults than in the younger population. The newer cyclooxygenese-2 (COX)-2 inhibitor NSAIDs are believed to be associated with a lower side effect profile in older adults [41]. COX-2 inhibitor NSAIDs has been linked to an increased incidence of acute coronary syndrome, although there is evidence that cardiovascular-related adverse events are not limited to the selective COX-2 inhibitors. Additionally, chronic use of either APAP or NSAIDs has been associated to elevations in blood pressure [47].

Data was collected from 428 patients aged ≥50 years with non-inflammatory musculoskeletal pain during a consultation with their general practitioner (GP). In cases, where a prescription is issued, this is more strongly influenced by previous NSAID prescriptions than the patient's pain level. Researchers concluded that GPs mostly adopt an individualized approach to the treatment of musculoskeletal pain in older adults [48]. A survey of inpatients' drug knowledge showed that 66–90% of older adults did not know which of several medicines contained APAP, and only 7% knew the maximum daily dose. Therefore close monitoring of pain medication use is necessary in older patients, particularly those with cognitive impairment. According to the 2009 guidelines for pharmacologic management of persistent pain in older persons published by the AGS, NSAIDs should be used only with extreme caution in highly selected individuals once other safer therapies have failed. Absolute contraindications for NSAIDs use in older adults are chronic kidney disease, heart failure, and active peptic ulcer disease [16,46,49].

7.2. Opioids

Worries connected to taking opioids and a reluctance to report pain have caused inefficient pain management with opioids in older patients. In reality, addiction risk with opioids is low (<0.1%) when analgesics are used for acute pain in patients who are not substance abusers [4]. Opioids are one of the pharmacologic classes recommended for treatment from moderate to severe pain in guidelines released in 2009 by the AGS. According to the AGS, opioids should be considered for patients who have pain related functional impairment or diminished quality of life due to pain [23,50].

Within this population, short-acting opioids can be used in treatment of patients with intermittent pain, whereas sustained-release opioids should be given for continuous pain (with short-acting preparations available for breakthrough pain). Once total daily dose requirements have been determined, a long acting agent may be used. Sustained-released opioids should be used for the treatment of continuous pain while using short-acting preparations for breakthrough pain. Both morphine and oxycodone are commonly used and available in both short-acting and sustained-release preparations. For patients who may not be able to take oral preparations periodically, opioids are available as parenteral, sublingual (buprenorphine hydrochloride), suppository (oxymorphone hydrochloride), and transdermal (eg, fentanyl patch) products. Long-acting opioids should seldom be initiated in opioid-naive older patients [7,46].

Patient-controlled analgesia (PCA), whether using oral or parenteral agents, can be most beneficial in a cognitively intact population, with the likelihood of the best pain control in conjunction with the least amount of opioid needed to control musculoskeletal pain [4].

An oral long-acting agent such as morphine (the oral dose required is usually about 3 to 4 times greater than the parenteral dose needed for the same duration) or oxycontin in conjunction with a similar short-acting agent can also be used. Some people will metabolize the medication more quickly, and if breakthrough pain occurs after 8 hours of adequate pain relief, therefore the solution would be to increase the frequency of dosing to every 8 hours from every 12 hours rather than to increase the 12-hour dosage. A controlled-release morphine or controlled-release oxycodone should never be prescribed more frequently than every 8 hours [4].

Meperidine hydrochloride should not be used because of the accumulation of a nephrotoxic metabolite. Benzodiazepines have also been used in the treatment of a variety of painful conditions, particularly muscle spasms related to pain crises. Transdermal fentanyl patches should generally be avoided as a first-line agent in older patients, because absorption is unpredictable, being affected by differences in body temperature and subcutaneous fat and water in older patients as compared with younger adults studied in clinical trials [23]. Trescot et al reported that long-term effectiveness of 6 months or longer use of opioids is variable with evidence ranging from moderate for transdermal fentanyl and sustained-release morphine with a Level II-2, to limited for oxycodone with a Level II-3, and indeterminate for hydrocodone and methadone with a Level III [51].

Although opioid therapies may have a lower risk for organ failure than other therapies, confusion, dizziness, nausea, sedation, constipation, impaired balance, falls and hip fractures, depression, and agitation are other potential related side effects that can affect this population in particular. Finally, older adults with CMP taking opioid analgesics should be reassessed for ongoing attainment of therapeutic goals, adverse effects, and safe and responsible medication use [46].

7.3. Adjuvant analgesics

Adjuvant medications, while not classically categorized as analgesics, may be effective in treating certain CMP syndromes in older adults. Steroids, anticonvulsants, topical local anesthetics, and antidepressants are adjuvant agents. Depression/anxiety is often unnoticed in older patients and requires consideration when managing patients with pain [4,23,41]. The study of the relationship between depression and pain complaints in older patients has revealed that initial control of depression greatly facilitates pain management. If depression is not addressed aggressively, interventions to manage pain are unlikely to be successful [7]. Tertiary amines (e.g., amitriptyline, imipramine, trimipramine, doxepin, clomipramine, should be avoided in older patients because of greater anticholinergic side effects, including sedation, delirium, urinary retention, constipation, glaucoma exacerbation, and dizziness and, for amitriptyline, especially, the risk of cardiac arrhythmia. By contrast, secondary amines (nortriptyline, desipramine, protriptyline, amoxapine) tend to have better adverse event profiles in older patients [41].

Tramadol is another agent available to help control mild to moderate pain and, except in a substance-abuse population. It should have a low tolerance problem and may be beneficial in a variety of pain situations [23].

In about 90% of cases, additional adjuvant medications will be needed to control pain. Vitamin D is also likely to be helpful in some pain situations. Vitamin D and calcium have also been shown to decrease fracture rates, which are a source of pain themselves. Lower concentrations of 25(OH)D are associated with significant back pain in older women, but not men. Because vitamin D deficiency and CMP are fairly prevalent in older adults, these findings suggest it may be worthwhile to query older adults about their pain and screen older women with significant back pain for vitamin D deficiency [52]. Calcitonin has been shown in clinical trials to relieve pain associated with vertebral compression fractures. Topical agents are also available for site-specific pain. Also, topical treatments can be useful for patients who have difficulty swallowing pills and for patients taking multiple medications. The safety of topical lidocaine has been established as well. Topical capsaicin should be started at the lowest dose recommended. However the burning sensation associated with capsaicin application during the chemical desensitization phase makes for poor tolerability; many older patients are not able to endure the treatment long enough to achieve therapeutic effects [4,41,50].

Adverse drug reactions occur more than twice as frequently among older adults than younger ones and increase as the number of medications increases. On average, a 70-year-old takes seven different medications. A high prevalence of medication errors in older adults results from accumulation of factors that contribute to medication errors in all age groups, such as polypharmacy, polymorbidity, enrollment in several disease-management programs, and fragmentation of care [53]. The essential approach to treating older adults is not necessarily to find a set number of medications and try to stay below it, but to find the right medication at the right dosage and for the shortest possible duration on a case-by-case basis. This individualized approach to treating patients will provide a much safer and more effective means of practicing and will improve patients' quality of life [54]. In general, as specific initial and titrating dosage regimens for the elderly are not readily available, the "start low and go slow" approach to drug prescribing in the elderly is particularly important as it applies to pain management (AGS 2002) [16,21,42].

8. Non-pharmacological approaches

8.1. Physical therapy

Ideally, first-line interventions should directly address the source of pain in older adults with CMP. A comprehensive examination of the patient to identify impairments associated with the painful condition will direct those interventions. Physical therapy interventions reduce stress and correct malalignments of joint structures, correct muscle imbalances, and enhance the shock absorption capacity of tissue structures. Selection of appropriate treatments must include consideration of contraindications associated with the patient's comorbid conditions (e.g., osteoporosis or osteopenia) [10,20,57].

Passive treatment modalities focused solely on temporarily decreasing pain symptoms (e.g., heat treatments, cryotherapy, transcutaneous electrical nerve stimulation [TENS]) should be used sparingly as part of the physical therapy intervention [1,2]. These modalities should be a means to an end, the end being decreasing pain to a sufficient extent to allow patients to participate in subsequent active treatments aimed at positively affecting functional abilities [20,50,55-57].

8.1.1. Thermal agents

Superficial heating agents (e.g. hot packs, warm hydrotherapy, paraffin, fluidotherapy and infrared) or deep heating agents (e.g. short-wave and microwave diathermy, and ultrasound) can be used to increase blood flow, membrane permeability, tissue extensibility and joint range of motion in ways that can contribute to decreasing pain. Heat and cold alter both peripheral and central nervous system excitability, and can thus serve as a means of modulating pain [20,58].

Although thermal agents are frequently used in the physical therapy treatment of patients with pain, the literature on the effects of thermal agents on pain in older adults is limited. Thermal agents are commonly used in the self-management of chronic pain [55]. In a study of 235 (mean age of 82 years) community-dwelling adults, Acetaminophen, regular exercise, prayer, and heat and cold were the most frequently used pain management strategies (61%, 58%, 53%, and 48%, respectively). 272 community-dwelling older adults aged 73 years or older reported hot and/or cold modalities (28%) as a pain-reduction strategy [59]. Chatap et al conducted a study to determine the effects of hyperbaric CO(2) cryotherapy in older adults with pain whose origin was usually musculoskeletal (80.3%). They found that the pain scores decreased significantly after four sessions, from 45mm to 13mm on visual analog scale ($P<0.001$) in those with chronic pain. They concluded that hyperbaric CO(2) cryotherapy is an innovative tool that should be incorporated within the non-pharmacological armamentarium for achieving pain relief in older patients [60].

8.1.2. Manual therapy

Although there is scant evidence on the use of joint mobilization and manipulation specifically for older adults, research has addressed the use of these treatments for knee and hip osteoarthritis (OA), conditions common in older adults [20]. A recent qualitative systematic review aimed to determine if manual therapy improves pain and/or physical function in people with hip or knee OA. Four RCTs were eligible for inclusion (280 subjects), three of which studied people with knee OA and one studied those with hip OA. There is silver level evidence that manual therapy is more effective than exercise for those with hip OA in the short and long-term. The researchers concluded that due to the small number of RCTs and patients, this evidence could be considered to be inconclusive regarding the benefit of manual therapy on pain and function for knee or hip OA [61].

A Cochrane systematic review concludes that manual therapy alone is insufficient in the management of persistent neck pain. However, there is strong evidence that either manipulation or mobilization combined with exercise is effective in reducing pain. This review also concluded that manual therapy with exercise improves function and the patients' global perceived effect of treatment [62]. The Philadelphia Panel (2001) concluded that there were insufficient data for the general population to reach a conclusion about the effect of massage for low back pain, neck pain, and shoulder pain. A systematic review by Harris et al [63], determined that slow-stroke back massage and hand massage showed statistically significant improvements on physiological or psychological indicators of relaxation in older people. A limited number of studies on massage have been conducted exclusively with older individuals. Hawk et al compared the clinical outcomes of spinal manipulation and a non-manipulative mind-body approach (Bioenergetic Synchronization Technique) for patients with chronic musculoskeletal pain in older adults. They reported that for this particular group of patients, both groups demonstrated similar improvement scores on the Pain Disability Index [64].

8.1.3. Protective and supportive devices

Protective and supportive devices assist a decrease in pain and increase in function for patients with joint instability or malalignment. Therapeutic taping for patellar realignment is effective in reducing pain and improving function in patients with osteoarthritis of the knee. Recently introduced kinesiotaping method helps to increase blood circulation, decrease pain and relaxation on fascia, tendon and muscles regarding painful musculoskeletal conditions. Impact-absorbing shoes may help to relieve foot, ankle, knee and hip pain from osteoarthritis. Patients with metatarsalgia associated with rheumatoid arthritis experienced decreased pain using custom-fitted foot orthotics. Besides supportive and protective devices, ambulation devices like wheelchair, cane, crutch etc. can help to relieve stress from lower extremity especially during immobilization period after musculoskeletal injuries in older adult. Therefore appropriate device selection and measurements are important in order to improve efficiency. Decisions regarding the use of protective or supportive devices should therefore be individualized to the patient based on the information gained in the examination [20,57,58].

8.1.4. Transcutaneous electrical nerve stimulation

Despite positive conclusions regarding the use of transcutaneous electrical nerve stimulation (TENS), methodological weaknesses of published studies limit the ability to conclusively support the use of TENS for chronic pain conditions in older adults. High-frequency TENS appears to be the most effective TENS application for postsurgical pain and can be used with modulating frequencies to control neurologic accommodation. A recent systematic review of TENS for persistent pain concluded that an insufficient number of high-quality randomized clinical trials existed to evaluate the use of TENS for the management of persistent pain. To date, only a small number of studies have been found that examined the effect of TENS exclusively with older adults [57,58].

Most recently, van Middelkoop M et al found no difference in effectiveness of TENS and sham TENS and no difference between TENS and active treatments. The data provided low quality evidence for TENS versus sham-TENS and very low quality evidence that percutaneous electrical nerve stimulation (PENS)/acupuncture is more effective than TENS for post-treatment and short-term pain relief [65]. They concluded that application of TENS attenuates blood pressure and vasoconstrictor responses during exercise and metaboreflex activation, associated with improved sympatho-vagal balance in healthy young and older individuals [66]. A recent study by Weiner et al provides some support for the use of percutaneous electrical nerve stimulation (PENS) for low back pain in older adults. Subjects randomized to PENS plus physical therapy intervention had significantly greater reductions in pain intensity measures at the end of the 6 weeks ($P<.001$). These pain reduction effects were maintained at 3-month follow-up [67].

In evidence-based meta analysis by Zhang W et al in 2008, authors search recommendations for the management of hip and knee osteoarthritis (OA). Recommendations cover the use of 12 non-pharmacological modalities: education and self-management, regular telephone contact, referral to a physical therapist, aerobic, muscle strengthening and water-based exercises, weight reduction, walking aids, knee braces, footwear and insoles, thermal modalities, TENS and acupuncture [68]. Same author groups made similar meta-analysis in 2010 and reported that among non-pharmacological therapies, effect size for pain relief was unchanged for self-management, education, exercise and acupuncture. However, with new evidence the effect size for pain relief for weight reduction reached statistical significance [69].

8.2. Complementary and alternative therapies

Complementary and alternative medicine is most often used to treat painful musculoskeletal conditions as well as conditions that are comorbid with pain in older adults as a holistic therapy. [70]. Molton et al researched the pain coping strategies among older, middle-aged, and younger adults living with CMP. They reported older adults report a wider range of frequently used strategies and significantly more frequent engagement in activity pacing, seeking social support, and use of coping self-statements than did younger or middle-aged adults [71]. Self-management programs for pain have particular relevance for the field of geriatric pain management [56,71]. Despite their documented efficacy in young to middle aged samples cognitive-behavioral and self-management pain therapies have been little-studied in elderly populations. A variety of self-management programs aim to enhance the ability of patients to successfully self manage their pain, using a variety of techniques [72,73]. The most common behavioral modes of therapy include self-regulation strategies such as relaxation, biofeedback, hypnosis, imagery, and meditation. Although there are variations among these approaches, they share some or all of the following components: 1) education about pain and its consequences; 2) relaxation skills training (e.g., progressive muscle relaxation); 3) cognitive coping skills training; 4) problem solving (e.g., addressing problems with homework exercises or goals that are proposed to be met after each class); and 5) communication skills training (e.g., how to talk to physicians or health care providers about pain). In pain management, self management therapy serves to focus a patient's attention to exercise control in decreasing sympathetic arousal [37,74]. Besides patient education caregiver education is especially important for caring in the elderly. Both one-on-one as well as group programs can be effective [3,7].

8.2.1. Cognitive-behavioral therapy

The American Psychological Association recognizes cognitive-behavioral therapy (CBT) as an empirically supported intervention in management of chronic musculoskeletal pain; including rheumatoid arthritis, osteoarthritis, fibromyalgia, and low back pain. Its foundation is the gate control theory integrating the sensory, affective, and cognitive components of pain. Cognitive processes are thoughts, self-statements, or evaluations about the pain and beliefs, interpretations, or attributions regarding this condition [37,75]. 10-session psychosocial (i.e. cognitive behavioral orientation) pain management program that was specifically designed for older adults was used in ninety-five community dwelling seniors with at least one chronic musculoskeletal pain condition. Although decreases in pain intensity were observed in both the treatment and wait-list control groups, the intervention was found to result in fewer maladaptive beliefs about pain and greater use of relaxation, which is considered to be an adaptive coping strategy [76]. Beissner et al reported if physical therapists incorporate CBT techniques (eg, relaxation, activity pacing) when treating older patients with chronic pain. Commonly used CBT interventions included activity pacing and pleasurable activity scheduling [75].

8.2.2. Mind-body therapies

The National Center for Complementary and Alternative Medicine defines mind–body medicine in the following way: Mind-body medicine focuses on the interactions among the brain, mind, body, and behavior, and the powerful ways in which emotional, mental, social, spiritual, and behavioral factors can directly affect health. It regards as a fundamental approach that respects and enhances each person's capacity for self-knowledge and self-care, and it emphasizes techniques that are grounded in this approach [72]. Morone et al conducted a structured review of eight mind–body interventions: biofeedback, progressive muscle relaxation, meditation, guided imagery, hypnosis, tai chi (TC), qi gong, and yoga for older adults with chronic nonmalignant pain. He reported that there is some support for the efficacy of progressive muscle relaxation plus guided imagery for osteoarthritis pain. There is limited support for meditation and TC for improving function or coping in older adults with low back pain or osteoarthritis. TC, yoga, hypnosis, and progressive muscle relaxation were significantly associated with pain reduction in these studies [72].

It is reported that prevalent coping strategies included analgesic medications (78%), exercise (35%), cognitive methods (37%), religious activities (21%), and activity restriction (20%) for older adults with chronic pain due to a musculoskeletal cause [77]. Reid et al suggested in their review (N = 27) that a broad range of self-management programs (yoga, massage therapy, TC, and music therapy) may provide benefits for older adults with CMP highlighting the need for research to establish the efficacy of the programs in different age and ethnic groups of older adults and identify strategies that maximize program reach long-term participation [74].

8.2.3. Biologically based therapies

Biologically based therapies, one of the major categories of complementary and alternative therapies, according to the federal National Institutes of Health (NIH), involve supplementing a person's normal diet with additional extracts, nutrients, herbs and/or certain foods. Among older adults, glucosamine sulfate and chondroitin sulfate are popular supplements used for the treatment of osteoarthritis and are among the most well studied biologic alternative medicines. Glucosamine and chondroitin are components of the extracellular matrix of articular cartilage; glucosamine is a substrate required to synthesize glycoproteins and glycosaminoglycans, components of synovial fluid, ligaments, and other cartilaginous joint structures, and chondroitin is a glycosaminoglycan that functions as a building block for joint matrix structure. Another commonly used biological agent for arthritis is S-adenosyl L-methionine (SAMe). This is a synthetic version of a naturally occurring coenzyme that is produced by the liver from methionine SAMe has been attributed with analgesic and antiinflammatory properties, and can stimulate articular growth [50].

8.3. Exercise

In recent years exercise, which is one of the non-pharmacological approaches, is getting the most important component of CMP management. Regular exercise, interventions to increase physical activity, strengthening the muscles, accompanied with weight loss are effective methods in the management of CMP such as OA, low back pain etc. in older adults. Regular moderate level exercise training or increased physical activity does not aggravate pain and joint symptoms as expected in OA according to RCTs and elicit significant health benefits. But pain, swelling, fatigue and weakness during activity or lasting more than 1-2 hours after exercise should be always considered as sign of excessive stress. Any activity that worsens pain or the other symptoms, and in acute flare-up periods of rheumatoid arthritis should be discontinued [78,79].

The most studied CMP among older adults in literature belongs to knee OA. High and low-intensity aerobic exercises are equally effective in improving pain in persons with knee OA [80]. Specifically, aerobic exercise, water-based (aquatic) and land-based exercises, aerobic walking, quadriceps strengthening, and resistance exercise, physiotherapy-based exercise modalities reduce knee pain in older adults [80-84]. But a recent systematic review states that there are few RCTs recommending the use of exercise in reducing pain related to hip and knee OA and the content, duration and frequency of the exercise sessions is very heterogeneous [85].

8.3.1. Benefits of exercise in chronic musculoskeletal pain

Regular exercise also as an important adjunct to other interventions (e.g. thermal agents, patient education, etc.) is the most frequently preferred pain management strategies after medication in some older adult populations [55,58].

Various forms of exercise can modulate pain either directly or indirectly. Passive or active exercise has a direct effect on pain through increasing input from joint mechanoreceptors. Indirect effects of exercise on pain may be related to increased blood flow, decreased edema, inhibition of muscle spasm, enhanced ROM, flexibility, strength and weight loss which may improve biomechanical factors and decrease joint stress, and provide [58,81,86,87]. Improved sleep, enhanced mood, relaxation, reduction in anxiety and general well-being following regular exercise also can alter pain sensitivity positively in same way. After a single exercise session pain tolerance increases significantly [58,88].

Another benefit of exercise is its effect on risk of falling among older adults with CMP. Older adults with CMP are at increased risk of falling because of pain related muscle weakness, increased body sway and impaired balance [33,89,90]. Primarily strengthening program and physical agents as an adjunct are recommended for joint pain management among this population [90]. The most effective physical therapy approach for the prevention of falls is a combination of balance and strength training [91] in addition to aerobic training such as walking, aerobic dance, circuit training, aquatics and active lifestyle [92]. RCTs are needed to learn whether pain reduction with exercise could affect fall risk in older adults with CMP.

8.3.2. Types of exercise used in chronic musculoskeletal pain

An exercise program should address primer functional problems and impairments (pain, limited joint range of motion, muscle weakness) for functional independence. After relieving from these impairments or reducing them exercise program can begin [78]. A physical therapist has the primary responsibility to plan an exercise program accommodating pain or other disabilities [93]. Flexibility, strength and aerobic endurance are the basic components for exercise programs aiming to control pain. Time needed for adaptation to exercise stress may be 2 to 3 months for older arthritic adults with low physical capacity [78].

Exercise sessions should have three phases: The first phase, a warm-up period lasting 5-10 minutes, involves repetitive low-intensity range-of-motion exercises. The second phase, the training period, includes range of motion, strength, or aerobic capacity exercises, or a combination of these. The final phase, cool-down period lasting 5 minutes, involves flexibility exercises [78,94]. In addition the time of the exercise during the day can change according to the chronic condition. Older adults with OA better perform exercise in the morning, whereas older adults with rheumatoid arthritis may be better several hours after awakening. Low-impact, non-weight-bearing exercises and exercise machines distributing the load to all limbs usually recommended for artritic patients [79].

8.3.3. Flexibility exercises

Flexibility exercise should begin at the beginning of an exercise program during the warm-up, preferably cool-down period. Static stretching is recommended during cool down period for the osteoartritic older adults at as full as possible pain-free range for the greatest improvements [95]. Stretching exercises must be modified when the joint is inflamed or painful. Painful joints should not be over stretched and superficial heat application, relaxation prior to stretching helps reduce pain [78]. Older adults tend to have some movement patterns and positioning, which causes joint movement limitation resulting in painful movement patterns. Consideration of the potential for future painful conditions also should be treated by stretching [96].

Stretching exercises should be performed at least 3 times per week or daily if the pain and stiffness are minimal or must be modified when the joint is inflamed or painful. The progression should be gradual from one stretching to 4-10 repetitions for each major muscle group. The stretch position should be hold 10-30 seconds. [78]. Effective stretching exercises require longer holding times with increasing age and loss of extensibility, so if there is no pain,

60 seconds is necessary for older adults to achieve a long-term effect. Four repetitions of a 60-second hold performed regularly, 5 to 7 days a week, appear to be most effective [96].

8.3.4. Aerobic exercises

Aerobic exercise programs aiming improvement in strength and proprioception reduce pain in OA patients. Examples of aerobic exercise are bicycling (stationary bike, recumbent-type bike etc.), walking, dance, Tai-Chi and aquatic exercises such as swimming, Ai-Chi etc. Daily activities and some hobbies like walking the dog, mowing the lawn or playing golf, are also considered as aerobic exercise [78,92]. To prevent overuse of specific joints and to elicit long-term participation, activity selection for aerobic exercise is important and depends on the patient's current disease state, joint stability, opportunities, individual's preference and abilities [96].

There are few studies addressing effect of aerobic exercise on CMP in older adults [97, 98]. A 14-year prospective longitudinal study showed that regular aerobic exercise over the long period in physically active seniors was associated with about 25% less CMP than reported by more sedentary ones [97].

The aerobic exercise intensity should range between 50%-60% of HRmax (220 - age in years), 10-12 point in rating of perceived exertion (an ordinal scale, 6 to 20), or be positive on the "talk test" [78]. The talk test represents the ability to engage in a conversation during exercise. When the exerciser reaches an intensity at which he or she can "just barely respond in conversation," the intensity is considered to be safe and appropriate for cardiovascular adaptation [96]. The initial intensity may be 9-11 point in rating of perceived exertion for frail and sedentary older adults [92]. A 2.5% increase in the intensity or volume weekly is appropriate for adaptation and prevention of musculoskeletal injuries among arthritic older adults [78].

The ideal volume for the beginner is 20 to 30 minutes per day but for sedentary, frailer or more deconditioned older adults, it would be easier to begin with one to five exercise bouts of 3-5 minutes in a day and gradually reach to ideal length. Totally 60 and 90 minutes of moderate level physical activity during a week is recommended by the ACSM (American Colleges of Sports Medicine) [78,92].

The initial frequency of exercise training is recommended 3 [78,92] and later maximum 4 days a week in order not to cause injury according to ACSM [78].

8.3.5. Strengthening exercise

Joint pain can limit older adults from contracting multiple muscles to provide a cardiovascular stimulus during aerobic exercise and causes muscle weakness. In those cases and for frail older adults, it is sensible to add aerobic activity following strengthening and balance exercise to stabilize or support the joint and decrease pain followed by functional improvement [15,82,83,92,96]. Both high and low intensity resistive training significantly reduces pain [99]. A Cochrane systematic review showed that there was evidence for modest reduction in pain following progressive resistive training. It is also reported that there was no significant difference in reducing pain between progressive resistive training with functional, aerobic and flexibility training [100,101].

Because low articular pressures during isometric contractions can be well tolerated, isometric strengthening with a few repetition should be given if the joints are inflamed, unstable, swollen, painful or if it is initial phase of strengthening program [78,79]. Isometric strength training should target the major muscle groups. The intensity should gradually increase to 75% from approximately 30% of the maximal voluntary contraction; the number of repetitions to 8-10 from one; number of sessions to 5-10 from 2 times throughout the day. During a contraction held for maximum 6 seconds (20 seconds resting between contractions), older adults should keep on breathing. Contractions should be performed at different muscle lengths or joint angles, too [78]. As soon as possible, when it is tolerated, isotonic training involving 8-10 major muscle groups should begin to improve overall function maximum of 2 days a week. The intensity should gradually increase to 80% from 40% of 1RM (repetition maximum) for adaptation [78]. 1RM is the weight a person can lift one time with good form. The ACSM recommends no more than three trials with a 30- to 60-second rest between trials to find out the most accurate 1 RM, but older adults may have a better response with a multiple RM of 6 to 10 because they need experience to learn to generate that type of force. Elastic bands or tubing, cuff and hand weights, barbells, dumbbells, hand-held blades, fixed weights, medicine and stability balls etc. can be used as equipment [96,102].

For safety reasons, older adults especially those with cardiovascular problems adults should not perform more than two to three sets of a given exercise and repetition number must be carefully determined. For muscular endurance sets of 12-15 repetitions with lighter resistances, for strength development 8-12 repetitions with higher resistance should be used [78].

Another option for exercise is stabilization exercises, which target co-activation of specific muscles and provide joint stability based on the spine [103]. Increased strength and cross-sectional area of the vertebral muscles reduces CLBP by maintaining muscle balance [102].

8.3.6. Tai-Chi

Tai-Chi [TC], shortly defined as a traditional Chinese mind-body exercise, has recently become popular worldwide because more people with musculoskeletal problems are looking for complementary and alternative treatments [104,105]. TC gives emphasis to diaphragmatic breath, relaxation and composed of slow, gentle, smooth, harmonic and coordinated movements of different body parts, and weight shifting [104,106]. TC involves routines or "forms" ranging from the classic 109 postures to as few as 42 and now has multiple styles modified from the original form. In addition to physical benefits, the focus required to complete these routines elicits mental and cognitive benefits [96].

TC is a moderate-intensity exercise, so it is suitable for physically frail older adults. Besides reducing the pain, people practice TC for also improving physical condition, muscle strength, coordination, flexibility, balance, decreasing risk for falls, stiffness, fatigue, improving sleep, cardiovascular and respiratory function, mood, depression, anxiety, self-efficacy, health-related quality of life and overall wellness in both eastern and western populations [103,104,106,107]. The therapeutic benefits of TC for chronic conditions have been showed in researches recently.

TC is common in older adults especially those with OA, because it is shown to improve pain [103,108], although it is stated that the methodological quality of TC research is generally less than strength and aerobic training research [84]. The physical component of TC provides current recommendations for OA (strength, balance, flexibility, and aerobic cardiovascular exercise) and the mental component could contribute to chronic pain reduction by modulating complex factors of OA pain [104].

Significant pain-relieving effect is shown especially at knee rather than other joints like in the upper extremities where less weight-carrying activity involved in TC [109-111]. It is believed that weight-carrying TC footwork provides pain-relieving effects on knee OA [106]. TC also showed no significant difference in pain reduction of older adults with knee and hip OA compared to hydrotherapy, where there is less knee joint stress than TC [112].

A systematic review and meta-analysis suggested that TC had a small positive effect on pain in people with arthritis and the extent to which it benefits other forms of CMP is unclear but the review also reported that the studies included were low-quality [108]. However a more recent study indicates that water- or land-based exercise, aerobic walking, quadriceps strengthening, resistance exercise, and TC reduce pain and disability from knee OA with evidence rating of A category [80].

There is another discussion about TC that if its benefit increases when combined with the other exercise types or not. Yip YB et al showed that self-management exercise program including stretching, walking, and TC types of movement, had positive effect in reducing pain [113] but a recent systematic review concluded that TC based exercise programs elicited better outcomes than mixed ones but without clear differences [85].

Among different TC styles (Chen, Yang, Wu styles…ect.) the "Sun" style is the most studied one. Sun style TC requires higher stance with bending knees less than other types, so it is more comfortable. In fact in all styles the patient can prefer high or low stance [106]. Song R et al reported that a Sun-style TC exercise could be applied to OA patients in outpatient clinics or public health centers if they are not in acute inflammatory stage to reduce arthritic symptoms [114]. Simplified Yang-style TC is also shown to be effective in osteoartritic knee pain [115,116].

Beside osteoartritis, benefits of TC have been found in some other musculoskeletal problems such as fibromyalgia [6], rheumatoid arthritis [117] and nonspecific CLBP [118].

8.3.7. Aquatic exercise

Aquatic exercise is another good option for the treatment of musculoskeketal problems because water is a safe exercise environment and its temperature provides analgesia for painful muscles and joints [78,119]. The water temperature is recommended between 85 and 90 Fahrenheit (29-32 Celsius) for artritic older adults [79].

The buoyancy of water causes less impact or compressive forces on the joints and therefore allows pain-free motion without the biomechanical stress experienced on land [119]. Older adults with OA or history of surgery may benefit from aquatic exercise. Water resistance can be used for strengthening to progress to land-based exercise among older adults with arthritis. Moreover aquatic exercise, usually practiced with a group, motivates practitioners [78,96]. It is reported that among older adults class attendance is higher for hydrotherapy compared with TC [112] because it provides a playful environment, many social and psychological benefits for them [119]. It also should be considered that heart rate is lower than heart rates when performing at the same level of oxygen consumption on land. "Aquatic heart rate reduction" should be included in the formula while determining target heart rate or it is sensible to use rating of perceived exertion when determining aquatic exercise intensity [96,119].

8.3.8. Exercise adherence in older adults with chronic musculoskeletal pain

Chronic pain has been found to be associated with difficulty in exercising regularly [120]. Motivation has a key role for older adults to participate in exercise willingly. Older adults' outcome and self-efficacy expectations, negative sensations associated with physical activity, such as fear of pain especially back pain or falling influence motivation to engage in physical activities [121]. These negative sensations and related beliefs must be eliminated through facilitating appropriate use of pain medications before exercise or alternative measures such as heat/ice before or after exercise to relieve activity related pain, use of braces or straps, or isolating the damaged joint during exercise. Additionally positive reinforcement and self-management interventions including explaining to older adults how exercise will help reduce pain, cognitive-behavioral therapy, relaxation and distraction techniques and graded exposure to overcome fear of falling or pain can improve participation to exercise among older adults with arthritic pain. Even pain should be minimized in every way possible, the older adult may have to learn to tolerate some pain or discomfort [73,79,86,121].

The use of supervised exercise sessions such as classes in the initial exercise period followed by home exercises and calling patients back for intermittent consultations, or "refresher" group exercise classes may also assist long-term adherence [83]. Generally older adults are interested in self-managing their chronic pain but can't find opportunity. Austrian et al indicated that 73% of the 68 patients (70 years of age and over with chronic pain) included in his study were willing to participate in an exercise program for pain management but 16% of them had this opportunity [40].

Most types of exercise with some evidence are frequently preferred for pain management in older adult populations with CMP especially for arthritis, mostly knee OA, and secondly CLBP. Exercise content, time and frequency are very heterogeneous in RCTs, so it is hard to determine the best exercise structure. At that point individualized approach to exercise prescription is required.

9. Conclusion

Because aging is an extremely variable process, older adults require more individualized management than younger individuals. Treatment decisions should weigh the risks of pain with the risks of treatment. In order to provide the most efficient and safest therapy approach in the older adults with musculoskeletal pain, the identification and frequent re-evaluation of the cause of the chronic pain and the impact on the patient's general medical state are crucial.

The high cost and adverse side effect profiles associated with many analgesic treatments, as well as the potential for drug-drug interactions, operate as significant barriers to the use of standard pharmacologic treatments in older adults [19,74]. Based on studies conducted to date, combined pharmacologic and non- pharmacologic therapies give the best results for pain relief. Regardless, alternative or complementary medical interventions should be recognized as options for older adults with chronic musculoskeletal pain [4,56]. While some studies have demonstrated that integrating complementary medicine into the care of older patients can yield promising results. Additionally, some of the challenges encountered with conventional pain management of older adults can be ameliorated by integrating complementary and alternative medicine approaches [56].

Author details

Ayse Ozcan Edeer
Adjunct Faculty, Doctoral Program in Physical Therapy, Dominican College, NY, USA

Hulya Tuna
School of Health, Department of Physiotherapy and Rehabilitation, Izmir University, Izmir, Turkey

10. References

[1] Ferrell BA, (2001) Pain management in the elderly. Clin Geriatr Med. 17:417-615.
[2] Keefe FJ, Beaupre PM, Weiner DK, Siegler IC (1996) Pain in older adults: a cognitive-behavioral perspective. In: Ferrell BR, Ferrell BA. Pain in the Elderly. Wash: IASP Press. Pp:11-19.
[3] Cavalieri TA (1999) Pain management at the end of life. J Am Osteopath Assoc. 99(6): 16-21.
[4] Gloth MJ and Black RA (2011) The Role of Rehabilitation in Managing Pain in Seniors. In Gloth FM (2011) Handbook of pain relief in older adults: an evidence-based

approach (1-60761-617-3, 978-1-60761-617-7), 2nd ed. DOI 10.1007/978-1-60761-618-4. P:45

[5] Schofield P, Black C, Aveyard B (2011). Management of Pain in Older People. Humana Press.

[6] Brown ST, Kirkpatrick MK, Swanson MS, McKenzie IL (2011) Pain experience of the elderly. Pain Manag Nurs. 12(4):190-6.

[7] Cavalieri TA (2002) Pain management in the elderly. JAOA. 102(9):481-485

[8] http://www.dh.gov.uk/en/Publicationsandstatistics/Publications/PublicationsPolicyAndGuidance/DH_4010161

[9] D'Astolfo CJ and Humphreys BK (2006) A record review of reported musculoskeletal pain in an Ontario long term care facility. BMC Geriatrics. 6:5. doi:10.1186/1471-2318-6-5.

[10] Williams AK (1999) Geriatric Rehabilitation Manual, In: Kaufman TL editor. Pain. Churchill Livinstone. pp:359-362.

[11] Cowan DT, Fitzpatricka JM, Robertsa JD, Whileb AE, Baldwin J et al. (2003) The assessment and management of pain among older people in care homes: current status and future directions. International Journal of Nursing Studies. 40 291–298.

[12] Arnstein P (2010) Balancing analgesic efficacy with safety concerns in the older patient. Pain Manag Nurs. 11(2 Suppl):11-22.

[13] Gloth F (2001) Pain Management in Older Adults: Prevention and Treatment. J Am Geriatr Soc. 49:188–199.

[14] http://www.iasp-pain.org,

[15] Tse MM, Wan VT, Ho SS (2011) Physical exercise: does it help in relieving pain and increasing mobility among older adults with chronic pain? J Clin Nurs. 20(5-6):635-44.

[16] AGS Panel on Persistent Pain in Older Persons. The management of persistent pain in older persons. (2002) J Am Geriatr Soc. 50(6 Suppl):205-224.

[17] Herr KA, Garand L (2001) Assessment and measurement of pain in older adults. Clin Geriatr Med. 17:457-478.

[18] Herr K (2010) Pain in the older adult: an imperative across all health care settings. Pain Manag Nurs. 11(2 Suppl):1-10.

[19] Ersek M, Turner JA, Cain KC and Kemp CA (2004) Chronic pain self-management for older adults: a randomized controlled trial. BMC Geriatrics 4:7. doi:10.1186/1471-2318-4-7

[20] Beissner K (2012) Conservative Pain Management for the Older Adult. In: Guccione A, Wong R, Avers D, editors. Geriatric Physical Therapy. 3rd ed. Elsevier. Pp:395-411.

[21] Charlton JE (2005) Pain in Older Adults Core Curriculum for Professional Education in Pain, IASP Press, (4):1-4.

[22] Frondini C, Lanfranchi G, Minardi M, Cucinotta D (2007) Affective, behavior and cognitive disorders in the elderly with chronic musculoskelatal pain: the impact on an aging population. Arch Gerontol Geriatr. 44 (Suppl 1):167-71.

[23] Podichetty VK, Mazanec DJ, Biscup RS (2003) Chronic non-malignant musculoskeletal pain in older adults: clinical issues and opioid intervention. Postgrad Med J. 79(937):627-33.

[24] Yamada E, Thomas DC (2011) Common musculoskeletal diagnoses of upper and lower extremities in older patients. Mt Sinai J Med. 78(4):546-57. doi: 10.1002/msj.20274.

[25] Morone NE, Karp JF, Lynch CS, Bost JE, El Khoudary SR, Weiner DK (2009) Impact of chronic musculoskeletal pathology on older adults: a study of differences between knee OA and low back pain. Pain Med. 10(4):693-701.

[26] Weiner DK, Cayea D (2005) Low back pain and its contributors in older adults: a practical approach to evaluation and treatment. In: Gibson SJ, Weiner DK, eds. Pain in Older Persons, Progress in Pain Research and Management. IASP Press. (35)329-354.

[27] Rudy TE, Weiner DK, Lieber SJ, Slaboda J, Boston JR (2007) The impact of chronic low back pain on older adults: a comparative study of patients and controls. Pain. 131(3):293-301.

[28] Leveille SG, Zhang Y, McMullen W, Kelly-Hayes M, and Felson DT (2005) Sex differences in musculoskeletal pain in older adults. Pain. 116(3): 332–338.

[29] Shah RC, Buchman AS, Boyle PA, Leurgans SE, Wilson RS, Andersson GB, Bennett DA (2011) Musculoskeletal pain is associated with incident mobility disability in community-dwelling elders. J Gerontol A Biol Sci Med Sci. 66(1):82-8.

[30] Buchman AS, Shah RC, Leurgans SE, Boyle PA, Wilson RS, Bennett DA. (2010) Musculoskeletal pain and incident disability in community-dwelling older adults. Arthritis Care Res. 62(9):1287-93.

[31] Mitchell C (2001) Assessment and management of chronic pain in elderly people. Br J Nurs. 8-21;10(5):296-304.

[32] Leveille SG, Bean J, Bandeen-Roche K, Jones R, Hochberg M, Guralnik JM (2002) Musculoskeletal pain and risk for falls in older disabled women living in the community. J Am Geriatr Soc. 50(4):671-8.

[33] Leveille SG, Jones RN, Kiely DK, Hausdorff JM, Shmerling RH, Guralnik JM, Kiel DP, Lipsitz LA, Bean JF (2009) Chronic musculoskeletal pain and the occurrence of falls in an older population. JAMA. 25;302(20):2214-21.

[34] Mesrine S, Boutron-Ruault MC, Clavel-Chapelon F (2010) Chronic pain and risk of falls in older adults. JAMA. 24;303(12):1147-8.

[35] Wilber ST, Sullivan AF, Camargo CA Jr (2010) Chronic pain and risk of falls in older adults. JAMA. 24:303(12):1148-9.

[36] Lihavainen K, Sipilä S, Rantanen T, Sihvonen S, Sulkava R, Hartikainen S (2010) Contribution of musculoskeletal pain to postural balance in community-dwelling people aged 75 years and older. J Gerontol A Biol Sci Med Sci. 65(9):990-6.

[37] Golden BA (2002) A multidisciplinary approach to nonpharmacologic pain management. JAOA. Supplement 3 102(9):1-5.

[38] Cayea D, Perera S, Weiner DK (2006) Chronic low back pain in older adults: What physicians know, what they think they know, and what they should be taught. J Am Geriatr Soc. 54(11):1772-7.

[39] Leveille SG, Bean J, Ngo L, McMullen W, Guralnik JM (2007) The pathway from musculoskeletal pain to mobility difficulty in older disabled women. Pain. 128(1-2):69-77.

[40] Austrian JS, Kerns RD, Reid MC (2005) Perceived barriers to trying self-management approaches for chronic pain in older persons. J Am Geriatr Soc. 53(5):856-61.

[41] Bruckenthal P, Reid C, and Reisner L (2009) Special Issues in the Management of Chronic Pain in Older Adults. Pain Medicine. 10:67-78.

[42] Ballentine NH (2008) Polypharmacy in the elderly: maximizing benefit, minimizing harm. Crit Care Nurs Q. 31(1):40-5.

[43] McPherson ML and Uritsky TJ (2011) Pharmacotherapy of Pain in Older Adults: Nonopioid. In Gloth FM Handbook of pain relief in older adults: an evidence-based approach (1-60761-617-3, 978-1-60761-617-7), 2nd ed. DOI 10.1007/978-1-60761-618-4. P:57

[44] Saad M, Harisingani R, Katinas L (2012) Impact of geriatric consultation on the number of medications in hospitalized older patients. Consult Pharm. 27(1):42-8.

[45] Elliott AF, Horgas AL (2009) Effects of an analgesic trial in reducing pain behaviors in community-dwelling older adults with dementia. Nurs Res. 58(2):140-5.

[46] Kean WF, Rainsford KD, Kean IR (2008) Management of chronic musculoskeletal pain in the elderly: opinions on oral medication use. Inflammopharmacology. 16(2):53-75.

[47] Cooper JW, Burfield AH (2003) Assessment and management of chronic pain in the older adult. J Am Pharm Assoc. 2010 50(3):89-99.

[48] Muller S, Bedson J, Mallen CD (2012) The association between pain intensity and the prescription of analgesics and non-steroidal anti-inflammatory drugs. Eur J Pain. 19. doi: 10.1002/j.1532-2149.2011.00107.x.

[49] Taylor R Jr, Lemtouni S, Weiss K, Pergolizzi JV Jr (2012) Pain Management in the Elderly An FDA Safe Use Initiative Expert Panel's View on Preventable Harm Associated with NSAID Therapy. Curr Gerontol Geriatr Res. 2012:196159.

[50] Bruckenthal P (2010) Integrating Nonpharmacologic and Alternative Strategies Into a Comprehensive Management Approach for Older Adults With Pain. Pain Management Nursing. 11(2):23-31

[51] Trescot AM, Helm S, Hansen H, Benyamin R, Glaser SE, Adlaka R, Patel S, Manchikanti L (2008) Opioids in the management of chronic non-cancer pain: an update of American Society of the Interventional Pain Physicians' (ASIPP) Guidelines. Pain Physician. 11(2 Suppl):5-62.

[52] Hicks GE, Shardell M, Miller RR, Bandinelli S, Guralnik J, Cherubini A, Lauretani F, Ferrucci L (2008) Associations between vitamin D status and pain in older adults: the Invecchiare in Chianti study. J Am Geriatr Soc. 56(5):785-91.

[53] Fialová D, Onder G (2009) Medication errors in elderly people: contributing factors and future perspectives. Br J Clin Pharmacol. 67(6):641-5.

[54] Planton J, Edlund BJ (2010) Strategies for reducing polypharmacy in older adults. J Gerontol Nurs. 36(1):8-12. doi: 10.3928/00989134-20091204-03.

[55] Kemp CA, Ersek M, Turner JA (2005) A descriptive study of older adults with persistent pain: use and perceived effectiveness of pain management strategies. BMC Geriatr. 8:5:12 doi:10.1186/1471-2318-5-12.

[56] Bruckenthal P (2010) Integrating nonpharmacologic and alternative strategies into a comprehensive management approach for older adults with pain. Pain Manag Nurs. 11(2 Suppl):23-31.

[57] Komp-Webb M (2008) Physical Therapy. In ed MP Jansen. Managing pain in the older adult. Ed Springer Pub. Co. P:93-117

[58] Barr JO (2007) Conservative interventions for pain control. In: Kauffman TL, Barr JO, Moran ML (eds). Geriatric Rehabilitation Manual (2nd ed), Churchill Livingstone.P:449-455

[59] Barry LC, Gill TM, Kerns RD, Reid MC (2005) Identification of pain-reduction strategies used by community-dwelling older persons. J Gerontol A Biol Sci Med Sci. 60(12):1569-75.

[60] Chatap G, De Sousa A, Giraud K, Vincent JP (2007) Acute Pain in the Elderly Study Group. Pain in the elderly: Prospective study of hyperbaric CO2 cryotherapy (neurocryostimulation). Joint Bone Spine. 74(6):617-21.

[61] French HP, Brennan A, White B, Cusack T (2011) Manual therapy for osteoarthritis of the hip or knee – A systematic review. Manual Therapy. 16(2):109-117.

[62] Miller J, Gross A, D'Sylva J, Burnie SJ, Goldsmith CH, Graham N, Haines T, Brønfort G, Hoving JL (2010) Manual therapy and exercise for neck pain: A systematic review. Manual Therapy.15:33-35.

[63] Harris M, Richards KC (2010) The physiological and psychological effects of slow-stroke back massage and hand massage on relaxation in older people. J Clin Nurs. 19(7-8):917-26.

[64] Hawk C, Rupert RL, Colonvega M, Boyd J, Hall S (2006) Comparison of bioenergetic synchronization technique and customary chiropractic care for older adults with chronic musculoskeletal pain. J Manipulative Physiol Ther. 29(7):540-9.

[65] van Middelkoop M, Rubinstein SM, Kuijpers T, Verhagen AP, Ostelo R, Koes BW, van Tulder MW (2011) A systematic review on the effectiveness of physical and rehabilitation interventions for chronic non-specific low back pain. Eur Spine J. 20(1):19-39.

[66] Vieira PJ, Ribeiro JP, Cipriano G Jr, Umpierre D, Cahalin LP, Moraes RS, Chiappa GR (2012) Effect of transcutaneous electrical nerve stimulation on muscle metaboreflex in healthy young and older subjects. Eur J Appl Physiol. 112(4):1327-34.

[67] Weiner DK, Rudy TE, Glick RM, Boston JR, Lieber SJ, Morrow LA, Taylor S (2003) Efficacy of percutaneous electrical nerve stimulation for the treatment of chronic low back pain in older adults. J Am Geriatr Soc. 51:599-608.

[68] Zhang W, Moskowitz RW, Nuki G, Abramson S, Altman RD, Arden N, Bierma-Zeinstra S, Brandt KD, Croft P, Doherty M, Dougados M, Hochberg M, Hunter DJ, Kwoh K, Lohmander LS, Tugwell P (2008) OARSI recommendations for the management of hip and knee osteoarthritis, Part II: OARSI evidence-based, expert consensus guidelines. Osteoarthritis Cartilage. 16(2):137-62.

[69] Zhang W, Nuki G, Moskowitz RW, Abramson S, Altman RD, Arden NK, Bierma-Zeinstra S, Brandt KD, Croft P, Doherty M, Dougados M, Hochberg M, Hunter DJ, Kwoh K, Lohmander LS, Tugwell P (2010) OARSI recommendations for the management of hip and knee osteoarthritis: part III: Changes in evidence following systematic cumulative update of research published through January 2009. Osteoarthritis Cartilage. 18(4):476-99.

[70] Barnes PM, Bloom B, Nahin RL (2008) Complementary and Alternative Medicine Use Among Adults and Children: United States, 2007, National Health Statistics Reports Number 12, December 10.

[71] Molton I, Jensen MP, Ehde DM, Carter GT, Kraft G, Cardenas DD (2008) Coping with chronic pain among younger, middle-aged, and older adults living with neurological injury and disease. J Aging Health. 20(8):972–996. doi:10.1177/0898264308324680.

[72] Morone NE, and Greco CM (2007) Mind–Body Interventions for Chronic Pain in Older Adults:A Structured Review. Pain Medicine. 8(4):359-75.

[73] Nour K, Laforest S, Gauvin L, Gignac M (2006) Behavior change following a self-management intervention for housebound older adults with arthritis: an experimental study. It J Behav Nutr Phys Act. 30:3:12.
[74] Reid MC, Papaleontiou M, Ong A, Breckman R, Wethington E, Pillemer K (2008) Self-management strategies to reduce pain and improve function among older adults in community settings: a review of the evidence. Pain Med. 9(4):409-24.
[75] Beissner K, Henderson CR Jr, Papaleontiou M, Olkhovskaya Y, Wigglesworth J, Reid MC (2009) Physical therapists' use of cognitive-behavioral therapy for older adults with chronic pain: a nationwide survey. Phys Ther. 89:456–469.
[76] Green SM, Hadjistavropoulos T, Hadjistavropoulos H, Martin R, Sharpe D (2009) A Controlled Investigation of a Cognitive Behavioral Pain Management Program for Older Adults Behavioral and Cognitive Psychotherapy. 37:221–226.
[77] Barry LC, Kerns RD, Guo Z, Duong BD, Iannone LP, Reid MC (2004) Identification of strategies used to cope with chronic pain in older persons receiving primary care from a Veterans Affairs Medical Center. J Am Geriatr Soc. 52(6):950-6.
[78] American Geriatrics Society Panel on Exercise and Osteoarthritis. Exercise prescription for older adults with osteoarthritis pain: consensus practice recommendations (2001) A supplement to the AGS Clinical Practice Guidelines on the management of chronic pain in older adults. J Am Geriatr Soc. 49(6):808-823.
[79] Rimmer JH (2005) Exercise Considerations for Medical Conditions. In: Jones CJ, Rose DJ, editors. Physical Activity Instruction of Older Adults. Human Kinetics. pp. 336-349.
[80] Ringdahl E, Pandit S (2011) Treatment of knee osteoarthritis. Am Fam Physician. 83(11):1287-1292.
[81] Bosomworth NJ (2009) Exercise and knee osteoarthritis: benefit or hazard? Can Fam Physician. 55(9):871-878.
[82] Ettinger WH, Burns R, Messier SP, Applegate W, Rejeski WJ, Morgan T, Shumaker S, Berry MJ, O'Toole M, Monu J, Craven T (1997) A randomized trial comparing aerobic exercise and resistance exercise with a health education program in older adults with knee osteoarthritis. The Fitness Arthritis and Seniors Trial (FAST). JAMA. 277(1):25-31.
[83] Roddy E, Zhang W, Doherty M (2005) Aerobic walking or strengthening exercise for osteoarthritis of the knee? A systematic review. Ann Rheum Dis. 64(4):544-548.
[84] Bennell KL, Hinman RS (2011) A review of the clinical evidence for exercise in osteoarthritis of the hip and knee. J Sci Med Sport.14(1):4-9.
[85] Escalante Y, Saavedra JM, García-Hermoso A, Silva AJ, Barbosa TM (2010) Physical exercise and reduction of pain in adults with lower limb osteoarthritis: a systematic review. J Back Musculoskelet Rehabil. 23(4):175-186.
[86] Resnick B (2001) Managing arthritis with exercise. Geriatr Nurs. 22(3):143-150.
[87] Messier SP, Loeser RF, Miller GD, Morgan TM, Rejeski WJ, Sevick MA, Ettinger WH Jr, Pahor M, Williamson JD (2004) Exercise and dietary weight loss in overweight and obese older adults with knee osteoarthritis: the Arthritis, Diet, and Activity Promotion Trial. Arthritis Rheum. 50(5):1501-1510.
[88] Bartholomew JB, Lewis BP, Linder DE, Cook DB (1996) Post-exercise analgesia: replication and extension. J Sports Sci.4(4):329-334.

[89] Downton JH. Why do old people fall? Falls in the elderly. Great Britain: Hodder and Stoughton Limited; 1993: 1-77.

[90] Alghwiri AA, Whitney SL (2012) Balance and Falls. In: Guccione A, Wong R, Avers D, editors. Geriatric Physical Therapy. 3rd ed. Elsevier. pp. 331-353.

[91] Karinkanta S, Piirtola M, Sievänen H, Uusi-Rasi K, Kannus P (2010) Physical therapy approaches to reduce fall and fracture risk among older adults. Nat Rev Endocrinol. 6(7):396-407.

[92] Dinan S, Skelton D, Malbut K (2005) Aerobic Endurance Training. In: Jones CJ, Rose DJ, editors. Physical Activity Instruction of Older Adults. Human Kinetics. pp. 191-210.

[93] Brown M, Avers D, Wong RA (2012) Wellness for the Aging Adult-Special Populations and the Continuum of Care. In: Guccione A, Wong R, Avers D, editors. Geriatric Physical Therapy. 3rd ed. Elsevier. pp. 446-456.

[94] Norman KV (2005) Principles of The Warm-Up and Cool-Down. In: Jones CJ, Rose DJ, editors. Physical Activity Instruction of Older Adults. Human Kinetics. pp. 141-153.

[95] Brown M, Rose DJ (2005) Flexibility Training. In: J ones CJ, Rose DJ, editors. Physical Activity Instruction of Older Adults. Human Kinetics. pp. 156-174.

[96] VanBeveren PJ, Avers D (2012) Exercise and Physical Activity for Older Adults. In: Guccione A, Wong R, Avers D, editors. Geriatric Physical Therapy. 3rd ed. Elsevier. pp. 64-85.

[97] Bruce B, Fries JF, Lubeck DP (2005) Aerobic exercise and its impact on musculoskeletal pain in older adults: a 14 year prospective, longitudinal study. Arthritis Res Ther.7(6):1263-1270.

[98] Fries JF, Singh G, Morfeld D, O'Driscoll P, Hubert H (1996) Relationship of running to musculoskeletal pain with age. A six-year longitudinal study. Arthritis Rheum. 39(1):64-72.

[99] Jan MH, Lin JJ, Liau JJ, Lin YF, Lin DH (2008) Investigation of clinical of high and low resiztance training for patients with knee osteoarthritis: a randomized controlled trial. Phys Ther. 88(4):427-436.

[100] Barrett CJ, Smerdely P (2002) A comparison of community-based resistance exercise and flexibility exercise for seniors. Aust J Physiother. 48(3):215-219.

[101] Liu CJ, Latham NK (2009) Progressive resistance strength training for improving physical function in older adults. Cochrane Database Syst Rev. 8(3):CD002759.

[102] Kraemer WJ, French DN (2005) Resistance Training. In: Jones CJ, Rose DJ, editors. Physical Activity Instruction of Older Adults. Human Kinetics. pp. 176-189.

[103] Christiansen C (2012) Impaired Joint Mobility. In: Guccione A, Wong R, Avers D, editors. Geriatric Physical Therapy. 3rd ed. Elsevier. Pp: 248-262.

[104] Wang C (2011) Tai Chi and Rheumatic Diseases. Rheum Dis Clin North Am. 37(1): 19-32.

[105] Hawker GA, Mian S, Bednis K, Stanaitis (2011) I. Osteoarthritis year 2010 in review: non-pharmacologic therapy. Osteoarthritis Cartilage. 19(4):366-374.

[106] Chyu MC, von Bergen V, Brismée JM, Zhang Y, Yeh JK, Shen CL (2011). Complementary and alternative exercises for management of osteoarthritis. Arthritis. 2011:364319.

[107] Ho TJ, Liang WM, Lien CH, Ma TC, Kuo HW, Chu BC, Chang HW, Lai JS, Lin JG (2007) Health-related quality of life in the elderly practicing T'ai Chi Chuan. J Altern Complement Med. 13(10):1077-1083.
[108] Hall A, Maher C, Latimer J, Ferreira M (2009) The effectiveness of Tai Chi for musculoskeletal pain conditions: a systematic review and meta-analysis. Arthritis Rheum. 61(6):717-724.
[109] Song R, Lee EO, Lam P, Bae SC (2003) Effects of tai chi exercise on pain, balance, muscle strength, and perceived difficulties in physical functioning in older women with osteoarthritis: a randomized clinical trial. J Rheumatol. 30(9):2039-2044.
[110] Wang C, Schmid CH, Hibberd PL, Kalish R, Roubenoff R, Rones R, McAlindon T (2009) Tai Chi is effective in treating knee osteoarthritis: a randomized controlled trial. Arthritis Rheum. 61(11):1545-1553.
[111] Brismée JM, Paige RL, Chyu MC, Boatright JD, Hagar JM, McCaleb JA, Quintela MM, Feng D, Xu KT, Shen CL (2007) Group and home-based tai chi in elderly subjects with knee osteoarthritis: a randomized controlled trial. Clin Rehabil. 21(2):99-111.
[112] Fransen M, Nairn L, Winstanley J, Lam P, Edmonds J (2007) Physical activity for osteoarthritis management: a randomized controlled clinical trial evaluating hydrotherapy or Tai Chi classes. Arthritis Rheum. 57(3):407-414.
[113] Yip YB, Sit JW, Fung KK, Wong DY, Chong SY, Chung LH, Ng TP (2007) Effects of a self-management arthritis programme with an added exercise component for osteoarthritic knee: randomized controlled trial. J Adv Nurs. 59(1):20-8.
[114] Song R, Lee EO, Lam P, Bae SC (2007) Effects of a Sun-style Tai Chi exercise on arthritic symptoms, motivation and the performance of health behaviors in women with osteoarthritis. Taehan Kanho Hakhoe Chi. 37(2):249-56.
[115] Ni GX, Song L, Yu B, Huang CH, Lin JH (2010) Tai chi improves physical function in older Chinese women with knee osteoarthritis. J Clin Rheumatol. 16(2):64-67.
[116] Field T (2011) Tai Chi research review. Complement Ther Clin Pract. 17(3):14-6.
[117] Uhlig T, Fongen C, Steen E, Christie A, Odegard S (2010) Exploring Tai Chi in rheumatoid arthritis: a quantitative and qualitative study. BMC Musculoskeletal Disorders; 5:11-43.
[118] Hall AM, Maher CG, Lam P, Ferreira M, Latimer J. Tai chi exercise for treatment of pain and disability in people with persistent low back pain: a randomized controlled trial. Arthritis Care Res (Hoboken). 2011 Nov;63(11):1576-83.
[119] Sova R (2005) Aquatic Training. In: Jones CJ, Rose DJ, editors. Physical Activity Instruction of Older Adults. Human Kinetics. pp. 248-261.
[120] Krein SL, Heisler M, Piette JD, Butchart A, Kerr EA (2007) Overcoming the influence of chronic pain on older patients' difficulty with recommended self-management activities. Gerontologist. 47(1):61-8.
[121] Resnick B, Avers D (2012) Motivation and Patient Education: Implications for Physical Therapist Practice. In: Guccione A, Wong R, Avers D, editors. Geriatric Physical Therapy. 3rd ed. Elsevier. pp. 183-206.

Chapter 6

Shoulder Pain in Swimmers

Julio José Contreras Fernández, Rodrigo Liendo Verdugo,
Matías Osorio Feito and Francisco Soza Rex

Additional information is available at the end of the chapter

http://dx.doi.org/10.5772/51013

1. Introduction

Shoulder pain is the most important symptom that affects competitive swimmers, with a prevalence between 40 – 91% [1-3], and it constitutes a special syndrome called the "swimmer's shoulder".

This syndrome, described by Kennedy and Hawkins in 1974 [3] consists in discomfort after swimming activities in a first step. This may progress to pain during and after training. Finally, the pain affects the progress of the athlete [4]. Some researchers have demonstrated that an important proportion of competitive swimmers have shoulder pain that interferes with training and progress of their abilities. The percentage of athletes with swimmer's shoulder is proportional to the age, the years of practice and the level of competition. Swimmers with interfering pain might not progress in training and thus will not compete as effectively [5].

One of the first reports of this problem was in the 1972 Olympic Games in Munich; Kennedy noticed a high incidence of shoulder pain among swimmers of Canadian group: of 35 competitive swimmers, there were 43 orthopaedic consultations, with 16 specific-related to shoulder (37%), being the most frequent problem [4].

Kennedy had performed a cross-Canada survey involving all competitive swimmers (5000 yards per day). A total of 2496 swimmers were included, reporting a 3% (81 swimmers) shoulder complaints, caused primarily by the freestyle and butterfly strokes and occasionally by the backstroke [4].

2. Epidemiology of shoulder pain in competitive swimmers

The epidemiology of shoulder pain in competitive swimmers has been studied by many researchers. The estimation of prevalence of shoulder pain is very difficult because it is related with the subjective experience of pain, memory factors, level of training and the definition of pain considered by the researchers. It is important to establish the difference about the type of evolution of pain (acute, sub-acute, chronic or history of pain) and to differentiate pain of exercise-induced soreness.

As mentioned above, Kennedy et al [4] found a prevalence of 3% of anterior shoulder pain in competitive swimmers. In later surveys, the prevalence has been reported as much higher from 15% to 80% [1].

McMaster and Troup [5] in 1993 performed one of the largest descriptive studies on shoulder pain in competitive swimmers, consisting in a survey questionnaire self administered under classroom-style supervision to a group of 1262 USA swimmers. They included group demographics, training profiles and out-of-water training techniques. They clearly defined the pain as that which interfered with training or progress in training as opposed to post-exercise muscle soreness. Specifically, they questioned about the current experience of pain and the history of pain at any time during the swimming career. With these definitions, the prevalence of history of pain was 71% for male swimmers and 75% for female swimmers. The prevalence of actual pain is less than history of pain (17% in males and 35% in women) [Table 1].

Richardson et al [6] in 1978 performed a survey and physical examination to 137 competitive swimmers. They found a prevalence of history of pain of 52% in "elite" swimmers and 57% in "championship" group (World Champion Team group). In the overall group, a greater percentage of men, as compared to women, complained about shoulder problems (46 vs. 40%). When individual groups were considered, the "elite" women had the greater number of complaints [Table 1].

Bak et al [1] in 1994-1995 season performed detailed interviews and clinical examinations (probably, the most detailed descriptive study of shoulder pain in competitive swimmers) to 36 Danish swimmers. 33 swimmers had unilateral shoulder pain and 13 had bilateral pain. Thirteen swimmers were National Team members (half of the subjects with bilateral complaints were National Team swimmers).

Author - year	Participants (n)	Age	Gender (female - male)	Acute Pain	Sub acute pain (2-week)	History of pain
McMaster et al - 1993	1262	19,5	Not described	9,4 – 35%	Not described	38 – 75%
Richardson et al - 1980	137	14 – 23	83 - 54	Not described	Not described	52 - 57%
Bak et al - 1997	36	17 (12 - 23)	22 - 14	Not described	Not described	91,66%
Contreras et al - 2010	40	17,96 ± 4,11	16 - 24	20%	46,67%	80%

Table 1. Descriptive studies of shoulder pain prevalence in competitive swimmers.

Our research group performed a descriptive study in 2008-2009 [7] to a group of 40 competitive swimmers from the "Universidad de Chile". In our study, the prevalence of history of shoulder pain is 80%. A 20% presented actual pain and the 47% a two week pain. These results are comparable with the international surveys [Table 2].

Years of practice	Meters per day	Weight work hours per week	Stretching time (minutes)	Use of implements	Preferred stroke	Preferred contest
6,07 (3,69)	4716,67 (1297,77)	2,72 (0,96)	7,72 (6,67)	73,33%	Freestyle 73,33%	Sprint 56,67%

Table 2. Training data; the values are expressed in mean (SD) or as percentages.

The survey method for data collection has inherent limitations to correlate cause and effect relationships. But competitive swimmers are very sensitive to their shoulder problems and their ability to effectively train. They have the opportunities to compete against other swimmers and to perform timed trainings.

3. Shoulder Biomechanics in swimming

Swimming requires several different shoulder motions, most being performed during circumduction in clockwise and counter-clockwise directions with varying degrees of internal and external rotation and scapular protraction and retraction [8].

Competitive swimmers used four types of strokes: freestyle or front crawl stroke, breaststroke, backstroke, and butterfly stroke. The fastest, most popular and most widely used stroke for training is the freestyle stroke [9]. The power for this stroke comes 80% from the pull and 20% from the kick [9].

The freestyle stroke pull-cycle can be divided in four phases [10]:

1. Early pull-through: beginning with the hand entry into the water and ending when the humerus is perpendicular to the axis of the torso.
2. Late pull-through: beginning at the completion of early pull-through and ending as the hand leaves the water.
3. Early recovery: beginning at hand exit and ending when the humerus is perpendicular to the water surface.
4. Late recovery: beginning at the completion of early recovery and ending at hand entry.

During the entry and beginning of the pull phases, the glenohumeral joint is in forward flexion, and the humerus is in abduction and internal rotation [9]. During the end of the pull, the joint is extended and the humerus is in adduction and internal rotation [9]. During the recovery period, the arm is in abduction and internal rotation, moving from extension to flexion above the water [9].

The backstroke is considered the complement to the freestyle stroke, and the arm actions involve the same four phases; however, power comes 25% from the kick and 75% from the pull [9].

The butterfly stroke is performed with the arms in the same phase of the stroke at one time. During the entry, both shoulders are flexed, abducted, and internally rotated. During the pull-through phase, the shoulders move into extension, and in the recovery, the arms are brought above the water from extension to flexion while abducted and internally rotated. The power for this stroke comes 30% from the kick and 70% from the pull [9].

The breaststroke has a fifty-fifty split from where the power is initiated. In the pull phase, the arms move into adduction, internally rotated, and are always below the water surface. During the recovery, the arms return in a circular pattern, always under the water surface [9].

In 1991 Marilyn Pink performed the most detailed electromyographic and cinematographic analysis of freestyle stroke [10]. In the pull-through phase, they recognized three different phases: the first phase was reaching forward and gliding. From the point that the hand entered the water to the point of maximal elbow extension, there was no actual pulling. Pulling began after the reach.

Reach began as the hand entered the water (predominance of phasic activity in the upper trapezius, rhomboids, supraspinatus, and the anterior and middle deltoids). The serratus anterior was upwardly rotating and protracting the scapula while the upper trapezius was elevating it and the rhomboids were retracting it.

Therefore, the hand followed an S-shaped curve during the pull-through phase (pectoralis major is the responsible for the initial powerful adduction and extension of the humerus). When the humerus is perpendicular to the body, latissimus dorsi continued the pulling by shoulder extension (internal rotation is given by subscapularis). Also, the serratus anterior was acting to move the body over the arm and through the water and upwardly rotate the scapula to maintain glenohumeral joint congruency. When the latissimus dorsi finished its activity, the posterior deltoid fired to lift the shoulder out of the water.

Finally, in the recovery position (much shorter), the activity noted at the end of pull-through in the middle deltoid and supraspinatus is maintained. The rhomboids fired to retract the scapula.

Pink et al highlighted that the subscapularis and the serratus anterior continually fire above 20% MMT (manual muscle test). Thus, these two muscles would appear to be susceptible to fatigue [10].

4. Etiology

The term "swimmer's shoulder" covers a spectrum of consecutive or coexisting pathologies, with rotator cuff–related pain to be the most common finding [11].

Kennedy and Hawkins [4] proposed that the avascularity zones of the supraspinatus and bicipital tendon in the adducted position of the arm are the explanation of swimmer's shoulder. When the shoulders are abducted, all of the vessels of the tendons are almost completely filled. However, when the arm is at the side in the adducted position, there is a constant area of avascularity extending 1 cm. proximal directly to the point of insertion of the supraspinatus and in the intracapsular portion of the bicipital tendon when it passes over the head of the humerus [4].

Bak reported that the main factor in the development of a swimmer's shoulder seems to be the high training volume during growth in the absence of a well-designed and balanced dryland training program, affecting the muscular balance and the scapular motion [11].

A clear consensus is lacking as to the causes of shoulder pain in swimmers. A general medical assumption has been that swimmer's shoulder is a rotator cuff pathology [12]. Kennedy and Hawkins explain this phenomenon based on the differential vascularity of the supraspinatus and bicipital tendons [4]. Other reports suggest that the impingement is produced by glenohumeral instability or muscular imbalance of the scapular stabilizers (secondary impingement). [9,13,14] Indeed, the muscular electric activity is different in the shoulders with pain during the swimming [10,15].

Essentially, there are various causes or contributor factors accepted to cause shoulder pain in swimmers. The intrinsic mechanism has been defined as a tendon injury that originates within the tendon from direct tendon overload, intrinsic degeneration, or other insult. The extrinsic mechanism has been defined as tendon damage caused by injury of the tendon through compression against surrounding structures, specifically the coracoacromial arch. Among these are: overuse, overload, bony configuration, hypovascularity, muscular imbalance, scapular dyskinesis, joint stability, flexibility, stroke technique, training errors, performance level and coaching factors [9].

Brushøj et al [16] in 2007 reported the arthroscopic findings of 18 competitive swimmers. The most common finding at arthroscopy was labral pathology in 11 (61%) shoulders. Of these, five had signs of posterior superior impingement, two in combination with subacromial impingement. The second most common finding was subacromial impingement (28%). Only two swimmers had isolated inflammation of the bicipital tendon.

4.1. Overuse

The repeated movement of the shoulder can cause micro injury to different structures under risk during swimming. The elite swimmers may log up to 8000-20000 meters per day average using the freestyle arm stroke for most of the distance [9]. At an average of 8-10 arm cycles per 25 meters, a swimmer completes over one million shoulder rotations each week [17]. Richardson and Jobe [6] calculated 396000 strokes per season in male competitive swimmers and declared that it is remarkable to them that an even greater number of shoulder problems do not develop.

Murphy [18] calculated that swimming is equated to running for energy expenditure in a ratio 1:4 in that running 4 miles is equivalent to swimming 1 mile.

This type of training predisposes swimmers to overuse injuries of the shoulder. Consequently, shoulder pain is directly proportional to the age, volume of training, and the ability of the swimmer (level, training duration and years of practice) [6]. To maintain proficiency, swimming requires a great amount of work. Rest from training quickly translates into detraining [5]. Accordingly, the cause of pain is a combination of overuse and overload [11].

4.2. Impingement and supraspinatus tendinopathy

Swimming involves repetitive overhead movement [19]. Jobe et al [20] hypothesized that repetitive and forceful overhead activity causes a gradual stretching out of the anteroinferior capsuloligamentous structures leading to mild laxity, instability and impingement.

The supraspinatus is the major rotator cuff muscle responsible for securing the humeral head in the glenoid, and its tendon is susceptible to tendinopathy in swimming [19]. The normal tendon appears yellow-white. Microcopically, quiescent rows of tenocytes can be seen interspersed among the compact parallel bundles of collagen fibres. In supraspinatus tendinopathy, the tendon appears grey, dull and oedematous. Microscopically, the tissue appears disrupted and hypercellular with fibroblastic cells in varying states [19].

Sein et al [19] reported in a group of 52 competitive swimmers that were imaged by MRI a 69% supraspinatus tendinopathy with no association between preferred swimming stroke. Tears of the supraspinatus tendon were found in three swimmers: two were reported as having a delaminated intrasubstance tear, and one had a partial 3 mm articular side tear. The bicipital tendon was normal in 46 imaged shoulders (3 unstable bicipital anchor and 3 bicipital sheat effusion) and two had subscapularis tendinopathy. One had infraspinatus tendon thickening, but no change was reported for the teres minor tendon.

Seint et al [19] found that the swimmers' supraspinatus tendon thickness correlated significantly with their level of training, years in training and hours per week in training. Competitive swimmers who trained for more than 15 h/week were twice as likely to have tendinopathy as those who trained less. Similarly, elite athletes who swam more than 35 km/week were four times more likely to have tendinopathy as those who swam fewer kilometres. Also, all swimmers with increased tendon thickness had impingement pain and supraspinatus tendinopathy. In fact, a positive impingement sign correlated strongly with the presence of supraspinatus tendinopathy. A positive impingement sign had 100% sensitivity and 65% specificity for diagnosing supraspinatus tendinopathy and failed to correlate with other shoulder lesions.

Sein et al [19] based in the results of their research, proposed a new model for swimmer's shoulder. In this model, repetitive movement causes tendinopathy with an associated increase in tendon thickness. Tendinopathy leads to pain when the thickened tendon and associated bursa are repeatedly squashed under the bony arch of the acromion during swimming as in impingement testing.

4.3. Scapular dyskinesis, muscular imbalance and secondary impingement

Normal scapular motion is required for adequate shoulder function and to prevent the development of pain [21]. Visible alterations in scapular position and motion patterns have been termed scapular dyskinesis [22,23]. SICK scapula (Scapular malposition, Inferior medial border prominence, Coracoid pain and malposition, and dysKinesis of scapular movement) is a recently recognized muscular overuse syndrome and it is prevalent in sports like tennis, volleyball and baseball [22,23]. The biomechanics of this disorder is the unbalance of scapular stabilizers generated by the unappropiate overtraining of one arm. In sports like swimming, where both arms are used equally, this pathology must be uncommon, but in competitive swimmers with an overtraining of shoulder muscles, a small asymmetry factor (hand or breath side dominance) can establish a difference between sides. However, this problem is not yet clarified. In our study, we found an important prevalence of asymmetry factors in competitive swimmers [7].

Visually, findings of dyskinesis have been reported as winging or asymmetry [23]. The lateral displacement of the scapula from the thoracic midline has been considered as a marker of scapular dyskinesis [21]. However, clinical measures of scapular position based on side-to-side differences of linear measures have lacked reliability [24]. In the case of the compromise of both scapulas, these methods are less reliable. Our research team recently developed a new technique to evaluate the scapular position and rotation based on digital photography. The exactitude, precision and reliability obtained in the evaluation of this technique accomplished the highest clinical standards [Figure 1].

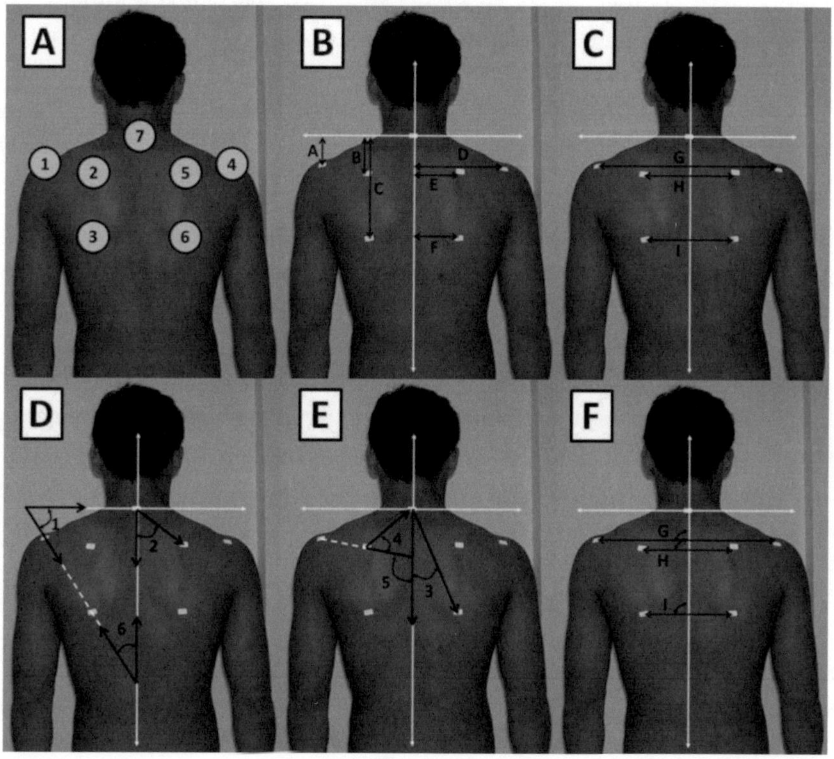

Figure 1. Digital photographic evaluation. (A)Anatomic points (B) Vertical and lateral movements (C) Interscapular distances (D,E,F) Rotation movements.

The relationship of scapular dyskinesis and swimmer's shoulder has been barely researched. Bak et al [1] had evaluated the scapulothoracic instability by observing the scapulohumeral rhythm. They found a severe lack of coordination in 33% of the symptomatic shoulders, compared with 9% of nonsymptomatic shoulders (statistically significant). Crotty et al [25] had evaluated swimmers pre-exercise and post-exercise with Kibler's Test, but there weren't significant differences. Madsen et al [26] evaluated the prevalence of scapular dyskinesis at 4 time intervals during a swim training session (scaption and wall push-up) in seventy-eight competitive swimmers with no history of shoulder pain; scapular dyskinesis was seen in 29 shoulders (37%) after the first time interval (1/4 of a training session), in another 24 (cumulated prevalence, 68%) after one-half of the training session, and in an additional 4 swimmers (cumulated prevalence, 73%) after three-quarters of the training session. During the last quarter of the training session, another 7 had dyskinesis, resulting in a cumulated prevalence of 82%.

The prevalence of asymmetry risk factors and scapular dyskinesis by visual and conventional clinical methods is high in competitive swimmers, considering that this sport presumably uses both scapulas equally. A large group is right-handed, and this correlates with right breathe side predominance, probably because it gives a longer and calmer breathe. This could be an explanation of the important prevalence of scapular asymmetry, because the one-sided movement of the head overuses the elevator muscles of scapula (upper trapezius, rhomboideus and sternocleidomastoideus), raising the risk to develop muscular unbalance. Concordantly, Smith et al [27] found higher electromyographic activity of upper fibers of trapezius than lower in competitive swimmers. However, the association of asymmetry and scapular dyskinesis in the development of shoulder pain is not clearly with this type of methods.

Competitive swimming predisposes to changes in the positioning of the scapula. Our research group found a protraction and lateral movement of the inferior angle of scapula with associated depression on both sides [Figure 2]. Kibler and McCullen [23] suggested that too much protraction will cause impingement as the scapula rotates down and forward. Also, the incapability to elevate the acromion can be a secondary source of impingement. Probably, the overdevelopment of internal rotators muscles (pectoralis major, pectoralis minor and serratus anterior) is the cause of these anatomical changes [7]. Also, scapular stabilizers fatigue reduces motion along two of three scapular axes [28], reducing retraction. This results in protraction and secondary impingement [29], because lower trapezius and serratus anterior muscle fatigue decrease acromial elevation. Su et al [14] suggest that the scapular kinematics of swimmers with shoulder impingement syndrome may not have changed until after they practiced swimming and fatigued the shoulder muscles. Kibler and McMullen [23] recognized this as possible muscular unbalance etiology the directly injured from direct-blow trauma; microtrauma-induced strain, leading to muscle weakness; become fatigued from repetitive tensile use; or are inhibited by painful conditions around the shoulder. In fact, they consider that the serratus anterior and the lower trapezius muscles, pivotal muscles in swimming, are the most susceptible to the effect of the inhibition.

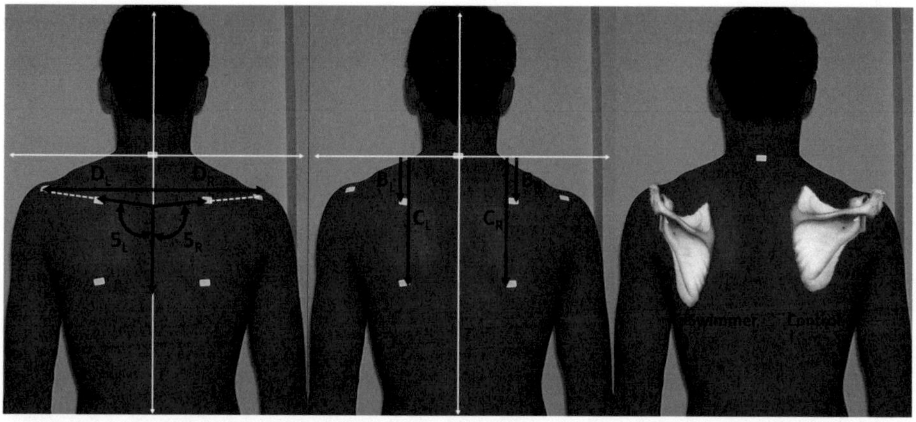

Figure 2. Significant differences between distances and angles of swimmers compared with control group.

Remarkable are the modifications in the positioning of the scapula in swimmers with shoulder pain. In our research, we have found differences in competitive swimmmers with control group and opposite variations in swimmers with and without shoulder pain. We found an elevation of both scapulas associated with retraction. Loss of protraction creates functional anteversion of the glenoid. This increases the degree of impingement between the posterior superior glenoid and posterior rotator cuff by moving the posterior aspect of the glenoid closer to the externally rotated and horizontally abducted arm [23]. Our data and other research suggest an association between scapular malposition and malrotation and swimmer's shoulder [Figure 3]. Pain has been shown to alter propioceptive input from Golgi tendon organs and muscle spindles, predisposing to muscular unbalance [23].

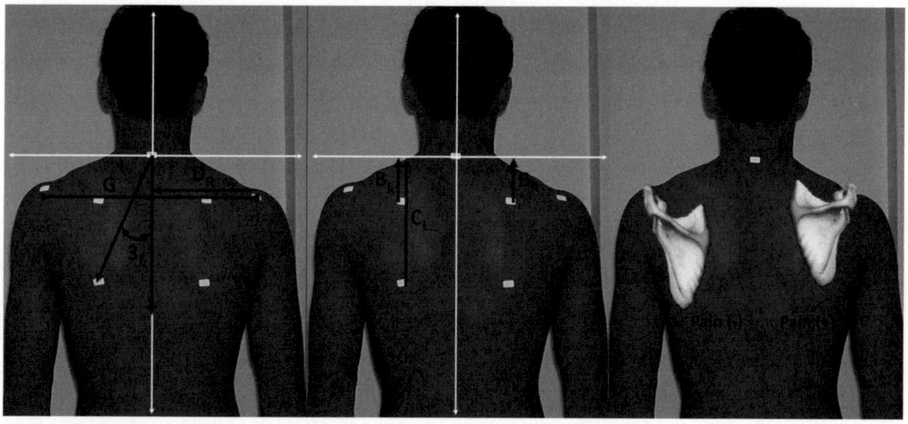

Figure 3. Significant differences between distances and angles of swimmers with pain compared with swimmers without pain.

4.4. Shoulder instability and range of motion

The primary stabilizer of the shoulder joint is the capsulolabral complex (static stabilizer). The rotator cuff muscles function dynamically as secondary stabilizers by contracting in a coordinated and synergistic fashion to contain the humeral head throughout abduction. The deltoid functions in a force-couple with the internal rotator and external rotator muscles to maintain the humeral head centered in the glenoid during arm elevation [30].

Imbalances of the rotator musculature, excess capsular laxity, or loss of capsular flexibility, have all been implicated as etiologic factors in both glenohumeral instability and impingement syndrome [30].

Warner et al [30] prospectively evaluated 53 subjects: 15 asymptomatic volunteers, 28 patients with glenohumeral instability, and 10 patients with impingement syndrome. They found that impingement syndrome is associated with posterior capsular tightness and a relative weakness of the external rotators and that anterior instability is associated with the findings of excessive external rotation, and a relative weakness of the internal rotators.

Bak and Magnusson [31] examined fifteen competitive swimmers allocated into two groups. The first group consisted of seven swimmers with unilateral shoulder pain related to swimming and the control group consisted of eight swimmers with no present or previous history of shoulder pain. They found that internal range of motion was reduced in painful shoulders compared with pain-free swimmers, although without significance. No differences in external range of motion were detected.

McMaster et al [32] evaluated shoulder laxity and interfering pain in competitive swimmers. The total study group of swimmers represented 80 shoulders at risk for possible pain. Fourteen swimmers (35%) noted significant interfering shoulder pain at the time of the assessment. Clinical examination assessed the sulcus sign and anterior and posterior manual provocation tests in the sitting and recumbent positions. The statistical analysis revealed a positive correlation at the 95% confidence level between the clinical examination score and the presence of interfering shoulder pain. McMaster proposed that the shoulder laxity may be a common denominator in the causation of significant interfering shoulder pain in the swimming athlete [32].

Burkhart et al [33] proposed that the essential lesion that affects these athletes is an acquired loss of internal rotation resulting from tightness of the posteroinferior capsule. They called it glenohumeral internal rotation deficit (GIRD) and defined it as "the loss in degrees of glenohumeral internal rotation of the dominant shoulder compared with the nondominant shoulder." Torres and Gomes [34] found that competitive swimmers mean GIRD was 12 degrees ± 6.8 degrees.

The main finding of our study is the decrease in the range of internal and external rotation of the glenohumeral joint of competitive swimmers compared to a healthy control group [Table 3]. This could be explained by repeated microtrauma in the soft tissues, which can ultimately lead to failure of the supporting structures. In fact, it has been shown that alterations in the glenohumeral rotation range, in addition to the continuous and ongoing training an elite athlete, can be modified with only one training season. In female athletes, there was a significant decrease in internal rotation after one season [35].

Variable	Competitive	Control group
IR Right	62,47 ± 12,4*	73,2 ± 9,74*
IR Left	67,3 ± 12,36*	76,87 ± 12,03*
ER Right	86,47 ± 14,72*	105,6 ± 10,24*
ER Left	84,67 ± 13,8*	107,2 ± 12,13*

Table 3. Glenohumeral rotation. The values are expressed in mean ± SD. * $p < 0,05$.

However, the etiologic impact of shoulder instability always has been discussed. Borsa et al [36] evaluated with ultrasound the glenohumeral joint displacement under stressed and non-stressed conditions in 42 competitive swimmers. They were unable to identify significantly greater glenohumeral joint displacement in elite swimmers compared to controls, and elite swimmers with a history of shoulder pain were not found to have significantly more glenohumeral joint displacement compared to swimmers without a history of shoulder pain.

4.5. Impingement, overuse, scapular dyskinesis, shoulder instability and supraspinatus tendinopathy: Biomechanical and molecular pathways to explain "swimmer's shoulder".

The biomechanics of the glenohumeral joint is the most complex and least understood of all joints. Allows range of motion than any other joint can be achieved, but with a cost: instability. Throughout this chapter, has given extensive and relevant evidence about the delicate muscular balance and the impact of instability on optimum performance of this joint. However, we face a difficult problem: swimming. This sport represents a challenge to both the glenohumeral joint stability and muscle balance, but certainly the most important problem is the overuse.

In the past ten years, many studies have tried to elucidate this problem, using rat models of supraspinatus muscle overuse, which is the most injured muscle in this sport. This animal model has been used to evaluate the role of intrinsic injury factors (acute insult) and extrinsic injury factors (subacromial impingement) on rotator cuff injury. The overuse exercise rat model consisted of treadmill running at 17 meters per minute, at a 10° decline, for 1 hour per day, 5 days per week, resulting that approximately 7500 strides per day is consistent with the number of strokes an competitive swimmer may take during a typical training protocol [37,38].

Soslowsky and Carpenter [37] with the use of a rat model, designed one of the first studies to elucidate the pathophysiology of the effect of overuse in the supraspinatus muscle. They measured the effects of an overuse running regimen on 36 rats after 4, 8, or 16 weeks of exercise and compared them with a control group who were allowed normal cage activity.

Histologically, cellularity was increased, and cell shape changed from elongated spindle shaped cells to more rounded plump cells; collagen fibers in the overuse groups were less aligned with respect to the longitudinal axis of the tendon.

Geometrically, cross-sectional area was significantly greater and continued to rise over time. The cross-sectional area increased significantly between 4 weeks and 16 weeks.

In a previous research, Carpenter et al [38] evaluated intrinsic (acute injury: bacterial collagenase) and extrinsic factors (impingement: Achilles tendon allograft was passed underneath and wrapped around the acromion) with overuse of supraspinatus tendon in the same model. The supraspinatus tendons which were subjected to a combination (intrinsic or extrinsic factor) plus overuse, exhibited an increase in histologic grade compared with overuse alone. Also, the shoulders that received the combination of alterations had an increased supraspinatus tendon area with respect to the contralateral overuse-alone tendons. This study demonstrates that detrimental changes in the supraspinatus tendon can be incited by combinations of overuse and intrinsic injury, overuse and extrinsic compression, and overuse alone.

Changes in cell shape, organization of collagen and cross-sectional area are the result of the activation of molecular pathways in response to the mechanical stress generated by overuse.

Several studies have addressed the major biochemical changes in tendon matrix composition in human tendinopathy [39]. Predominantly consisting of collagen type I (95%), there are many other matrix constituents (proteoglycans and noncollagen glycoproteins). The called "minor" collagens are implicated in a number of important processes including collagen fibril formation, regulating the ultimate diameter of the fibrils and mediating interactions with the surrounding cells and matrix.

Riley et al [40] shown that degenerate tendons have a small but significant reduction in the total collagen content relative to the tissue dry weight. This was partly because of an increase in the non-collagen glycoprotein content, as well as increases in matrix proteoglycan [40]. The type and distribution of collagen also changed, with an increase in the proportion of type III collagen, which was found associated with the type I collagen fibril bundles, thought to be intercalated into the fibrils, suggesting that the original fibrils had been extensively remodelled, resulting in a greater proportion of small diameter and randomly organized fibrils [39]. In tendinopathy, also there is a generalized increase in sulfated glycosaminoglycan, the majority of which was chondroitin sulfate [39]. Archambault et al [41] in the same rat overuse model found that supraspinatus tendon had increased expression of well-known cartilage genes such as Col2a1, Aggrecan and Sox9.

The tenocyte matrix equilibrium is regulated by the interaction of matrix-degrading matrix metalloproteinases (MMP) and tissue inhibitors of metalloproteinases (TIMPs) [39]. Most studies have focused on collagen degradation occurring in the extracellular environment mediated by MMP. Thornton et al [42] exposed a rat model to intermittent cyclic hydrostatic compression (to simulate impingement injury). Levels of MMP-13, MMP-3 and TIMP-2 mRNA were evaluated, finding increased expression of MMP-13 in the supraspinatus tendon. Ruptured human supraspinatus tendon have been demonstrated to have increased MMP-13 mRNA expression [43]; the unique upregulation of MMP-13 mRNA levels may be related to matrix turnover and, as such, could support the impingement injury theory for rotator cuff tendinopathy [42].

The balance of production and destruction found in the tendon matrix has been widely studied. However, as the mechanical stress is converted into biochemical signals that ultimately produce an imbalance at the level of MMP/TIMPs has been studied less. Szomor et al [44] evaluated the regulation of NOS (nitric oxide synthase), a potent regulator of tendon degeneration and healing. With the same animal model of supraspinatus tendon overuse, they found that the mRNA expression of all three NOS isoforms (inducible, endothelial and neuronal) increased in the supraspinatus tendons as a result of overuse exercise. Nitric oxide (NO) is a diatomic, highly reactive, free radical; high levels are often associated with degradative processes, including modulation of the activation of metalloproteinase enzymes, cytotoxicity (apoptosis, tenocyte death) and induction of pro-inflammatory cytokines [44].

De Castro Pochini et al [45] studied the effect of overuse with the same model of rat supraspinatus over the mechanoreceptors. On histologic evaluation, they found a typical response to overuse (cellularity was increased and cell shape changed from elongated spindle-shaped cells to more rounded plump cells). Supraspinatus tendons also were evaluated with immunohistochemistry using S100 protein antibodies, finding that the group of rats that ran showed significantly higher expression of proprioceptors than the group of rats that were not subjected to physical activity. They declared that the increase of mechanoreceptors for sure may not be indicated on increase of proprioception but is rather an indication of different pattern of tendon receptors following overuse physical activities.

It is important to consider, in addition to the response of the extracellular matrix, cell response to overuse. Research has found an imbalance between proliferation and apoptosis [46,47]. Scott et al [48] using the rat overuse model, found that tendinosis was present after 12 weeks of downhill running and was characterized by tenocyte rounding and proliferation, glycosaminoglycan accumulation and collagen fragmentation. His research group found a correlation between the proliferation index in tenocytes and local IGF-1 expression and phosphorylation of IRS-1 and ERK-1/2.

Apoptosis or programmed cell death is mediated by the activation of caspases (cysteine-containing aspartate proteases) and is involved in the stress-induced cascade of tendinopathy [49]. Yuan et al [49] studied the levels of apoptosis at the edges of torn supraspinatus rotator cuff tendons from patients with rotator cuff tear. Apoptosis was detected by in situ DNA end labelling assay and DNA laddering assay. The percentage of apoptotic cells in the degenerative rotator cuff (34%) was significantly higher than that in controls (13%).

Following oxidative and other forms of stress, one family of stress proteins that is often upregulated are heat shock proteins (HSPs). HSPs play a protective role as molecular chaperones in cells by facilitating the folding, intracellular transport, assembly, and disassembly of other proteins. In addition, HSPs protect cells from oxidative damage and protect cells from apoptosis [46,47]. Millar et al [46] found upregulation of HSP 27 and HSP 70, cellular FLICE-inhibitory protein receptor and caspase 8 while downregulation of Poly(ADP-ribose) polymerase, Type-2 angiotensin II receptor and Hypoxia inducible factor

1 occurred in rat supraspinatus tendon subjected to daily treadmill running for 4 weeks. Also, they found that the expression levels of caspases 3 and 8 and HSPs 27 and 70 was higher in the torn edges of supraspinatus of patients undergoing arthroscopic shoulder surgery when compared to matched subscapularis tendon.

Other researches have demonstrated different possible pathways to trigger apoptosis from overuse stimuli. Arnoczky et al [50] found that cyclic strain resulted in an immediate activation of JNK (c-Jun N-terminal kinase), which peaked at 30 min and returned to resting levels by 2 h. This activation was regulated by a magnitude-dependent but not frequency-dependent response and appeared to be mediated through a calcium-dependent mechanotransduction pathway. While transient JNK activation is associated with normal cell processes, persistent JNK activation has been linked to the initiation of the apoptotic cascade [50]. Also, JNK plays an important role in tendon matrix degradation, possibly through upregulating of MMP-1 [51].

In summary, in light of the evidence previously discussed, we can say that the swimmer's shoulder is a multifactorial disease. The main factor that differentiates the swimming of other predisposing factors for shoulder pathology is overuse. All other factors associated with shoulder pain in swimmers (scapular dyskinesis, shoulder instability, impingement syndrome) are secondary and modulate the final effect of overuse.

Sein et al [19] demonstrated that muscle supraspinatus tendinopathy is the pathological basis of swimmer's shoulder and associated factors that generate it.

Overuse, together with the effect of intrinsic and extrinsic factors are the etiology of muscle supraspinatus tendinopathy. Overuse and other factors activate different biochemical signals (HSP, JNK, mechanoreceptors, NO) to generate alterations in the balance between MMP/TIMPs, which in turn alter the composition and architecture of the tendon matrix. Furthermore, these biochemical signals affect the balance between cell proliferation and programmed cell death. If the stimulus produced by the overuse continues, it would develop muscle supraspinatus tendinopathy and finally shoulder pain [Figure 4].

5. Diagnosis and clinical management

5.1. Diagnosis

Kennedy and Hawkins [3] based their clinical syndrome named "Swimmer's shoulder" in the repetitive mechanical impingement of the supraspinatus and the bicipital tendon produced by pull and over-arm recovery. In their original paper [3], they reported that "...diagnosis is usually not difficult. Discomfort is first noticed only after swimming activities. This may progress to pain during and after training and even finally to pain which affects performance of the stroke..." In the physical examination, they described point tenderness over the great tuberosity and over the anterior acromion; a painful arc of abduction maximum at 90° degrees; and impingement signs (Neer or Hawkins). If the bicipital tendon is compromised, there will be tenderness to palpation and a positive Yergason and Speed tests.

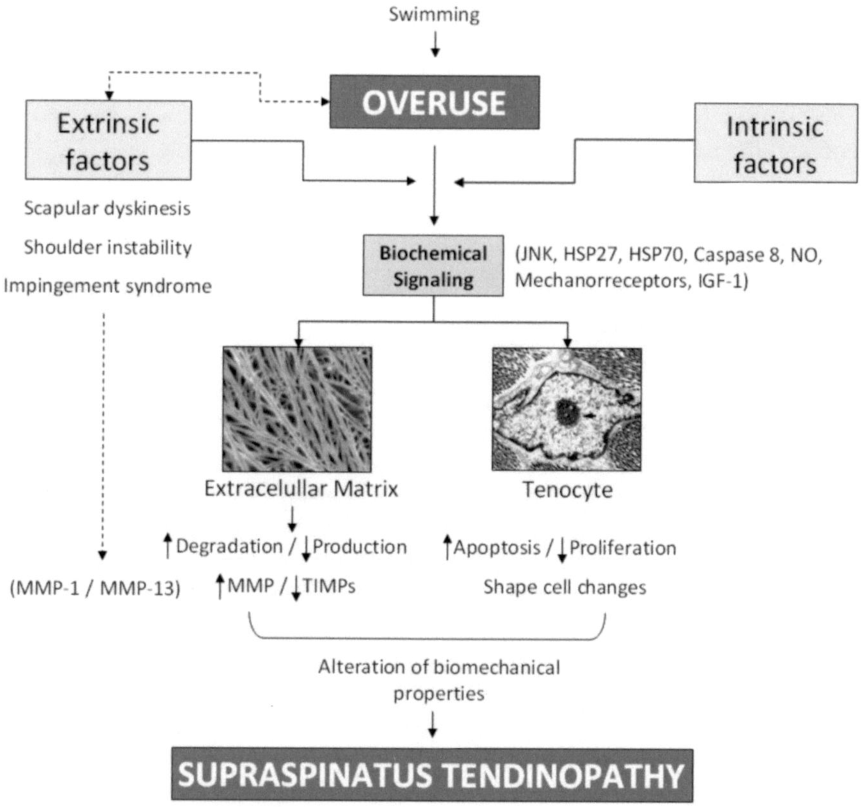

Figure 4. Etiology for supraspinatus tendinopathy.

Bak identified five main categories of swimmer's shoulder [11] [Table 4]. Types A, B, and C may represent different stages of the same condition. The first 4 types nearly always have scapular dyskinesis present.

Type A	Isolated external impingement with subacromial bursitis and increased amount of fluid in the supraspinatus tendon. Normal morphology of acromion. Possible enlarged coracoacromial ligament. No hyperlaxity or instability. Scapular dyskinesis present in most cases.
Type B	Isolated internal impingement without instability. Labral wearing/fraying and minor partial articular side supraspinatus tendon lesions. Scapular dyskinesis present in most cases.
Type C	Complex impingement with both extra-articular and intra-articular pathology. Nearly always minor instability. Scapular dyskinesis present in all cases.
Type D	Isolated minor instability. Often with bilateral hyperlax shoulders. Rarely pain. Scapular dyskinesis is always present.
Type E	Other pathologies, that is, acromioclavicular joint meniscus tear/arthritis (may be related to weight training). Scapular dyskinesis may be present.

Table 4. Types of Swimmer's Shoulder according to Bak's description.

5.2. Preseason assessment

The exact activities that predispose to altered shoulder biomechanics and tissue damage are not fully understood. Most of the research has been done in swimmers that already have the impairment, and the results are extrapolated to design preventive programs [8].

It is consensus that swimmers at high level that have more than five sessions per week should perform dry-land exercise in order to prevent lesions.

Some authors recommend a program to prevent shoulder injury that might lead to pain and dysfunction appears warranted and might include exposure reduction, cross-training, pectoral and posterior shoulder stretching, strengthening, and core endurance training [52].

5.3. Training errors

A rapidly increase in the hours or distance per day is a classic training error. The high level of repetitions can led to fatigue and is the start of the pathological way to swimmer's shoulder, so if the swimmer progression is too aggressive or if he has reached a plateau and some discomfort has appear. A modification of the swim distance may need to be done and/or an increase in the dry-land activities to prevent a progression of an injury. And in some cases a short period of rest out of the water is advisable.

Another training error is to gain more muscle abusing of hand paddles. The increased surface area and resistance tend to over stress the shoulder muscles leading to early fatigue and the imbalance discussed before. If a kickboard is thought to use to rest the pain in the shoulder, it is not a good idea, because they tend to put the shoulder in a disadvantage position for the subacromial space, which is in full elevation and internal rotation.

Yanai and Hay [53] propose: (a) decrease the amount of internal rotation of the arm during the pull phase. (b) Improve early initiation of external rotation of the arm during the recovery phase. (c) Improve the tilt angle of the scapula.

Improper techniques are a common cause of shoulder problems. The coach should seek for increased body roll with scapular retraction to aim optimal strength and endurance of rotator cuff and scapular stabilizers improving a flexibility of pectoral minor in the recovery phase an early pull-through [54].

It has been study that an excessive body roll led to cross the mid-line with the hand during the pull-through phase. This position tends to compress the subacromial space. The arm must stay close to the plane of the scapula in order to reduce the stress in that area [18]. The optimal body roll allows a greater length of the adductors, medial rotator, scapular protractors and abdominal oblique muscles in the beginning of the pull-through phase [55]. In the other hand, an absent body rolls forces the shoulder to a greater extension, abduction and medial rotation compromising the subacromial space.

In other sport and disorder of the shoulder there is a factor that should be considered in prevention and for intervention: improvement of core stability [56,57]. In swimming, the abdominal and lumbar muscles are the base of the kinetic chain for the propulsion, and should be exercise.

5.4. Treatment strategies

The first time the swimmers experience pain, usually complaints in the subacromial region. The symptoms are related to an inflammatory condition (bursitis, tendonitis) and labeled as impingement syndrome. As we have learned, impingement is a consequence of a subtle or evident imbalance in the shoulder that produces an antero/superior migration of the head by imbalance forces or tissues that can be corrected.

According to Bak [11], when the pain is only at swimming (phase 1), the first strategy is to active rest, reduce training and use icepack after training. The coach should look for technical stroke analysis and correction. Exercise directed toward specific dysfunction. The best documentation of scapular stabilizing exercises is for the low rows, lawn mower, robbery, shrugs and push-ups [57,58].

When the pain is daily and not related to swimming practice (phase 2), the strategy is to rest [11]. Swimming should not be allowed for 1 o 2 weeks. A short course of nonesteroidal anti-inflammatory drugs for 5 to 7 days may be prescribed. Injection of corticosteroid in the bursa is not advisable; this practice is at least controversial. Once the pain is tolerable, direct exercise can continue.

If the pain persist despite of the rest and treatment for more than 3 months [11]. Imaging and a complete study should be done and other strategies should be addressed. Surgical strategies should be considered.

An approach to the specific impairments associated with the symptoms should look for: impaired posture, tight posterior capsule, scapular stabilization and altered scapulohumeral rhythm, impaired rotator cuff strength and glenohumeral hypermobility or instability.

5.5. Impaired posture

Impaired posture are managed through joint and soft tissue mobilization, improve flexibility and strengthening of scapular retractors and deep cervical flexors. Lynch [59] demonstrated that an 8 week exercise program to correct posture and strength muscles result in a decrease in pain and dysfunction in elite swimmers.

The propose muscles that should be stretched are the pectoralis major [Figure 5 and 6], the pectoralis minor [Figure 7], the scalene muscles [Figure 8] and elevator scapula [Figure 9]. The scapular retractor muscles that should be strengthened are the middle/lower trapezius [Figure 10] and the rhomboid muscle [Figure 11 and 12].

Care must be taken to avoid overstretching the anterior capsule [Figure 13], because this could lead anterosuperior migration of the humeral head in swimmers with shoulder laxity.

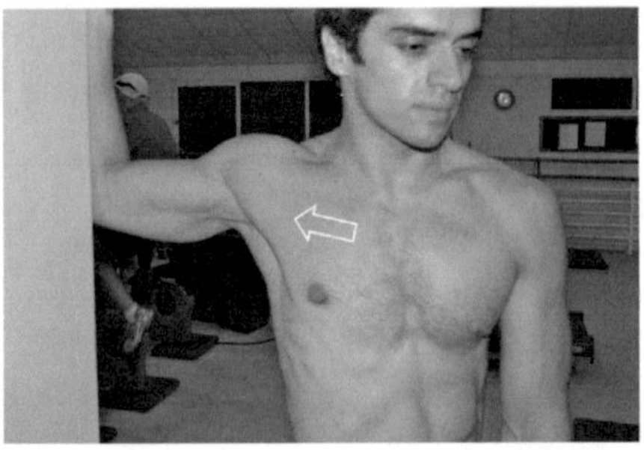

Figure 5. The shoulder is at 90° abduction and 90° external rotation and some extension, in swimmers with excessive shoulder laxity caution has to be taken to not overstretch the anterior capsule.

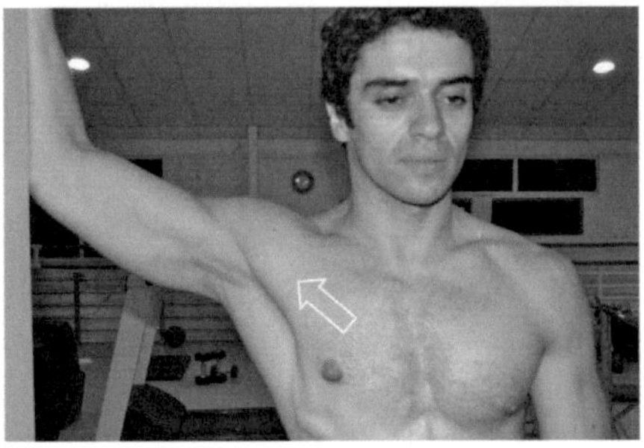

Figure 6. The shoulder is at 120° abduction and 90° external rotation and some extension, in swimmers with excessive shoulder laxity caution has to be taken to not overstretch the anterior capsule.

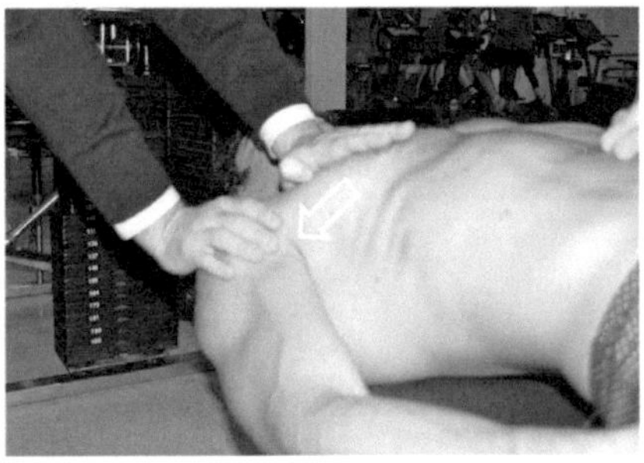

Figure 7. The pectoral minor is stretched in supine position when the scapula (coracoids) is mobilized superior and downwards.

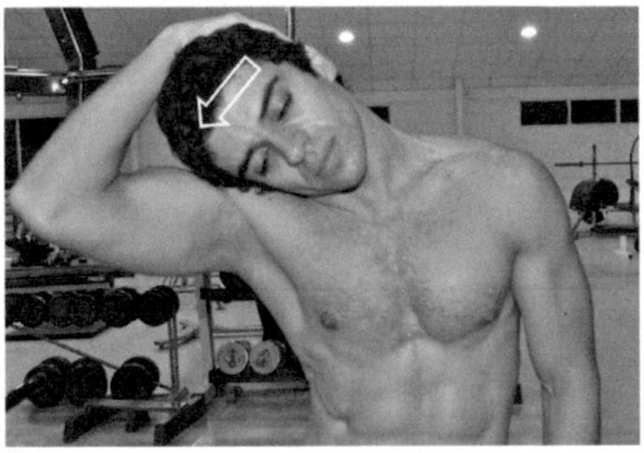

Figure 8. Self stretching of the scalene muscles.

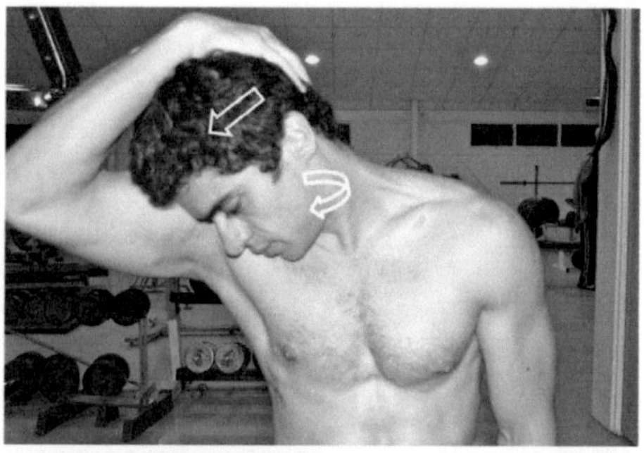

Figure 9. Self stretching of elevator scapula muscle.

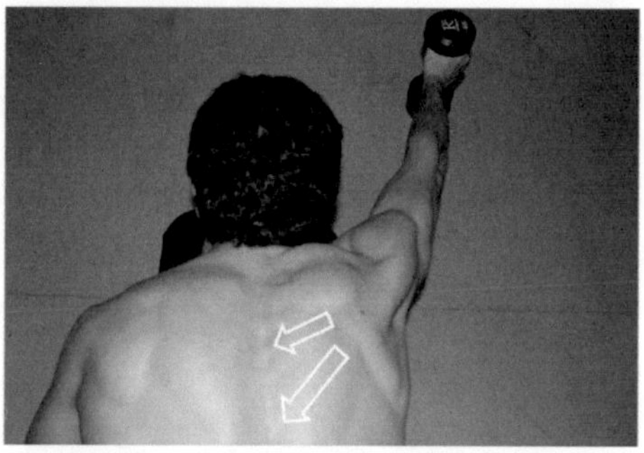

Figure 10. Recruitment of the middle/lower trapezius.

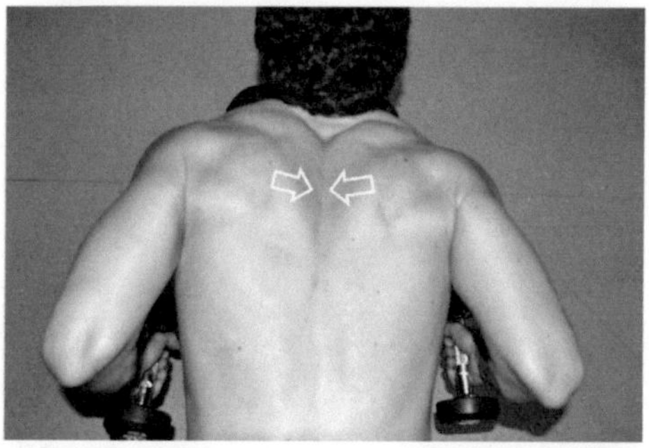

Figure 11. Strengthening of the rhomboid muscles.

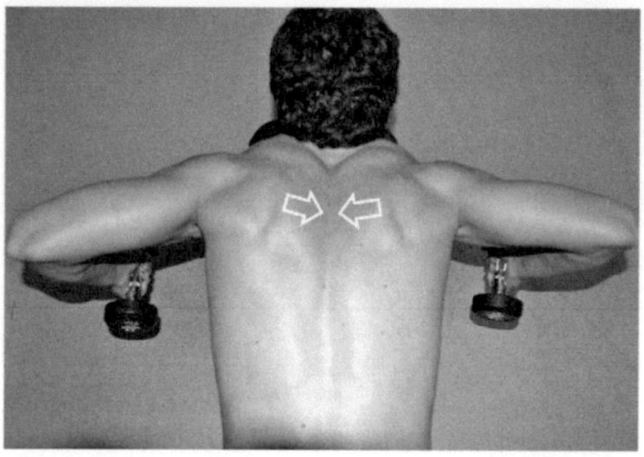

Figure 12. Strengthening of middle/lower trapezius and rhomboid muscles.

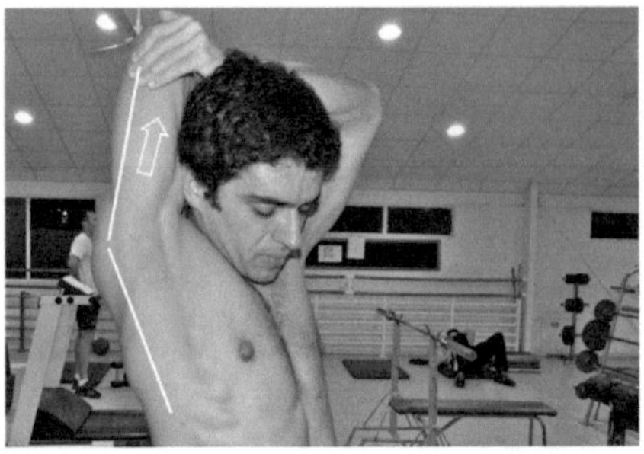

Figure 13. Care must be taken to stretch muscles without compromising the anterior capsule.

5.6. Tight posterior capsule

Posterior capsule tightness is associated with anterior shoulder laxity. Another clinical finding that is common seen is an external rotation and internal rotation deficit. Posterior capsule mobilizations can be performed [Figure 14] or manual self stretching also can be done [Figure 15].

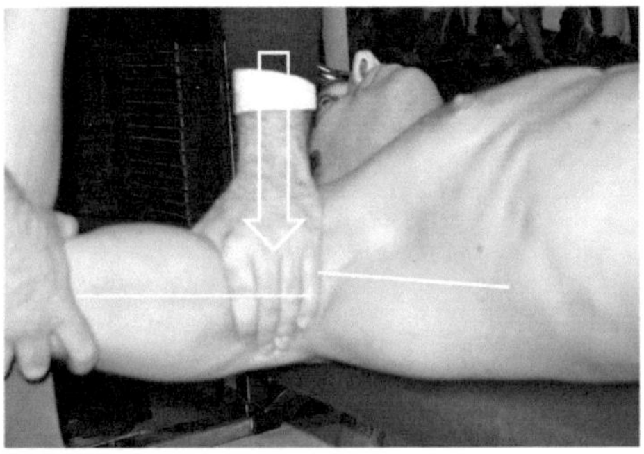

Figure 14. Downward forces are applied to the humerus in order to stretch posterior capsule.

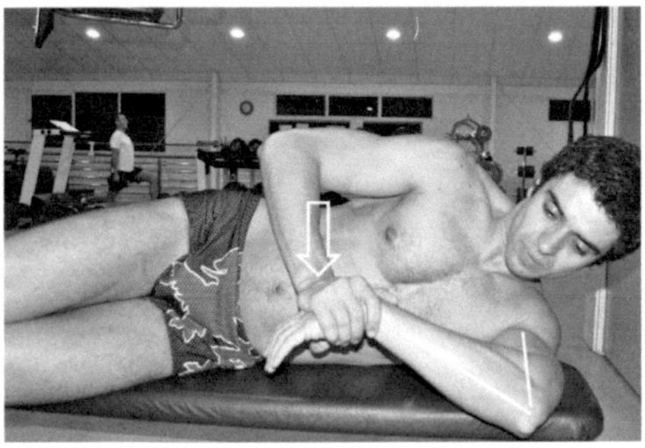

Figure 15. Self stretching posterior capsule.

5.7. Scapular stabilization

Scapular stability and scapulohumeral rhythm is essential in prevention and rehabilitation. The scapular position determines the strength of the rotator cuff and its ability to center the humeral head. The essential muscles to scapular stability are middle and lower trapezius, serratus anterior and rhomboids. In order to improve scapular movement, a soft tissue release and neuromuscular control must be achieved [Figure 16 and 17].

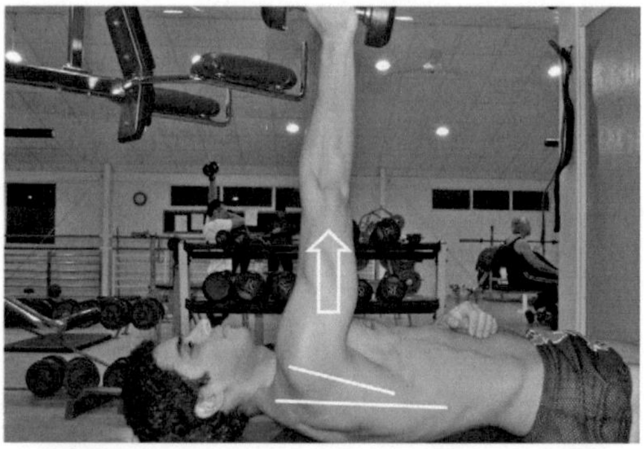

Figure 16. Serratus anterior exercises.

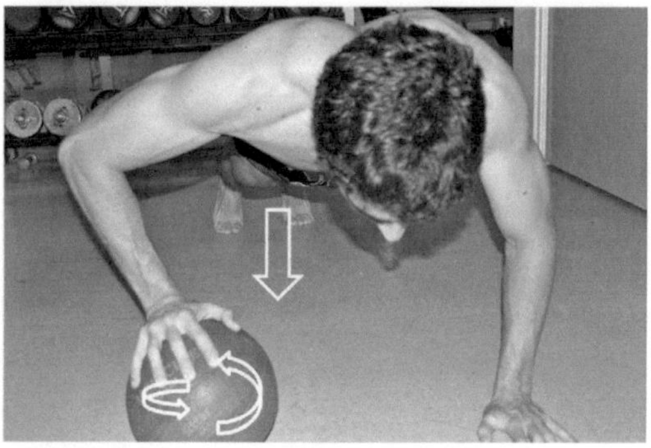

Figure 17. Push up one hand in a ball

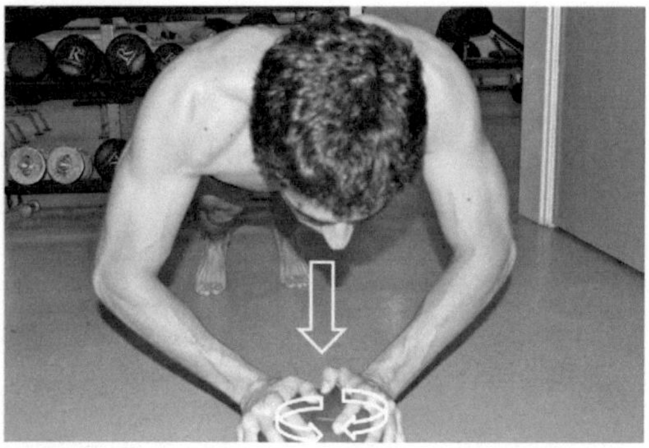

Figure 18. Push up both hands in a ball.

The clinician should instruct the patient to retract the scapula prior to and during the humeral motion. Scapular protraction and stabilization in the protracted position are trained through a series of exercises, an example is provided in figure 16, 17 and 18.

5.8. Rotator cuff strength

The range of rotator cuff strengthening exercises may include isometric, concentric, eccentric, and plyometric. Infraspinatus and teres minor are strengthen to counter force the translator forces of anterior muscles [Figure 19 and 20].

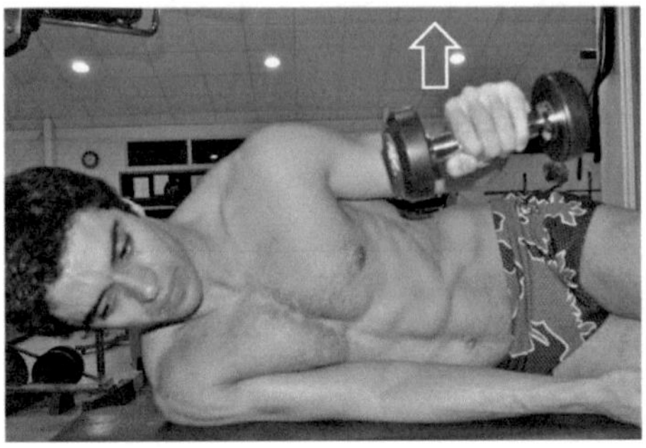

Figure 19. Isolated external rotator exercise.

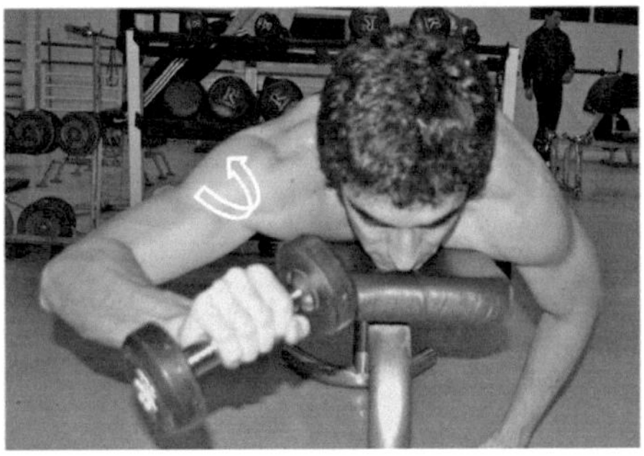

Figure 20. Scapular retraction should be addressed prior external rotation.

5.9. Hyperlaxity

This special condition is very common in swimmers. Hyperlaxity is often multidirectional in swimmers. The superior migration of the humeral head can cause impingement syndrome [32]. Only certain athletes who crossed the physiological laxity to instability are prone developing symptoms and should be treated. It is documented that heavy-resistance overhead weight training has on causing shoulder pain in swimmers [60]. This is presumably due to forced subluxation of the lax joint during the activity. There are protocols to ameliorate the rotator cuff strength ratio shifts that occur in swimmers and found that this can be helpful for symptomatic athletes but may not be universally effective [61].

Swimmers with a diagnose shoulder laxity and pain; a global training program must be emphasize. This includes strengthening external rotators and scapula stabilizers as lower trapezius.

Clinically, for swimmers with demonstrated pathologic shoulder laxity and pain, the exercise protocol, which emphasizes strengthening of the abductors, external rotators, and lower trapezius muscle, seems to be helpful. The efficacy of such a program may be multifactorial, including reducing fatigue in the external rotators and scapula stabilizers, and better centering the humeral head in the lax joint, thereby reducing subluxation potential.

Given the shoulder joint laxity of this population, caution should be exercised when prescribing certain training activities that may have a laxity-potentiating effect. Activities that need to be critically examined include passive stretching of the shoulder, especially when forced or causing discomfort, the use of hand paddles, and heavy-resistance overhead weight training. Any activity that promotes increased joint laxity and has the potential to move the situation from physiologic to pathologic laxity must be examined.

For the swimmer with painful shoulders, certain technical adaptations may be helpful. These include increasing body roll, maintaining a high elbow, and avoiding excessive elbow extension before beginning the hand insweep.

5.10. Surgical treatment

A failed conservative treatment is considered after 3 to 6 month, and when a pathological condition is found after a proper clinical and imaging study.

Return to competition after a surgical intervention is not very promising. In a series of anterior acromioplasty for impingement syndrome described by Tibone [15] only a 44% percent return to sport. Another study by Brushøj described returning rates of 56% at a mean of 4 month with labral debridement and subacromial bursectomy [16]. McMaster [63] described a bucket-handle labral tear like a meniscal pathology and labral fraying in an arthroscopic series of swimmers with shoulder problems.

In the other hand when a swimmer presents with pain, global shoulder laxity and failed conservative treatment the surgical results are very promising. Montgomery [64] demonstrated an 80% percent of return to sport when an arthroscopic capsular plication is done.

Author details

Julio José Contreras Fernández[1], Rodrigo Liendo Verdugo[2],
Matías Osorio Feito[2,3] and Francisco Soza Rex[1,2]
[1]*Traumatology and Orthopaedics Department, Universidad de Chile, Chile*
[2]*Shoulder and Elbow Department, Instituto Traumatológico, Santiago, Chile*
[3]*Universidad de Chile, Santiago, Chile*

Acknowledgement

To our families, to Instituto Traumatológico and Universidad de Chile for their support in all parts of this chapter.

6. References

[1] Bak K, Faunø P (1997) Clinical findings in competitive swimmers. Am J Sports Med. 25: 254–260.

[2] McMaster WC (1999) Shoulder injuries in competitive swimmers. Aquat Sports Inj Rehab. 18: 349–359.

[3] Kennedy JC, Hawkins RJ (1974) Swimmers shoulder. Phys Sports Med. 2:34–38.

[4] Kennedy JC, Hawkins R, WB Krissoff (1978) Orthopaedic manifestations of swimming. Am J Sports Med 6(6): 309-322.

[5] McMaster WC, Troup J (1993) A survey of interfering shoulder pain in United States competitive swimmers. Am J Sports Med. 21(1):67-70.

[6] Richardson AB, Jobe FW, Collins HR (1980) The shoulder in competitive swimming. Am J Sports Med. 8(3):159-63.

[7] Contreras JJ, Espinoza R, Liendo R, Torres G, Soza F (2010) Análisis de la rotación interna y externa de la articulación glenohumeral y su relación con el dolor de hombro en nadadores de élite. Rev Andal Med Deporte. 3(3):92-97.

[8] Tovin BJ (2006) Prevention and Treatment of Swimmer's Shoulder. N Am J Sports Phys Ther. 1(4):166-75.

[9] King D (1995) Glenohumeral joint impingement in Swimmers. J Athl Train. 30(4):333-337.

[10] Pink M, Perry J, Browne A, Scovazzo ML, Kerrigan J (1991) The normal shoulder during freestyle swimming. An electromyographic and cinematographic analysis of twelve muscles. Am J Sports Med. 19(6):569-76.

[11] Bak K (2010) The Practical Management of Swimmer's Painful Shoulder: Etiology, Diagnosis, and Treatment. Clin J Sport Med 20:386–390.

[12] Hawkins RJ, Kennedy JC (1980) Impingement syndrome in athletes. Am J Sports Med. 8:151-158.

[13] D Schmitt L, Snyder-Mackler L (1999) Role of scapular stabilizers in etiology and treatment of impingement syndrome. J Orthop Sports Phys Ther. 29:31-38.

[14] Su KP, Johnson MP, Gracely EJ, Karduna AR (2004) Scapular Rotation in Swimmers with and without Impingement Syndrome: Practice Effects. Med Sci Sports Exerc. 36:1117-1123.

[15] Scovazzo ML, Browne A, Pink M, Jobe FW, Kerrigan J (1991) The painful shoulder during freestyle swimming. An electromyographic cinematographic analysis of twelve muscles. Am J Sports Med. 19:577-582.

[16] Brushøj C, Bak K, Johannsen HV, Faunø P (2007) Swimmers' painful shoulder arthroscopic findings and return rate to sports. Scand J Med Sci Sports 17: 373–377

[17] Kammer CS, Young CC, Niedfeldt MW (1999) Swimming injuries and illnesses. Phys Sports Med. 27:51-60.

[18] T Murphy TC (1994) The athlete's shoulder. New York, NY: Churchill Livingstone Inc. pp. 411-424.

[19] Sein ML, Walton J, Linklater J, Appleyard R, Kirkbride B, Kuah D, Murrell G (2010) Shoulder pain in elite swimmers: primarily due to swim-volume-induced supraspinatus tendinopathy. Br J Sports Med 44:105–113

[20] Jobe FW, Kvitne RS, Giangarra CE (1989) Shoulder pain in the overhand or throwing athlete. The relationship of anterior instability and rotator cuff impingement. Orthop Rev 18:963–75.

[21] Kibler WB (1998) The role of the scapula in athletic shoulder function. Am J Sports Med. 26:325–337.

[22] Burkhart SS, Morgan CD, Kibler WB (2003) The disabled throwing shoulder: spectrum of pathology Part III: The SICK scapula, scapular dyskinesis, the kinetic chain, and rehabilitation. Arthroscopy. 19(6):641-61.

[23] Kibler WB, McMullen J (2003) Scapular dyskinesis and its relation to shoulder pain. J Am Acad Orthop Surg. 11(2):142-51.

[24] Odom C J, Taylor AB, Hurd CE, Denegar CR (2001) Measurement of scapular asymetry and assessment of shoulder dysfunction using the Lateral Scapular Slide Test: a reliability and validity study. Phys Ther. 81(2):799-809.

[25] Crotty NM, Smith J (2000) Alterations in Scapular Position with Fatigue: A Study in Swimmers. Clin J Sport Med. 10(4):251-8.

[26] Madsen PH, Bak K, Jensen S, Welter U (2011) Training Induces Scapular Dyskinesis in Pain-Free Competitive Swimmers: A Reliability and Observational Study. Clin J Sport Med. 21:109–113.

[27] Smith MJ, Sparkes V, Enright S (2007) Scapular rotator muscle imbalance in swimmers with subacromial impingement symptoms. Br J Sports Med. 41:118-124.

[28] McQuade KJ, Hwa Wei S, Smidt GL (1995) Effects of local muscle fatigue on three-dimensional scapulohumeral rhythm. Clin Biomech. 10:144–148.

[29] Solem-Bertoft E, Thuomas K, Westerberg C (1993) The influence of scapular retraction and protraction on the width of the subacromial space: an MRI study. Clin Orthop Rel Res. 296:99–103.

[30] Warner JJP, Micheli LJ, Arslanian LE, Kennedy J, Kennedy R (1990) Patterns of flexibility, laxity, and strength in normal shoulders and shoulders with instability and impingement. Am. J. Sports Med. 18(4):366-75

[31] Bak K, Magnusson P (1997) Shoulder Strength and Range of Motion in Symptomatic and Pain-Free Elite Swimmers. Am. J. Sports Med. 25(4):454-9.

[32] McMaster WC,Roberts A, Stoddard T (1998) A Correlation Between Shoulder Laxity and Interfering Pain in Competitive Swimmers. Am J Sports Med. 26(1):83-6.

[33] Burkhart SS, Morgan CD, Kibler WB (2003) The disabled throwing shoulder: spectrum of pathology. Part I: pathoanatomy and biomechanics. Arthroscopy.19:404-420.

[34] Torres RR, Gomes JL (2009) Measurement of glenohumeral internal rotation in asymptomatic tennis players and swimmers. Am J Sports Med. 37(5):1017-23.

[35] Borsa PA, Scibek JS, Jacobson JA, Meister K (2005) Sonographic stress measurement of glenohumeral joint laxity in collegiateswimmers and age-matched controls. Am J Sports Med. 33(7):1077-84.

[36] Thomas SJ, Swanik KA, Swanik C, Huxel KC (2009) Glenohumeral rotation and scapular position adaptations after a single high school female sports season. J Athl Train. 44(3):230-7.

[37] Soslowsky J, Thomopoulos S, Tun S, Flanagan CL, Keefer CC, Mastaw J, Carpenter JE (2000) Overuse activity injures the supraspinatus tendon in an animal model: A histologic and biomechanical study. J Shoulder Elbow Surg 9:79-84.

[38] Carpenter JE, Flonogon Cl, Thomopoulos S, Yion EH, Soslowsky LJ (1998) The effects of overuse combined with intrinsic or extrinsic olterotions in on onimol model of rotator cuff tendinosis. Am J Sports Med 26:80 l-7.

[39] GP Riley (2005) Gene expression and matrix turnover in overused and damaged tendons. Scand J Med Sci Sports 15: 241–251.

[40] Riley GP, Harrall RL, Constant CR, Chard MD, Cawston TE, Hazleman BL (1994) Glycosaminoglycans of human rotator cuff tendons: changes with age and in chronic rotator cuff tendinitis. Ann Rheum Dis 53: 367–376.

[41] Archambault JM, Jelinsky SA, Lake SP, Hill AA, Glaser DL, Soslowsky LJ (2007) Rat Supraspinatus Tendon Expresses Cartilage Markers with Overuse. J Orthop Res 25:617–624.

[42] Thornton GM, Shao X, Chung M, Sciore P, Boorman RS, Hart DA, Lo IKY (2010) Changes in mechanical loading lead to tendon-specific alterations in MMP and TIMP expression: influence of stress deprivation and intermittent cyclic hydrostatic compression on rat supraspinatus and Achilles tendons. Br J Sports Med 44:698–703.

[43] Lo IK, Marchuk LL, Hollinshead R, Hart DA, Frank CB (2004) Matrix metalloproteinase and tissue inhibitor of matrix metalloproteinase mRNA levels are specifically altered in torn rotator cuff tendons. Am J Sports Med 32:1223–9.

[44] Szomor ZL, Appleyard RC, Murrell GAC (2006) Overexpression of Nitric Oxide Synthases in Tendon Overuse. J Orthop Res 24:80–86

[45] de Castro Pochini A, Ejnisman B, de Seixas Alves MT, Uyeda LF, Nouailhetas VL, Han SW, Cohen M, Albertoni WM (2011) Overuse of training increases mechanoreceptors in supraspinatus tendon of ratsSHR. J Orthop Res. 29(11):1771-4

[46] Millar NL, Wei AQ, Molloy TJ, Bonar F, Murrell GA (2008) Heat shock protein and apoptosis in supraspinatus tendinopathy. Clin Orthop Relat Res. 466(7):1569-76

[47] Millar NL, Wei AQ, Molloy TJ, Bonar F, Murrell GA (2009) Cytokines and apoptosis in supraspinatus tendinopathy. J Bone Joint Surg Br. 91(3):417-24.

[48] Scott A, Cook JL, Hart DA, Walker DC, Duronio V, Khan KM (2007) Tenocyte Responses to Mechanical Loading In Vivo. Arthritis & rheumatism 56(3):871–881
[49] Yuan J, Murrell GA, Wei AQ, Wang MX (2002) Apoptosis in rotator cuff tendonopathy. J Orthop Res. 20:1372–1379.
[50] Arnoczky SP, Tian T, Lavagnino M, Gardner K, Schuler P, Morse P (2002) Activation of stress-activated protein kinases (SAPK) in tendon cells following cyclic strain: the effects of strain frequency, strain magnitude, and cytosolic calcium. J Orthop Res 20:947–52.
[51] Wang F, Murrell GA, Wang MX (2007) Oxidative stress-induced c-Jun N-terminal kinase (JNK) activation in tendon cells upregulates MMP1 mRNA and protein expression. J Orthop Res 25:378–89.
[52] Tate A, Turner GN, Knab SE, Jorgensen C, Strittmatter A, Michener LA (2012) Risk factors associated with shoulder pain and disability across the lifespan of competitive swimmers. J Athl Train. 47(2):149-58.
[53] Yanai T, Hay JG (2000) Shoulder impingement in front-crawl swimming: II.Analysis of stroking technique. Med Sci Sports Exerc. 32:30–40.
[54] Weldon EJ III, Richardson AB (2001) Upper extremity overuse injuries in swimming. Clin Sports Med. 2001 20:423–438.
[55] Shapiro C (2001) Swimming. In: Shamus E, Shamus J, editors. Sports injury prevention and rehabilitation. New York: McGraw-Hill. pp. 103-154.
[56] Kibler WB, Press J, Sciascia A (2006) The role of core stability in athletic function. Sports Med. 36:189–198
[57] Ludewig PM, Reynolds JF (2009) The association of scapular kinematics and glenohumeral joint pathologies. J Orthop Sports Phys Ther. 39:90–104
[58] Kibler WB, Sciascia AD, Uhl TL, Tambay N, Cunningham T (2008) Electromyographic analysis of specific exercises for scapular control in early phases of shoulder rehabilitation. Am J Sports Med. 36:1789–1798.
[59] Lynch SS, Thigpen CA, Mihalik JP, Prentice WE, Padua D (2010) The effects of an exercise intervention on forward head and rounded shoulder postures in elite swimmers. Br J Sports Med. 44(5):376-81.
[60] Greipp JF: Swimmer's shoulder: The influence of flexibility and weight training (1985). Physician Sportsmed 13(8): 92–105.
[61] McMaster WC (1994). Assessment of the rotator cuff and a remedial exercise program for the aquatic athlete. In: Miyashita M, Mutoh Y, Richardson AB, editors. Medicine and Science in Aquatic Sports. Volume 39. Basel, S. Karger AG Pub. pp. 213–217.
[62] Tibone JE, Jobe FW, Kerlan RK, Carter VS, Shields CL, Lombardo SJ, Yocum LA (1985) Shoulder impingement syndrome in athletes treated by an anterior acromioplasty. Clin Orthop Relat Res 198:134–140.
[63] McMaster WC (1986) Anterior glenoid labrum damage: a painful lesion in swimmers. Am J Sports Med 14(5):383-7.

[64] Montgomery SR, Chen NC, Rodeo SA (2010) Arthroscopic capsular plication in the treatment of shoulder pain in competitive swimmers. HSS J. 6(2):145-9.

Chapter 7

The Epidemiology of Shoulder Pain: A Narrative Review of the Literature

Mario Pribicevic

Additional information is available at the end of the chapter

http://dx.doi.org/10.5772/52931

1. Introduction

This chapter provides some findings from the literature on the prevalence of shoulder pain seen in clinical practice that may affect the general population. The findings include a literature-based discussion on risk factors associated with the onset of shoulder pain – including personal, occupational, and psychosocial working factors that may be related to symptomatology of the shoulder.

2. Epidemiology of shoulder pain

In obtaining epidemiological data relevant to the shoulder a number of difficulties exist. According to Bjelle [1] there are four methodological problems associated with epidemiological study of the shoulder:

- criteria and classification
- diagnostic procedure
- study design
- methods of measuring risk factors

An additional concern is the lack of homogenous terminology in identifying specific shoulder disorders in the literature. One disorder will often have several names or another too few.[2] This also relates to the complex structure of the shoulder and close functional biomechanical association with adjacent areas, including the spine. These differences in the reporting of pain prevalence are, at least in part, a consequence of the different definitions of pain used in individual studies. However, other variability can be explained by differing study methodologies and groups, or pools of participants studied. For example, some studies ask participants whether they experienced shoulder pain, yet others use more specific questionnaires with the incorporation of time of pain and diagrams. A common finding from the literature is the use of a diagram that incorporates the anterior, posterior and lateral aspects of the shoulder including the cervical spines and scapulae in order to define shoulder pain (Figure 1).

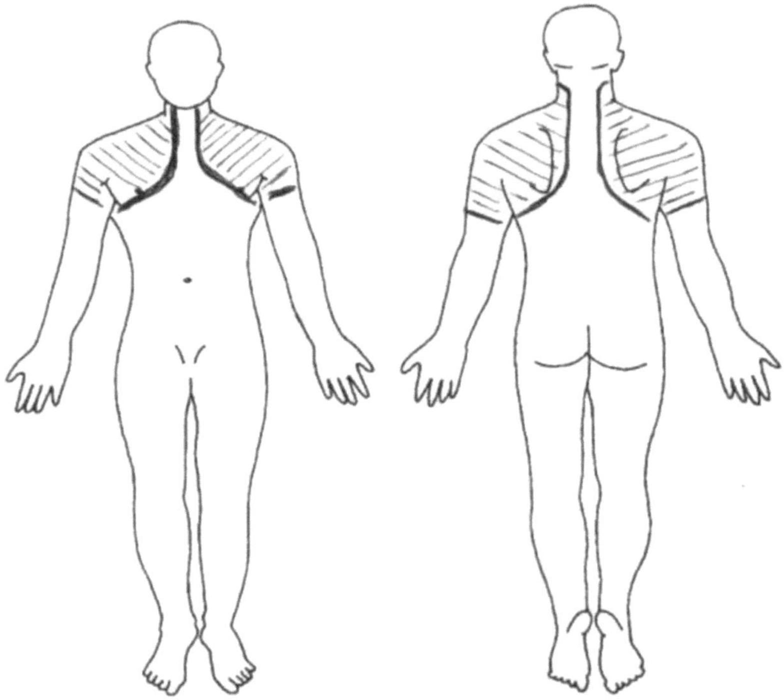

Figure 1. Diagrammatic representation of shoulder pain

Some further causes of variability in reporting relate to that fact that the shoulder may be a primary or secondary source of pain, so many authors and clinicians tend to summarise such a presentation simply as shoulder pain syndrome or just shoulder pain.[3] In order to properly define the anatomical source of pain a thorough history is required, including a detailed physical and orthopaedic examination and possibly the use of diagnostic imaging. As a consequence, by following these standard clinical procedures, it becomes impractical for large-scale epidemiological studies, mainly due to questionable repeatability and validity of certain orthopaedic diagnostic procedures and the cost to image everyone. Therefore, many clinicians and researchers generally use the all-encompassing term of shoulder pain in studies of shoulder pain occurrences.

Many studies have asked directly about the presence of pain in the shoulder.[1,2,3] This relies on the respondents' perceptions as to the anatomical origin of their symptoms. Pain can arise from structures around the shoulder complex and can be felt in a wider area, for example the neck, upper arm or upper trunk, and thus may be undetected with a 'self-perceived' definition.

In spite of the complications with obtaining epidemiological data, the focus of this chapter will be to report some findings from the literature with regards to the prevalence of shoulder pain in the general population, age distribution, occupational and psychosocial risk factors associated with the onset of shoulder-related pain symptoms.

3. The prevalence of shoulder pain

Shoulder pain is a difficult area to research as there are a number of different measures that are used in reporting rates. McBeth et al. discuss the difference between incidence and prevalence of pain and indicate that the incidence may represent the first ever episode (incident) when the patient experienced pain.[4] Shoulder pain can be episodic and large proportions of patients report symptoms that may resolve, only to be experienced again some time in the near (or distant) future. Accordingly as some researchers do report "incident" cases of shoulder pain it is safe to assume that those cases are probably new episodes of pain that have been identified among individuals who were symptom-free at the time of recruitment into the study. Therefore, the following findings will be a report on the prevalence of shoulder pain.

3.1. Prevalence of shoulder pain in the general population

Chronic shoulder pain has large health care costs and a major impact on the health of affected individuals, including absence from work and disability. Shoulder complaints may have an unfavourable outcome, with only about 50% of all new episodes of shoulder complaints presenting in medical practice showing a complete recovery within 6 months.[5,6] After 1 year this proportion increases to 60%.[6] Most of the shoulder pain prevalence data is derived from population-based research. The easiest method for obtaining information about musculoskeletal pain and syndromes is via the use of specially designed self-administered questionnaires that seek specific information from the responding participants. One of the largest and earliest population-based studies that used a self-administered questionnaire was conducted by Hasvold et al.[7] The aim of the study was to determine the prevalence of neck or shoulder pain as part of a general health screening procedure in Norway, and also the direct consequences of these complaints. The sample size was 29,026 with a 75% response rate. The prevalence of shoulder pain was estimated to be 15.4 % in men and 24.9% in women who reported weekly episodes of pain. The study also reported a significant increase in pain prevalence or severity with age most significantly in the 50–56 year age bracket. The study determined that as many as 30% of participants from both sexes reported being significantly disadvantaged at work and unable to perform simple tasks.

Similar prevalence estimations of shoulder pain were also determined by Pope et al.[8] with the total level of suffering in the community from shoulder pain to be as great as 20% of the population. Pope et al. further suggest that most of these will not seek help for their condition so it is important to determine shoulder pain prevalence in order to discuss its impact on the population. Shoulder pain can be influenced by the case definition,[8] as there are numerous sources of shoulder pain. In order to investigate the influence of case definition the authors of this publication compared estimates of shoulder pain prevalence (based on different definitions of shoulder pain), and restricted the definition of shoulder pain to include only those conditions with associated disability in a cross-sectional population survey of patients registered with a general practice in England. The patients were randomly selected from the sample from either sex with an age distribution between 18–75 years. These participants were asked to fill out a questionnaire. The initial response rate was 312(66%) to the postal survey sent out to the sample. Of the responders 232(74%) underwent an interview. The questionnaire used four definitions of shoulder pain; two were based on questions asking directly about pain in the shoulder or upper trunk and neck region, while the other two involved marking a pain drawing of the shoulder or upper trunk. Those that were interviewed also marked a shoulder pain drawing. If the interviewees were experiencing current pain, they were asked specific questions about the pain plus any associated disability. The study found that prevalence was inversely proportional to the case definition. That is, the prevalence increased as the specificity of the definition decreased. Thus a broader definition to incorporate the upper trunk and neck as well as the shoulder had a higher prevalence compared with a prevalence that was based entirely on a specific gleno-humeral cause of shoulder pain.

The study recommended using a pain drawing-based definition restricted to an area of the shoulder complex when conducting prevalence surveys of shoulder pain in the general community. Studies focusing on shoulder pain report the presence or absence of symptoms, but there is limited information from the literature about the extent to which the pain troubles the individual, or as to the severity of the pain. A recent study by Parsons et al. in 2007 measured the prevalence and troublesomeness or burden of musculoskeletal pain, including the shoulder, in different age groups by means of a cross-sectional postal survey of 4,049 adults registered with 16 Medical Research Council General Practice Research Framework practices.[9] The survey achieved a response rate of 60% with 2,504 participants replying to the survey. Frequency of chronic pain overall and troublesome pain by location and age was calculated. The level of pain was measured using the concept of troublesomeness using the following categories — 'not at all troublesome', 'slightly troublesome', 'moderately troublesome', 'very troublesome' and 'extremely troublesome'. The prevalence of chronic pain was 41%. The prevalence of chronic pain rose from 23% in 18–24-year-olds reaching a peak of 50% in 55–64-year-olds. Moderately troublesome pain over the last four weeks was commonest in the lower back (25%) and shoulder (17%). Troublesome shoulder pain was most prevalent in the 45- to 64-year-age groups. The response rate for this survey was adequate (60%) with some 2,504 participants replying to the survey, which is comparable to other published epidemiological studies. The study provides valuable information on the health impact of pain on the participants with the potential to guide future delivery of health care by assisting health professionals' decision-making based on patients' symptoms rather than a diagnosis. The only flaw of the study relates to the reliability of retrospective reports. The questionnaires used may be unreliable because of recall and social desirability biases with the prevalence figures based on those participants who replied.

The findings from this survey with respect to the shoulder data concur with two previously published studies investigating the prevalence of chronic pain and its effect on the general population.[10,11] A large European-based survey from 15 countries measured chronic pain prevalence, intensity of pain and duration of pain symptoms.[11] In addition to these basic variables the survey also attempted to determine the impact of chronic pain on psychological wellbeing of participants, effect on work and daily living, and methods of management of the pain. Some findings from the study include that one third of the chronic pain sufferers were currently not being treated, two thirds used non-medication treatments such as massage, acupuncture or physiotherapy, with almost half of the participants taking non-prescription analgesics, and two thirds prescription medicines. According to the authors, 19% of adult Europeans suffer from moderate to severe pain including the shoulder, which has a detrimental effect on their working and daily lives.

In order to provide insight in the prevalence of musculoskeletal health problems of different anatomical sites including the shoulder, in 2003 Picavet et al. carried out a similar population-based survey on musculoskeletal pain in the Netherlands.[12] This survey, besides prevalence figures, sought to determine the direct consequences of pain in the form of health care consultations, time off work, effect on daily life and identifiable risk groups based on general sociodemographic characteristics.

A random sample of 8,000 persons aged 25 years and over was chosen by the authors, with the survey achieving a response rate of 46.9%. The findings from the study found that almost three quarters (74.5%) of the Dutch population aged 25 years and over reported musculoskeletal pain during the past 12 months, 53.9% reported musculoskeletal pain during the survey (point prevalence) and 44.4% reported musculoskeletal pain lasting longer than three months. The majority of those reporting pain, reported pain at more than one site; roughly two thirds for the period prevalence over 12 months and more than half at the time of the survey (point prevalence) which was present greater than three months (chronic pain). The shoulder was the second most commonly affected site behind low back pain with the period prevalence (12 months) of shoulder pain being 30.3%, and point prevalence 20.9 %. The prevalence of chronic shoulder pain was determined to be 15.1%.

Some interesting findings from the study include that 30% of the complaints were described as continuous pain and 55% as recurrent pain. Severe pain was reported in 15% of the study population and mild pain was present in 70%. A third of the study population consulted a general practitioner, medical specialist or physiotherapist, and reported the use of medication for the pain — with 30% reporting limitation in daily life due to their shoulder pain. Some risk factors presented include a greater prevalence of shoulder pain reported in women (26%) compared to men (16%), age, especially those in middle age from 45–64 years, and those participants living by themselves. The differences in male/female prevalence rates for the 25–44 year age group were (23/13%), 44–65 year age group (21/31%) and over 65 years (13/23%). This study provided a valuable insight in the effect and risk factors associated with musculoskeletal pain including the shoulder, with prevalence figures comparable with the previously cited studies.[10,11,12] The major limitations of this study include the possibility of selective non-response — although the authors state that the general characteristics of the responding and non-responding participants were similar — and the methods used in measuring pain. The prevalence of pain data derived from population-based surveys is determined by the methods used, including the definitions used for the pain, the wording of the questions in the questionnaire, and the length of survey instrument.[8] Hence, the figures derived from this study may be slightly overestimated.

A number of other community-based studies have been cited in the literature with sound methodological quality. These include a study from Finland that demonstrated a shoulder pain prevalence of 17% over a 12-month period in a mixed population of adults from the age of 40–64 years.[13] The definition of shoulder pain used in this study included ache or stiffness in the shoulder or upper arm and a difficulty in movement. A study from the US determined a prevalence of 7%, from a pool of 6,913 participants aged 29–74 years who reported pain in their shoulder for most days over a period of one month.[14]

Two studies from Sweden measured the prevalence of shoulder over two different time frames.[15,16] The first study showed a prevalence of shoulder pain of 13% for males and 15% for females for those who reported shoulder pain for at least one day over the last month.[15] The second study showed that among a group aged between 25–74 years, there was a male prevalence of 18% and female prevalence of 22% for participants who reported pain in the shoulder in the last three months.[16]

A number of further studies report a prevalence of shoulder pain of 16% in participants who have had pain in the shoulder for more than one week over a one-month period,[17] 30% in an adult population over the age of 30 years,[18] 7% from a pool of 21,889 households or 42,826 people over the age of 15 years [19], and 26% in a community survey of the elderly aged 70 years or older.[20]

In the UK, symptoms associated with shoulder problems are a significant cause of morbidity and disability in the general population. The reported overall prevalence of shoulder pain in the UK population is estimated at 7%,[21] which increases according to some authors to 26% in the elderly.[20] Shoulder problems can lead to an inability to work and perform domestic and social activities, as well as leading to serious economic hardship for affected individuals and their families. During 1995, musculoskeletal disorders accounted for 9.9 million days of sick leave in the UK, of which 4.2 million (42%) were related to the upper limb and neck area.[22] Shoulder disorders represent the third most common musculoskeletal presentation to general practice,[23] yet many more patients do not consult their general practitioner (GP). Thus, in the UK, the estimated proportion seeking treatment is between 20 and 50%.[24,25]

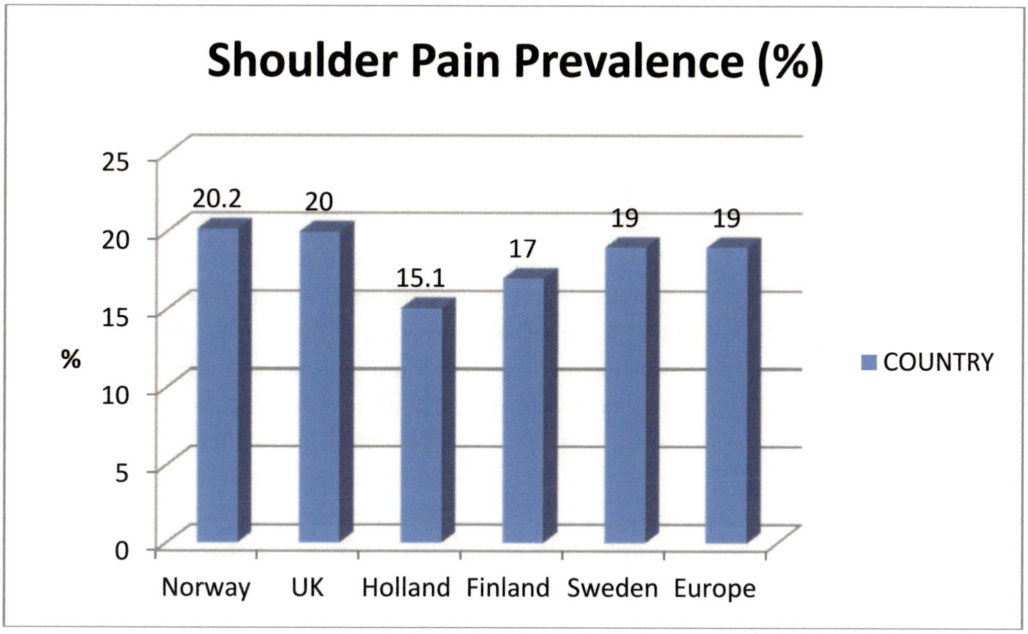

Figure 2. The prevalence of chronic shoulder pain based upon the country of origin of the epidemiological data.

3.2. Prevalence of shoulder pain in medical practice

The prevalence of shoulder pain has been studied in medical practice and represents a common reason for consulting a GP. Data derived from the Netherlands demonstrates a prevalence of 30.3% during a 12-month period during which 30–40% of people reported musculoskeletal pain (including shoulder) during the past year and indicated that they had contacted their GP for these complaints.[12] However, the finer details about these presentations are scarce in the literature, including the nature of the presenting complaints. More detailed research about the prevalence of shoulder pain in general practice is required in order to determine the burden of these complaints on the general population — in other words, the number of people with shoulder complaints that are serious, painful, or annoying enough to seek medical care. Prevalence data on shoulder complaints also helps identify the patient categories that are responsible for the main primary care practitioner workload caused by these complaints.

With respect to chiropractic practice the data is limited, with very few studies citing prevalence figures for shoulder pain presentations. The only data from the profession has been provided by the National Board of Chiropractic Examiners,[26] which conducted a survey of the job analysis of chiropractors in the US, in order to provide a comprehensive source of information about the scope of chiropractic practice (response rate 26%). The survey demonstrated a prevalence of upper extremity presentations, including the shoulder at 8.3%. A very important finding of the survey was that most chiropractors use a multimodal management approach to manage extremity conditions.

One of the first investigations into the prevalence of shoulder pain in medical practice was conducted in the Netherlands by van der Windt et al.[27] who studied the incidence of shoulder disorders in Dutch general practice by means of an observational study. Eleven general practices participated in the study with a total of 35,150 registered patients. All shoulder complaints were recorded over a 12-month period. The term shoulder complaint describes four intrinsic shoulder syndromes, according to the Dutch College of General Practitioners guidelines. These include capsular syndrome, acute bursitis, acromioclavicular syndrome and subacromial syndrome. In the recording period, 754 consultations were recorded in 472 patients with the presence of shoulder pain confirmed in 392 patients. The cumulative incidence varied slightly between practices, but was estimated to be 14.7 per 1,000 per year on average. The incidence was also greater for women (11.1/1000/year) than men (8.4/1000/year) who made up 44 and 56% of the sample size respectively. A previous history of shoulder pain was noted in 54% of men and 46% of women, and the disorder most commonly diagnosed was rotator cuff tendinitis at 29%.

A more recent study in 2005 conducted by Bot et al. collected data from 195 general practitioners (GPs) from 104 practices across the Netherlands in order to record all contacts with patients during 12 consecutive months to determine the prevalence of neck and upper extremity musculoskeletal complaints.[28] The total number of GP contacts during the registration period of one year was 1,524,470. The most commonly reported complaint was neck symptoms (incidence 23.1 per 1000 person-years), followed by shoulder symptoms (incidence 19.0 per 1000 person-years), which translates to approximately 8% of all people registered consulting their GP at least once with a shoulder complaint. The number of consultations for a shoulder complaint/complaint was higher in females (31.4 per 1000) and 23.2 for males. The prevalence of shoulder complaints also increased with age, peaking in the 40–49 and 50–59 year age brackets with a higher ratio of female compared to male presentations.

The prevalence of shoulder pain has also been investigated in a community-based rheumatology practice.[29] Eleven thousand patients from a large general practice were referred for assessment over a nine-month period. Each patient underwent a pain history, shoulder examination — including passive, active and resisted — as well as an assessment of the cervical spine. Diagnosis was based on an accurate history with a directed examination. The most common source of pain in the shoulder was found to be soft tissue lesions (81%), of which the bulk were lesions of the rotator cuff (65%), peri scapular soft tissue (11%), acromioclavicular joint pain (10%) and cervical referred pain (5%). Shoulder pain forms a large part of a specialist rheumatologist's new patient workload.

These prevalence findings are in contrast to a large-scale population-based study recently conducted in the UK.[30] This study attempted to estimate the national prevalence and incidence of adults consulting for a shoulder condition and to investigate patterns of diagnosis, treatment, consultation and referral three years after the initial presentation. Prevalence and incidence rates were estimated for 658,469 patients aged 18 years and over in the year 2000 using a primary care database – the International Medical Statistics (IMS) Disease Analyzer-Mediplus UK. A cohort of 9,215 incident cases was followed-up prospectively for three years beyond the initial consultation. The results demonstrate the annual prevalence and incidence of people consulting for a shoulder condition was 2.36% and 1.47% respectively.

Prevalence increased linearly with age while incidence peaked at around 50 years then remained static at around 2%. Around half of the incident cases consulted once only, while 13.6% were still consulting with a shoulder problem during the third year of follow-up. During the three years following initial presentation, 22.4% of patients were referred to secondary care, 30.8% were prescribed non-steroidal anti-inflammatory drugs and 10.6% were given an injection by their general practitioner (GP). The authors conclude that the prevalence of people consulting for shoulder problems in primary care is substantially lower than community-based estimates of shoulder pain with most referrals occurring within three months of initial presentation, but only a minority of patients are referred to orthopaedic specialists or rheumatologists. GPs may lack confidence in applying precise diagnoses to shoulder conditions.[30] In the United Kingdom it is estimated that approximately 1% of adults will consult a medical practitioner for a new episode of shoulder pain during the course of a year.

In summary, shoulder pain is a common musculoskeletal pain syndrome seen in medical practice, however, the available data demonstrate significant variability in cited prevalence levels. These differences are mainly due to the different definitions of pain used in the individual studies, but may also be explained by differing methodologies used in the various studies and the groups studied. The broader the definition used in the studies yielded a higher prevalence level, however once the definition was reduced to point prevalence the levels were significantly reduced. Future research should define an area, and include all pain in this area as shoulder pain, even though pain from the shoulder may be felt or referred to a wider area distal to the shoulder, or pain may be referred from the spine or internal organs to the shoulder.

Across the cited studies a number of different questionnaires and tests were used for the physical examination, with very little discussion on the validity and reliability of these tests; unfortunately, due to the lack of availability of gold standard diagnostic tests, this may also influence the cited prevalence levels.

The number of consultations for shoulder pain in medical practice may also be influenced by the level of individual insurance coverage.[28] In some countries, such as Holland and even Australia, individuals with public health insurance are reimbursed in full, whereby individuals with private insurance need to pay a gap fee. Hence, the greater numbers of medical consultations occur in individuals with public insurance, so accordingly this has the potential to influence prevalence levels.[28]

Very little research has been conducted with respect to the prognosis and treatment of shoulder pain in medical practice and including chiropractic clinical practice, therefore more research is needed for this clinically challenging area.

In the author's opinion, all of the above comments would also apply for chiropractic, physiotherapy and manipulative therapy clinical practice. Prevalence information for shoulder pain would be useful to estimate the demand for management of shoulder and upper extremity complaints, and possibly determine a further need for chiropractors to undergo additional training in managing these complaints.

4. Features associated with the prevalence of shoulder pain

Features that may be associated with the development or perpetuation of a health problem are represented by the term "risk factors". The presence of risk factors may predispose a person to developing a particular problem and continuing to suffer from it over a long period of time. A number of risk factors that may predispose a person to developing shoulder pain have been cited and studied in the literature. Risk factors for shoulder pain are usually subdivided in to personal risk factors, work-related physical risk factors and work-related psychosocial risk factors.

4.1. Personal risk factors

4.1.1. Age and gender

Age and gender represent personal risk factors that may be associated with shoulder pain, with the presence of pain increasing with an advancing age. Shoulder pain is particularly prevalent in the adolescent age group. A recent study that examined chronic pain prevalence (regardless of location) in children and adolescents (age birth to 18 years) reported that prevalence increased with age, peaking in the 12–15-year-old group, with 33% of adolescents reporting chronic pain.[31]

Siivola et al. conducted a longitudinal study to estimate the prevalence and incidence of neck and shoulder pain in young adults based on a seven year follow up.[32] In the study a random sample of 826 high school students was investigated when they were 15 to 18 years old and again at 22 to 25 years of age. Altogether, 394 (48%) patients participated in both surveys. The outcome variable was weekly neck and shoulder pain during the past 6 months in adulthood, and the explanatory variables included some sociodemographic factors, leisure time activities, self-assessed physical condition, psychosomatic stress symptoms, and symptoms of fatigue and sleep difficulties. In 7 years, the prevalence of weekly neck and shoulder pain increased from 17% to 28%.

Among those who were asymptomatic at baseline, 6-month incidence of occasional or weekly neck and shoulder pain was 59% 7 years later. In females, neck and shoulder pain in adolescence was associated with prevalent neck and shoulder pain in adulthood. Psychosomatic stress symptoms predicted neck and shoulder pain in adulthood. The authors conclude that the prevalence of shoulder pain is high with a multifactorial association of symptom development. The correlation with gender and shoulder pain in the adolescent age group does not appear to be a significant factor as there is a lack of population-based research in this area. Yet some publications demonstrate a higher prevalence of shoulder pain among girls when compared to boys,[33] and a significantly higher prevalence of chronic pain in adolescent females when compared to males.[29] This was also confirmed in a recent study by Vikat et al. who investigated the prevalence and determinants of self-reported neck or shoulder pain (NSP) among 12–18-year-olds by mailing a questionnaire to a nationally representative sample of 11,276 12-, 14-, 16- and 18-year-olds.[34] Shoulder pain was perceived at least once a week by 15% of 12–18-year-olds with symptoms more prevalent among girls than among boys, with the prevalence increasing with age. Participants with shoulder pain also demonstrated perceived psychosomatic symptoms. The study concludes that shoulder pain is frequent among 16–18-year-old girls and, due to the strong association of psychosomatic symptoms, the results suggest that the pain state could be more psychosomatic than nocieceptive in character. A further study correlated gender and age in a biennial cross-sectional survey conducted amongst Finnish adolescents.[35] Pain was more common among girls and older groups: pain of the neck and shoulder affected 24% of girls and 12% of boys in 14-year-olds, 38% of girls and 16% of boys in 16-year-olds, and 45% of girls and 19% of boys in 18-year-olds. Data from this cross-sectional survey has been tracked over a 15-year period with findings suggesting pain in the neck and shoulder is becoming more common in Finnish adolescents, which may suggest a new disease burden of degenerative musculoskeletal disorders in future adults.

The onset of shoulder pain has a strong correlation with adult age, possibly due to the fact that aging is associated with degenerative processes and changes of the shoulder and rotator cuff tendon, which may explain the increase in symptom reporting as we age. With age, repetitive shoulder pain episodes may lead to the accumulation of symptoms and therefore the development of chronic pain. Prevalence of shoulder pain in adults has been extensively studied in the literature and it is accepted that the prevalence of shoulder pain increases with age.[36]

Gender also plays a prominent role in the prevalence of shoulder pain and pain in the upper extremity in general, with the presence of shoulder symptoms more prevalent in females as opposed to men.[37–39] Data from a recent population-based survey showed an increase in shoulder pain prevalence with age, especially in the middle-age group, but also a strong gender correlation.[12] In the age range of 25–44 years the demonstrated prevalence of shoulder pain was 13.3% for men and 22.8% for women, a peak prevalence of 21.4% in men and 30.9% in women in the 45–64 years age group, and for the 65 years plus age group a prevalence of 13.2% in men and 23.1% in women. A prevalence of shoulder pain of 17% in the middle-age bracket of 40–64 years was also demonstrated in a study by Takala et al. in 1982[13] and Parsons et al. in 2007 [9] who also determined the highest prevalence of shoulder pain (17%) in the middle-age group from 45–64 years of age. This age group also reported the pain to be the most troublesome, with the greatest impact on daily and working life. The prevalence of chronic pain rose from 23% in 18–24-year-olds reaching a peak of 50% in 55–64-year-olds. Once again, prevalence and chronicity of shoulder pain increase with advancing age especially in the middle-age bracket.

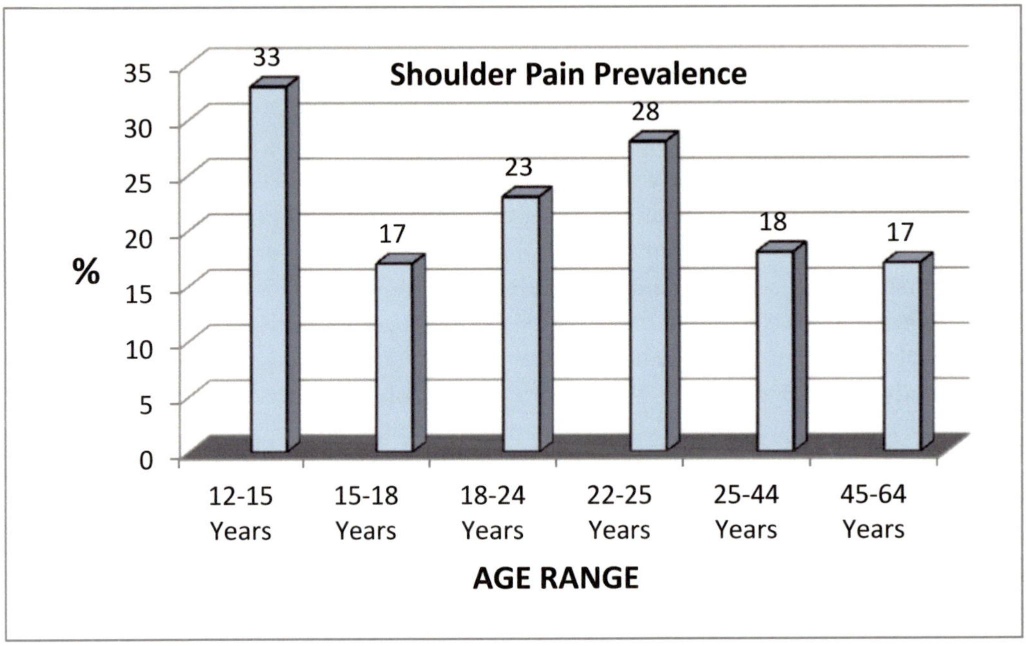

Figure 3. The prevalence of chronic shoulder pain based upon the age range.

A number of hypotheses potentially explain why shoulder symptoms may be more prevalent in women, with one explanation being that women's jobs, more often than men's, involve work tasks with static load on the neck and shoulder muscles, high repetitiveness, low control and high mental demands that maybe potential risk factors for neck or shoulder pain.[40] Some further citations from the literature that may explain excess symptom reporting by women include a tendency to label stimuli as more noxious,[41] an increased sensitivity to pain and significant differences between genders in mean pain thresholds, with women recording lower pain thresholds[42] and an increased exposure to risk factors for symptom onset.[43] Reports in the literature have correlated also gender as a risk factor for the development of shoulder pain, with females particularly at risk, according to two large epidemiological surveys.[44,45]

In the older age group there is a tendency of decreasing shoulder symptoms that could be attributed to a change in those risk factors associated with further symptom onset or persistence, such as a change in workplace risk factors after retirement.[4] Although a reduced prevalence of shoulder pain in the older age group, compared to the middle aged group is evident a number of studies have still demonstrated a reasonably high prevalence. Chard et al. conducted a hospital-based survey and found that 21% of patients presenting to an acute care geriatric clinic had a symptomatic shoulder disorder.[46] A later study by Chard et al.,[20] was based on a community survey to try to discover the true prevalence of shoulder disorders in the elderly. A random sample of 644 individuals over the age of 70 was selected from two general medicine practices. The conditions diagnosed after examination included rotator cuff tendinitis, 'frozen shoulder' (adhesive capsulitis), chronic rotator cuff rupture or impingement, A-C joint arthritis, glenohumeral joint rheumatoid or osteoarthritis, and shoulder pain without obvious shoulder pathology that represented referred pain. Of the participants, 27 % reported shoulder pain with 21% having an identifiable disorder present. The gender differences were male17% and female 25%. This study also confirmed that the female gender appears to be a risk factor associated with the development of a shoulder problem in the elderly age group.

In at least 70% of shoulder disorders the rotator cuff was primarily involved with the most frequent condition being rotator cuff tendinopathy. At least 50% of conditions involved chronic rotator cuff rupture or impingement. Duration of pain varied from one month to many years dependent on the disorder. The impact of shoulder pain as reported by the patients was disability in personal care (washing) and with household chores, and difficulty in lifting and doing tasks above the level of the shoulder. In the older age group more than 40% of patients consulted their GP with their pain, however more than 50% generally have had previous undocumented episodes of shoulder pain.[20]

A recent study of shoulder pain in the elderly age group attempted to determine the prevalence of shoulder pain and identify factors associated with this pain, to assess the pattern of coexisting joint pain and to evaluate the impact of this pain on physical functioning.[47] The study was a cross-sectional study of Black and White men and women aged 70–79 years. The results demonstrated a shoulder pain prevalence of 18.9% with Black women having the highest prevalence of shoulder pain (24.3%). The correlates of both neck and shoulder pain were female gender, no education beyond high school, poorer self-rated health, depressive symptomatology and a medical history of arthritis, heart attack, and angina. Increasing severity of both neck and shoulder pain was associated with an increased prevalence of joint pain at other body sites and with poor functional capacity. Measures of physical performance involving the upper extremity were also decreased. The authors conclude that neck and shoulder pain, either alone or in conjunction with pain in other joints, has a substantial impact on the function and wellbeing of the older adults in this cohort.

Some further personal risk factors derived from epidemiological studies from America and Europe have demonstrated sleep disturbances, smoking and the consumption of caffeine to be associated with shoulder pain.[45,48,49] Immigrant status is another factor that can be associated with shoulder pain, which was demonstrated by Ekberg et al. in an epidemiological survey conducted in 1995.[44] A small amount of evidence is emerging in the literature demonstrating a correlation between race, ethnicity and pain. A study from the US demonstrated when Caucasian populations are compared with participants from African American and Hispanic groups they report more severe pain levels, have a lower tolerance to pain stimuli, and are more likely to seek health care for their symptoms.[50] All these citations from the literature represent personal risk factors associated with the development of shoulder pain.

The cited publications demonstrate a correlation with age and gender with respect to the onset of shoulder pain, with prevalence densities increasing with age especially in the age bracket above 40 years. Women appear to be more affected by shoulder pain — often due to jobs characterised by static loads on shoulder musculature, monotonous and repetitive tasks, but also due to additional stresses from unpaid work such as child minding and household duties. However, strong conclusions cannot be drawn from the available research due to the significant differences in methodology between the studies with respect to lack of uniform criteria for describing shoulder pain and poor diagnostic uniformity.

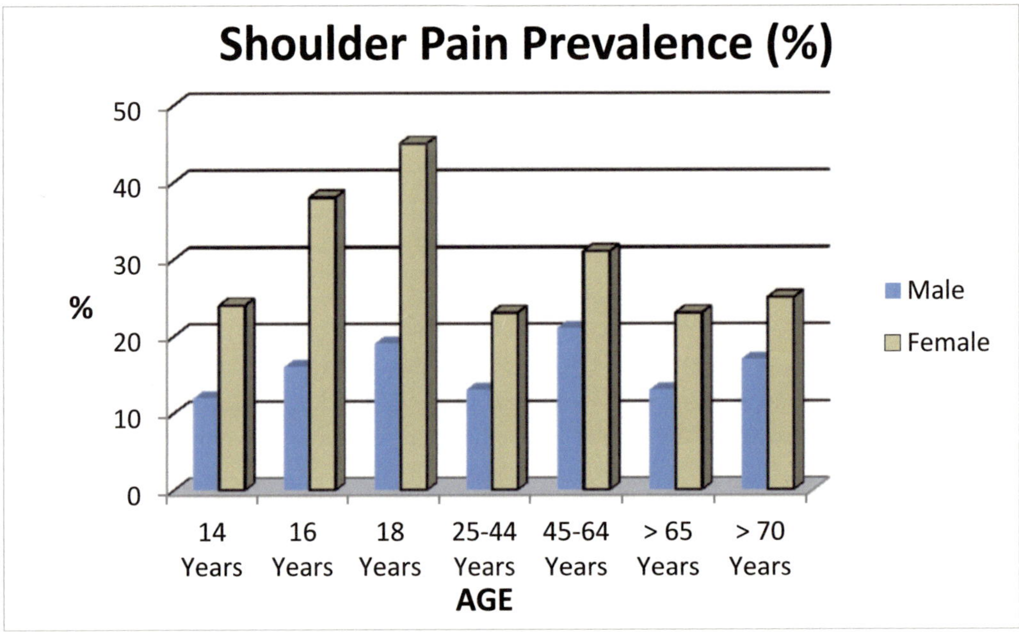

Figure 4. The prevalence of chronic shoulder pain based upon gender.

Shoulder pain also appears to have a relatively high prevalence in the younger population especially in the age group from 12–18 years, particularly in teenage girls. The data derived from the Finnish studies with sound methodology suggest that shoulder pain is becoming more frequent, which has the potential to cause further long-term and chronic musculoskeletal disorders in their adult lives.[34,35] The increasing pain levels appear to correlate with the substantial changes seen in western societies today with respect to increased level of computer usage, access to internet, and high usage of computer games. The high level of shoulder pain symptoms may relate to risk factors such as repetitive movements, static postures and static muscular activation patterns as seen with computer mouse usage.[51]

4.2. Occupational factors

Numerous studies in an occupational setting have demonstrated work-related physical risk factors associated with the development of shoulder pain. The transition from no or minor pain to more severe pain was influenced by physical and psychosocial workplace factors together with individual and health-related factors.[52] Work-related risk factors associated with the onset of shoulder pain have been cited in the literature including: repetitive work, high force demand and vibration, work-related posture, computer work and psychosocial factors.

4.2.1. Repetitive work

The correlation between repetitive work and the onset of shoulder pain has been cited in a number of studies. In 2004, Leclerc et al. conducted a study to determine the predictiveness of personal and occupational factors for the onset of shoulder pain in occupations requiring repetitive work from a sample of workers in five activity sectors who completed a self-administered questionnaire in 1993–94 and again three years later.[53] Both questionnaires included questions about shoulder pain. The associations between various factors at baseline and subsequent shoulder pain were studied among participants free from shoulder pain at baseline. The results show the incidence of shoulder pain was associated with several independent risk factors: depressive symptoms, low level of job control, and biomechanical constraints. After adjustment for other risk factors, the presence of depressive symptoms predicted occurrence of shoulder pain. A low level of job control was also associated with the onset of shoulder pain in both sexes. For men, repetitive use of a tool was a strong predictor, while the two most important biomechanical risk factors for women were use of vibrating tools and working with arms above shoulder level. The results confirm the role of several biomechanical constraints in developing shoulder pain with psychological symptoms and a low level of job control also playing an important role. Two systematic reviews also demonstrate a significant relationship between repeated movements and upper extremity disorders in general and also a consistent relationship specifically between neck or shoulder pain and repeated movements.[54,55]

Van der Windt et al. systematically reviewed the literature for occupational risk factors of shoulder pain.[55] The review determined potential risk factors related to physical load and included heavy work load, awkward postures, repetitive movements, vibration and duration of employment, with consistent findings found for the latter three items. Nearly all studies that assessed psychosocial risk factors reported at least one positive association with shoulder pain, but the results were not consistent across studies for either high psychological demands, poor control at work, poor social support, or job dissatisfaction. The authors conclude that it seems likely that shoulder pain is the result of many factors, including physical load and the psychosocial work environment.

4.2.2. High force demands (physical demands) and vibration

Occupation is a very important factor in the aetiology of shoulder pain. The occurrence of pain is generally more common in participants with moderate to heavy physical demands, and the pain tends to occur during the course of the working day (i.e., it is occupationally dependant).[56] Bergenudd et al. classified participants according to occupational workload into three groups: light physical demands (teachers, clerks), moderate physical demand (Nurses, light industry workers), and heavy physical demands (carpenters, bricklayers).[56]

The findings from the study showed a relationship between shoulder pain prevalence and occupational workload. It demonstrated that participants in the moderate to heavy physical demand groups were more likely to have pain and require sick leave due to disability. Factors that may contribute to increased shoulder pain are muscle loading, prolonged static work, repetition and working with hands at or above shoulder level. The major psychosocial factor that was affected by the pain sufferers was poor job satisfaction.

In 2000, Ariens et al. conducted a systemic review of the literature and determined some evidence for a correlation between the work-related force requirements in the arms and neck or shoulder pain, as well as between heavy lifting (arm force), arm posture, vibration and workplace design on the development of neck or shoulder pain.[57] These findings were also confirmed by Malchaire et al. who found a correlation between forceful hand and wrist work on the development of shoulder pain.[58]

A recent prospective cohort study conducted by Grooten et al. in 2007 demonstrated that three simultaneous work-related exposures influenced the development of shoulder pain; these included manual handling (physical load), working with the hands above shoulder level, and working with vibrating tools.[59] The presence of any of these three variables also influenced the long-term prognosis of workers with shoulder pain.

A most recent investigation by Miranda et al. investigated whether occupational physical load predicted subsequent chronic shoulder disorders.[60] A comprehensive national survey was carried out among a representative sample (n = 7,217) of the Finnish adult population in 1977–80. Twenty years later, 1,286 participants from the previous survey were invited to be re-examined, and 909 (71%) participated. After excluding those with diagnosed shoulder disorders at baseline, 883 participants were available for the analyses. The prevalence of shoulder pain at follow-up was 7%. Work exposure to repetitive movements and vibration at baseline increased the risk of a shoulder disorder. The adverse effects of physical work were seen even among those older than 75 years at follow-up. These statistically and clinically significant risk factors differed between genders: for men vibration and repetitive movements, and for women lifting heavy loads and working in awkward postures. This is the first prospective study in a general population showing that occupational physical loading increases the risk of a subsequent clinical shoulder disorder and the effects seem to be long term. According to these results ergonomical assessment of the workplace and implementation of strategies that may reduce the exposure of the worker to the associated risk factors may have long-lasting health benefits for the shoulder and potentially reduce the prevalence and adverse effects of work-related shoulder pain.

Certain occupational groups have been studied in the literature – including manual handlers, delivery drivers, technicians, customer services computer operators, and general office staff – on reported physical and psychosocial working conditions and symptoms of neck and upper limb disorders by the use of a self-administered questionnaire.[60] The respondents from that survey were classified into one of four exposure groups: high physical and high psychosocial, high physical and low psychosocial, low physical and high psychosocial and low physical and low psychosocial. The definition of high physical exposure criterion is deemed as lifting greater than 16 kg more than or equal to once per hour would classify a worker as high physical exposure. A worker would also be classified as having high physical exposure if a 6–15 kg load was lifted more than or equal to once per hour and, additionally, vibration while sitting – for example, driving – was experienced for more than or equal to half the working day. The prevalence of shoulder pain among workers from the low physical and low psychosocial group was 39%, low physical and high psychosocial 34%, high physical and low psychosocial 57% and high physical and high psychosocial 69%. The study showed that workers highly exposed to both physical and psychosocial workplace risk factors were more likely to report shoulder symptoms than workers highly exposed to one or the other.

When certain occupations have been studied individually there is a strong correlation between manual work (physical demands) on the development of shoulder pain. In a study of Finnish forest workers,[61] the prevalence of mild or severe shoulder pain was 14% over a 12-month period. Higher age, obesity and mental stress as well as physically strenuous work and working with trunk forward flexed or with a hand above shoulder level increased the risk of incident shoulder pain. The findings from the study support the view that shoulder pain is the result of many factors, including occupational and individual factors such as heavy physical work with a heavy load, awkward work postures and mental stress. This study also linked obesity as a risk factor for the development of shoulder pain.

Stenlund et al. confirmed a relationship between shoulder tendinitis and heavy manual work and exposure to vibration.[62] The prevalence of shoulder pain in their study over the previous 12 months was 40% among the rock blasters and 8–15% among bricklayers. In 1999, Frost et al. investigated the association of shoulder impingement syndrome with shoulder-intensive work.[63] The prevalence of shoulder pain in slaughterhouse workers was 60%. The slaughterhouse worker activities included monotonous and manually intensive work with their upper arms raised to at least 30 degrees of shoulder abduction for half of the working day (48%), and raising the arms above 30 degrees of shoulder abduction at least 10 times per minute.

Similarly, some early investigations by Herbets et al. demonstrated the relationship between shoulder pain and heavy manual labour in shipyard welders.[64] According to their research, the general population demonstrates shoulder pain prevalence of 15–25% in persons between the ages of 40–50 years, and in shipyard industry the prevalence increases to 30–40%. Localised muscle fatigue appears to be a relevant factor in the onset of shoulder pain. It normally arises as a consequence of sustained muscle contractions in differing work situations with the arms at or above shoulder level, repetitive elevations or muscular work and generalised shoulder muscle load. The workers often work in situations aggravated by awkward posture and the use of heavy equipment, as well as the very difficult environment encountered in a shipyard when exposed to the climactic elements (heat and cold).

A number of other studies investigating heavy manual work and high physical demands also correlate a high prevalence of shoulder related disorders.[45,65–69]

4.2.3. *Work related posture*

Work-related posture is a well-documented risk factor associated with the development of shoulder-related disorders. This entails prolonged and/or repetitive periods of sustained shoulder or neck positions, either awkward or extreme.[40] such as severe shoulder flexion or abduction.[55,60]

In 2006, Sim et al. determined an age-standardised one-month period prevalence of neck and upper limb pain at 44% from a cohort of industrial and manual workers.[70] Significant independent associations for shoulder pain were demonstrated with actions involving repeated lifting of heavy objects, working with arms at/above shoulder height (postural position) and psychosocial variables including little job control and little supervisor support. The population attributable fractions were (24%) for exposure to work activities and (12%) for exposure to psychosocial factors. Some further findings show that the highest prevalence of shoulder pain was seen in the 55–64 year age group, and predominantly in women. The results of the study demonstrate a high prevalence of shoulder pain over a four-week period, which may be slightly inflated due to the preselected study. This category of workers are already exposed to risk factors, hence the results may not be a true reflection of the prevalence, as it may have been if the sample was chosen from the general population incorporating a large variety of occupations. Irrespective of the methodological weaknesses of this study the findings suggest that with modification of the work environment up to one in three cases of shoulder pain can be prevented.

From a population-based study of occupational risk factors for shoulder pain — including physical exposures, working conditions, and psychosocial aspects of the workplace — Pope et al. also identified some further risk factors, including those for workers who reported working with hands above shoulder level, using wrists or arms in a repetitive way, or stretching down to reach below knee level.[71] This action had about twice the risk of shoulder pain and disability. Leclerc et al. also confirmed a postural association (working with arms above shoulder level) with shoulder pain. This was particularly demonstrated in the female gender, with the use of vibrating tools an additional risk factor.[53]

Numerous other publications have confirmed posture as a risk factor for the development of shoulder pain among workers, as evident in a number of recent cross-sectional and case-controlled studies that have confirmed this correlation with shoulder pain.[72,73]

In 2000 van der Windt et al. conducted a systematic review of the literature in order to evaluate the available evidence on occupational risk factors of shoulder pain.[55] The review involved a search of databases so that details could be extracted on the study populations, exposures (physical load and psychosocial work environment), and results for the association between exposure variables and shoulder pain. According to the authors, the number of epidemiological studies reporting on potential risk factors for shoulder pain has greatly increased in the past decade, with work-related factors playing an important part in the development of shoulder pain with many studies conducted in various occupational settings. However, a number of the published papers did not consider shoulder pain specifically or did not use systematic methods for the selection of papers, assessment of methodological quality, or data extraction and analysis, hence with somewhat unreliable methodology. Therefore, after conducting a systematic review and laying down a standardised checklist for the assessment of methodological quality of cross sectional studies), case-control studies and prospective cohort studies the authors were able to identify six papers with good methodological quality that confirmed the relationship between awkward postures — including twisted postures, working with forward flexed trunk, and working with arms above shoulder — and shoulder pain, and three studies that identified conducting the same activity for a prolonged period—such as typing or driving a car and shoulder pain.

4.2.4. *Computer work*

With the rapid development of information technology a number of changes in working life have ensued. It is estimated that more than half of the working population in western societies currently use personal computers at work.[74] The time spent in front of the computer and the use of a computer mouse has also increased rapidly over the years. This entails prolonged and sustained postures, constant force and highly repetitive movements as well as psychosocial factors such as time constraints and high quantitative demands at work.[40] This has resulted in an increase in shoulder-related disorders especially amongst adolescents and the youth.[32–35]

This is exacerbated with ready access to the internet, mobile phone use, and playing of computer games that have all opened up a new pathway of risk factors associated with shoulder pain in adolescents. Hakala et al. recruited adolescents aged from 14–18 years in a study who reported a weekly prevalence of shoulder pain at 26%.[75] The authors conclude that daily use of computers exceeding two to three hours seems to be a threshold for neck or shoulder pain, which may explain why with an increase in computer-related activities there is an increase in shoulder-related pain among the youth. A further study also evaluated the prevalence of neck or shoulder, and arm pain with computer use in Dutch adolescents.[76] The survey was distributed to a pool of 12–16-year-olds attending a secondary school in Amsterdam. The study demonstrated an overall prevalence of neck or shoulder pain of 11.5%. The prevalence of pain was higher among girls and adolescents not living with both parents. The study also found a correlation with depressive symptoms and neck or shoulder pain.

In 2007, Eltayeb et al. conducted a study to investigate the prevalence of arm, neck and shoulder pain in a Dutch population of computer workers and also to develop a questionnaire aimed at measuring workplace physical and psychosocial risk factors for the presence of these complaints.[77] The authors used a questionnaire to determine sociodemographic characteristics (age, gender, and employment status) to assess potential risk factors with regard to (1) work station, (2) posture during work, (3) quality of break time, (4) job demands, (5) job control, and (6) social support. In addition, a number of items assess the quality of the work environment and the frequency and nature of extremity complaints, in the neck, shoulder, upper and lower arm, elbow, hand and wrist. The study demonstrated a prevalence of shoulder pain over the past 12 months that lasted for at least one week to be 31% overall, with a prevalence of 20% in males and 42% in females. A further study concentrated on determining factors of computer work that predict musculoskeletal symptoms in the shoulder, elbow, and low-back regions.[78] A questionnaire on ergonomics, work pauses, work techniques, and psychosocial and other factors was delivered to 5,033 office workers with the results showing the prevalence of shoulder pain at 18% with symptoms more prevalent among female workers. The authors conclude that work pauses, reduction of glare or reflection, and screen height are important factors in the design of future computer workstations. Previous symptoms were a significant predictor of recurrent symptoms in the shoulder.

There are few publications that have investigated prolonged or chronic shoulder pain and their association with the use of the computer. One study reported in a publication from Denmark evaluated the prevalence of moderate to severe neck and shoulder pain among frequent computer users, and the associated effect of mouse and keyboard use.[79] The study followed a pool of participants over a 12-month period determining a prevalence of moderate-to-severe pain in the neck and right shoulder at 4.1% and 3.4%, respectively, and the one-year incidence for no or minor baseline symptoms at 1.5% and 1.9%, respectively. These findings indicate that computer mouse use is associated with an increased risk of moderate-to-severe pain in the neck and right shoulder, especially with prolonged mouse and keyboard use.

In contrast to previous publications, Anderson et al. studied the effect of keyboard and computer mouse usage as a predictor for the onset of acute, prolonged and chronic pain in the neck and shoulder.[80] The study measured three different pain patterns, namely:

(1) acute pain (measured as weekly pain), (2) prolonged pain (no or minor pain in the neck and shoulder region over four consecutive weeks followed by three consecutive weeks with a high pain score), and (3) chronic pain (reported pain or discomfort lasting more than 30 days and ''quite a lot of trouble'' during the past 12 months). The study showed that in any one week during the study period, 9.8% males and 10.2% females reported severe shoulder pain. Risk for acute neck pain and shoulder pain increased linearly by 4% and 10%, respectively, for each quartile increase in weekly mouse usage time. Mouse and keyboard usage time did not predict the onset of prolonged or chronic pain in the neck or shoulder. Women had higher risks for neck and shoulder pain. The authors conclude that there seems to be no relationship between computer use and prolonged and chronic neck and shoulder pain. The major weakness of the study was the non-standard definition of shoulder pain, hence this may have contributed to the authors' conclusions. The cohort members were mouse users more than they were keyboard users. The mean mouse usage was around six hours per week and total computer use was 9.2 hours per week and was strongly correlated with mouse use Keyboard usage was at a low level, so the results for keyboard users should be cautiously interpreted and may not hold for heavy keyboard users.

The presence of shoulder pain and symptoms associated with dysfunction of the shoulder girdle in workers that use the computer on a daily basis can lead to sickness, absence and chronic disability, but also reduced work effectiveness.

The results of a British national survey in 1995 showed that musculoskeletal disorders of the neck and upper extremity were responsible for the loss of 4.2 million working days in a 12-month period, hence this represents a significant form for society.[81] Many workers still go to work despite the feeling that, in the light of their health, they should have taken sick leave. This phenomenon is known as sickness presenteeism.[82] Although the workers are physically present at work, their productivity could be reduced due to functional limitations. The extent of productivity loss while present at work is uncertain, but it has been suggested that it accounts for the majority of lost productivity costs associated with chronic pain.[83,84] A recent cross-sectional population-based study of computer workers investigated the effect of shoulder, neck pain and loss of productivity among the working population.[85] From the study population a total of 10% reported shoulder and neck symptoms and, on average, in 26% of the cases reporting symptoms, productivity loss was involved. If symptoms of the hand and arm were also present the productivity loss was 36%. The productivity loss was caused by sickness absence and by a decreased performance at work (decreased work speed and working hours but no sickness absence). In the study psychosocial load was defined as effort–reward imbalance and job satisfaction, which was strongly associated with productivity loss.

4.2.5. Psychosocial factors

A number of work-related psychosocial variables have been identified in the literature and appear to be linked with shoulder-related symptoms. Workers who are highly exposed to both physical and psychosocial workplace risk factors were more likely to report symptoms of musculoskeletal disorders, including the shoulder, than workers highly exposed to one or the other.[61] Devereux et al. defined psychosocial exposure criteria at work into high psychosocial exposure criteria, which represents high mental demands, low job control, and low social support; and low psychosocial exposure criteria, which is represented by low mental demands at work, high job control, and high social support.[61]

The results from the study demonstrate an interaction between physical and psychosocial risk factors in the workplace that increased the risk of reporting symptoms in the upper limbs. Symptoms of the shoulder are more prevalent in workers with high psychosocial exposure. Associations between both physical and psychosocial exposures in the work environment and seeking care for neck or shoulder pain have also been found in the literature. Long-term exposure to a hindrance at work, an increase of exposure to reduced opportunities to acquire or use new knowledge, or lack of opportunity to participate in planning of the work are associated with seeking care because of neck or shoulder pain. The presence of these factors in the work environment represented risk factors for the development of work-related shoulder pain.

In attempt to identify whether psychosocial and mechanical risk factors related to a new onset of shoulder pain, or whether these factors can predict onset of shoulder pain in newly employed workers, Harkness et al. conducted a two-year prospective study of newly employed workers from twelve diverse occupational settings.[86] New onset of shoulder pain was reported by 15% of participants at 12 months. An increased risk of symptom onset was found in participants reporting mechanical exposures involving heavy weights, including lifting with one or two hands, carrying on one shoulder, lifting at or above shoulder level, and pushing or pulling. Working with hands above shoulder level was also predictive of new onset shoulder pain. When considering psychosocial variables, participants were asked about the following with respect to their current job: job satisfaction, whether they felt their work was monotonous or boring, work pace, stress/worry, control over work, ability to learn new things, and support from work colleagues and supervisors. Most of the psychosocial factors were modestly associated with new onset shoulder pain. However, monotonous work was a strong risk factor for new onset shoulder pain. The strength of the study was its prospective cohort design following a pool of participants from a variety of occupations over a two-year period. Most available data on psychosocial variables has been obtained from cross-sectional studies,[55] hence the practical implications of this research are that by targeting the perception of monotonous or tedious work by applying more interesting or varied tasks in the workplace with more breaks and better job opportunities, the onset of shoulder pain may be reduced.

In a more recent study[70] of psychosocial factors related to work and the occurrence of shoulder pain the authors asked participants a number of questions a number of questions on a five-point adverbial scale ('none of the time' to 'all of the time'):

- Can/could you control the way you worked in this job?
- Is/was your work physically demanding in this job?
- Do/did the tasks and activities that you perform/performed in this job change during your time in the job?
- Do/did you get job satisfaction from your work in this job?
- On the whole, are/were your supervisors/managers supportive?

This method of collecting information on work-related psychosocial factors has been previously used.[87] The results demonstrate that factors such as little job control, physically demanding work, and little supervisor support were strongly associated with the occurrence of work related shoulder pain. High levels of psychological demand (hectic work and conflicting demands) and physical exertion in the workplace were significant predictors of work-related repetitive strain injury in the shoulder.[88]

These findings have also been confirmed in a prospective study of newly employed workers from 12 diverse occupational groups.[86] In addition to the above mentioned factors this study also identified a number of variables associated with the development of shoulder pain including: lack of control over work, seldom learning new things, and dissatisfaction with job and dissatisfaction with support from colleagues. Aspects of job demand, poor support from colleagues, and work dissatisfaction were all associated with increased odds of reported pain onset and presented very strong predictors for associated shoulder symptoms.

A recent systemic review of the literature of occupational risk factors for shoulder pain identified the following psychosocial factors including: duration of employment, psychological work demands, job control, social support, job satisfaction and stimulation at work.[55]

According to van der Windt et al. psychosocial factors seem to be important in both the development and maintenance of sub-acute and chronic shoulder problems.[55] Pain behaviour may be learned over time and may eventually cause the pain problem to persist, even after physical healing has occurred. In this model, pain is considered to be more than a neurophysiological entity, having both cognitive and behavioural dimensions. A poor social work environment, together with an inadequate personal capacity to cope with these factors, may increase work-related stress. The increase in stress may increase muscle tone directly, or strengthen the relation between physical work load and musculoskeletal symptoms. This may result in an enhancement of the perception or reporting of symptoms, or a reduction of the capacity to cope.

In summary, it is important to identify risk factors (physical and psychosocial) associated with the development of shoulder pain as a number of these variables can be controlled and, in some instances, significantly reduced, which may improve the health of the adult population including workers. Musculoskeletal disorders including the shoulder are some of the most frequent reasons for long-term absence from work, with a major impact on daily living and quality of life. From a public health perspective the information derived from these studies may contribute to reducing the population burden of shoulder and upper limb pain. Therefore, there may be appreciable scope for preventive modification of the physical and psychosocial work environment to reduce the impact of shoulder and upper limb pain.

From a research point of view it would be interesting to determine to what extent these identified risk factors are common across specific and non-specific disorders of the shoulder. Perhaps this maybe a new avenue of investigation for future prospective or longitudinal studies.

5. Predictors of outcome

In clinical practice it is important to know more about the prognostic value of clinical, psychosocial, and occupational factors in patients with shoulder disorders. It may help to provide patients with adequate information regarding the most likely course of their symptoms.

A number of recent studies have investigated the course and prognosis of patients presenting to a primary care practitioner with shoulder pain. In 2008, Reilingh et al. investigated the course and prognosis of shoulder pain in the first 6 months after presentation to the general practitioner.[89] The authors also separately studied patients with acute, sub-acute and chronic shoulder pain, as duration of symptoms at presentation has been shown to be the strongest predictor of outcome. A prospective cohort study was conducted with 6-month follow-up of a pool of patients with shoulder pain, which also included patients with a new episode of shoulder pain. Patients were categorised as having acute (symptoms <6 weeks), sub-acute (6–12 weeks) or chronic (>3 months) shoulder pain in predefined area of the shoulder. The course of shoulder pain, functional disability and quality of life was analysed over 6 months. Patient and disease characteristics, including physical and psychosocial factors, were investigated as possible predictors of outcome. The results demonstrated that acute shoulder symptoms showed the most favourable course over a 6-month follow-up, with more pain reduction and improvement of functional disability. Patients with chronic shoulder symptoms showed the poorest results. Predictors of a better outcome at 6 months for acute shoulder pain were lower baseline disability scores and higher baseline pain intensity scores. Predictors of a better outcome for chronic shoulder pain were lower scores on pain catastrophising scale at baseline. The authors conclude that, besides a different course of symptoms in patients presenting with acute or chronic shoulder pain, predictors of outcome may also differ with psychosocial factors being more important in chronic shoulder pain.

A similar observational, prospective cohort study was conducted in general practice to describe the clinical course and to identify predictors of recovery, changes in pain intensity, and changes in functional disability in patients with neck or shoulder symptoms at three, and 12-month follow-up.[90] The study involved 443 patients who consulted their general practitioner with neck or shoulder symptoms. Baseline scores of pain and disability, symptom characteristics, sociodemographic factors, psychological factors, social support, physical activity, general health, and co-morbidity were investigated as possible predictors of recovery, changes in pain intensity, and changes in functional disability using multiple regression analyses. The results showed a low recovery rate; 24% of the patients reported recovery at three months and 32% reported recovery at 12-month follow-up. This study also showed that duration of the symptoms before consulting the GP and also a previous history neck or shoulder symptoms increased the probability of an unfavourable outcome. A number of psychological variables were noted, including less vitality and more worrying, and were consistently associated with poorer outcome after three and 12 months. In conclusion, the results from the study indicate that besides clinical characteristics, psychological factors also predict the outcome of neck and shoulder symptoms.

In a narrative review of the literature a number of prognostic indicators of a favourable outcome within three months have been described including: mild trauma preceding symptoms, early presentation, preceding overuse and heavy and unusual activities of the upper extremity.[91] Factors that were reported to predict a poor outcome at 3 months were severe pain at first presentation, a prior episode, a severe restriction of the passive abduction range, concomitant neck pain, cervical spondylosis and radicular symptoms, higher age, involvement of the dominant side and sick leave from work. The reported evidence for these factors is weak and, according to the reviewers, is based on studies with weak methodology. However, a number of more recent studies suggest strong evidence for 'high pain intensity' as a predictor of poor outcome.[92,93]

Kuijpers et al. also found high pain intensity to be a strong predictor of persistent symptoms at short-term (six weeks) and long-term (six months) follow-up.[91] There is evidence that high pain intensity in primary care populations and middle age (45–54 years) in occupational populations are strong predictors for a poor prognosis; that long duration of complaints and high disability score at baseline are predictors for a poor prognosis in primary care populations.[92]

A number of psychological factors, such as inadequate pain cognitions and pain behaviour are likely to predict a poor outcome of painful musculoskeletal conditions.[91] In addition, psychosocial work environment (e.g., decision authority and job satisfaction) [55] and heavy physical work load (e.g., pushing and pulling, repetitive work) may be associated with an increased risk of new episodes of shoulder pain.[55, 94]

In summary, the major predictor of outcome for patients presenting with shoulder pain to primary care practitioners appears to be the level of pain intensity on the first consultation, and a previous history of shoulder problems. Due to the small number of studies available with heterogeneous methodologies strong conclusions cannot be drawn at this stage. This area of research necessitates further studies that will enable better decisions on the choice of interventions and help generate guidelines for indexing patients into high- or low- risk categories for persistent shoulder pain, which may allow caregivers to predict the likelihood of recovery. New focused studies should emphasise the importance of the predictive value of sociodemographic and clinical factors, but also psychological factors and work-related risk factors for shoulder pain.

6. Shoulder pain and sport

The prevalence of shoulder pain in sport is quite high, especially in overhead sports that require the repetitive overhead use of the shoulder – such as swimming, baseball, tennis and overhead athletes. Overhead sports subject the shoulder to stress, fatigue, microtrauma, laxity of static stabilisers, and muscular imbalances of shoulder dynamic stabilisers that can create altered mechanical functioning of the shoulder and predispose it to injury.

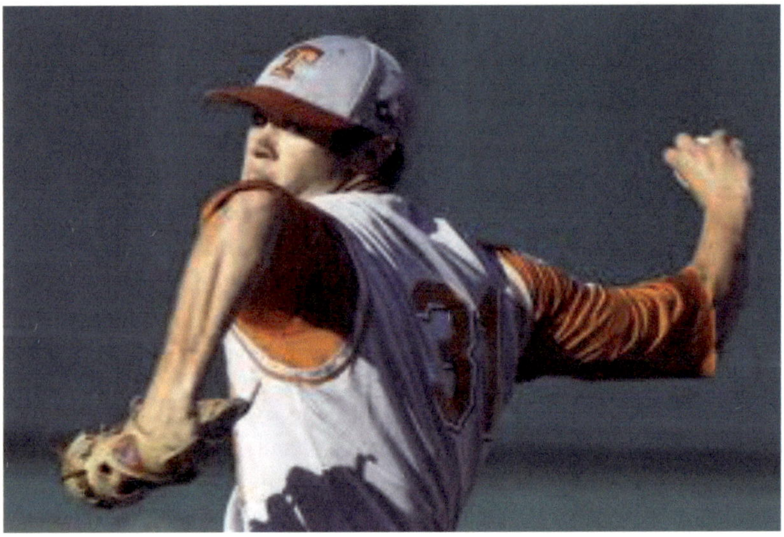

Numerous sports have been studied in the literature including swimming and activities involving overhead throwing. The cause of shoulder pain in the athlete involved in overhead sports (e.g., tennis, volleyball) or throwing (e.g., cricket, baseball) maybe due to the repetitive and high-energy forces going through the shoulder, leading to chronic stresses placed on the stabilising structures of the shoulder. When the stresses are applied to the shoulder at a rate that exceeds repair this will result in progressive damage to stabilising structures. With continued stress, the static stabilisers of the shoulder become hyperelastic, enabling anterior glenohumeral subluxation. Initially the dynamic stabilisers can compensate for this mild instability with increased muscle activity. However, with increased activity fatigue results, which in turn leads to overloading of these compensatory mechanisms. Consequently, the humeral head may sublux anteriorly, come in contact with the coracoacromial arch, ultimately leading to subacromial impingement. This form of athletic injury is known as anterior glenohumeral instability of the shoulder and, as such, can be a secondary cause of impingement. This mechanism of injury was first described by Jobe et al. in 1989.[95]

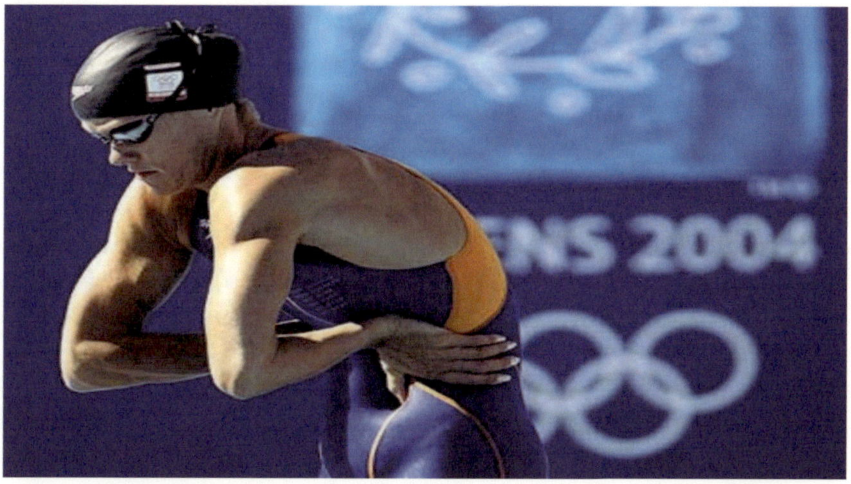

In the swimming population the shoulder joint is particularly vulnerable with 92% of propulsive forces coming from the upper extremity. The shoulder is the most injured area in swimmers with many publications citing different prevalence levels.[96–98] In a survey of 1,262 competitive swimmers from the United States the prevalence of shoulder pain ranged from 38–75%,[96] from a 1997 study up to 65% of swimmers reported shoulder pain.[97] A study on high-level swimmers demonstrated a prevalence of interfering pain necessitating a cessation or reduction of practice in 23% of athletes.[98] Signs of impingement with orthopaedic evaluation was revealed in 50% of the swimmers with pain, and a positive apprehension sign indicative of anterior instability was also seen in 50% of swimmers with pain. A study of collegiate and masters level swimmers reported a similar percentage prevalence of shoulder pain with 47 and 48%, respectively, experiencing shoulder pain lasting three weeks or more, despite the lesser distances and intensities associated with the latter group.[99]

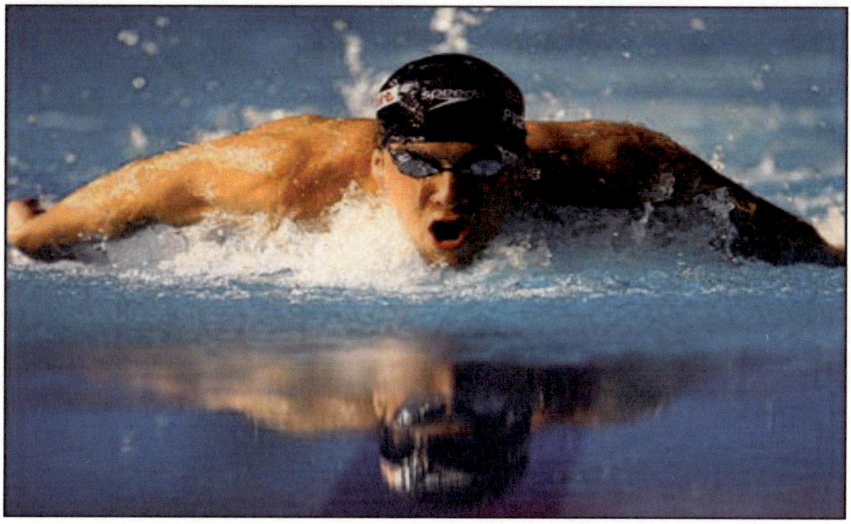

Other sports have also been extensively studied in the literature with volleyball players also reporting a high prevalence of shoulder pain. A recent study from The Netherlands investigated the epidemiology of injuries in volleyball players and determined a prevalence of 32% for overuse injuries of the shoulder, causing a mean absence from the sport of 9.4 weeks throughout a competitive year.[100] Shoulder pain syndromes represent the third most common injury among both female and male volleyball athletes and the second most common overuse-related condition, accounting for 8–20% of all volleyball injuries.[101] Elite volleyball players, but also baseball pitchers and tennis players are highly skilled sportspeople, but because of the intense practise, short recreational time, high intensity, and arm repetitive loads caused by specialisation on certain tasks in the game this will predispose the shoulder to injury. In volleyball the majority of the force imparted to the ball during a spike originates from the torso. It has been estimated that the elite volleyball athlete performs as many as 40,000 spikes in a season.[101] During a spike the scapula is involved in transferring kinetic energy to the upper limb and provides a stable base of support so that the upper limb can be correctly positioned in space during the performance of overhead skills. The dynamic stabilisers of the scapula and the humeral head are critical to maintaining the functional integrity of the glenohumeral joint; a change in one of the components of the shoulder girdle leads to a complete change in shoulder motion. This leads to depression and lateralisation of the dominant scapula compared with the non-dominant side.

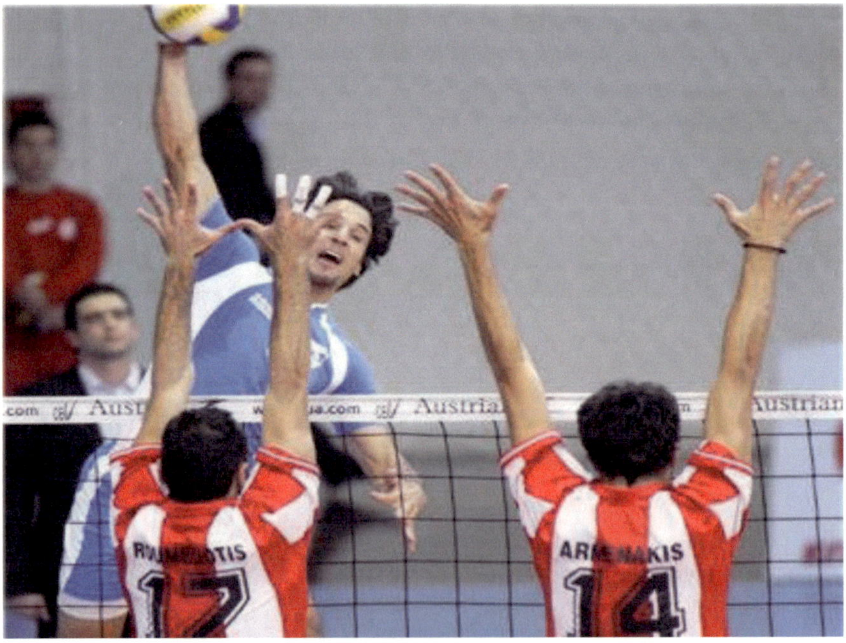

Interestingly, similar physical adaptations have subsequently been reported to occur among other overhead athletes, and the constellation of findings has been characterised in the literature as the 'SICK scapula' (scapular malposition, inferior medial border prominence, coracoid pain and malposition, and scapular dyskinesis).[102] The SICK scapula is associated with shoulder pain due to the spectrum of rotator cuff pathologies and functional instabilities.

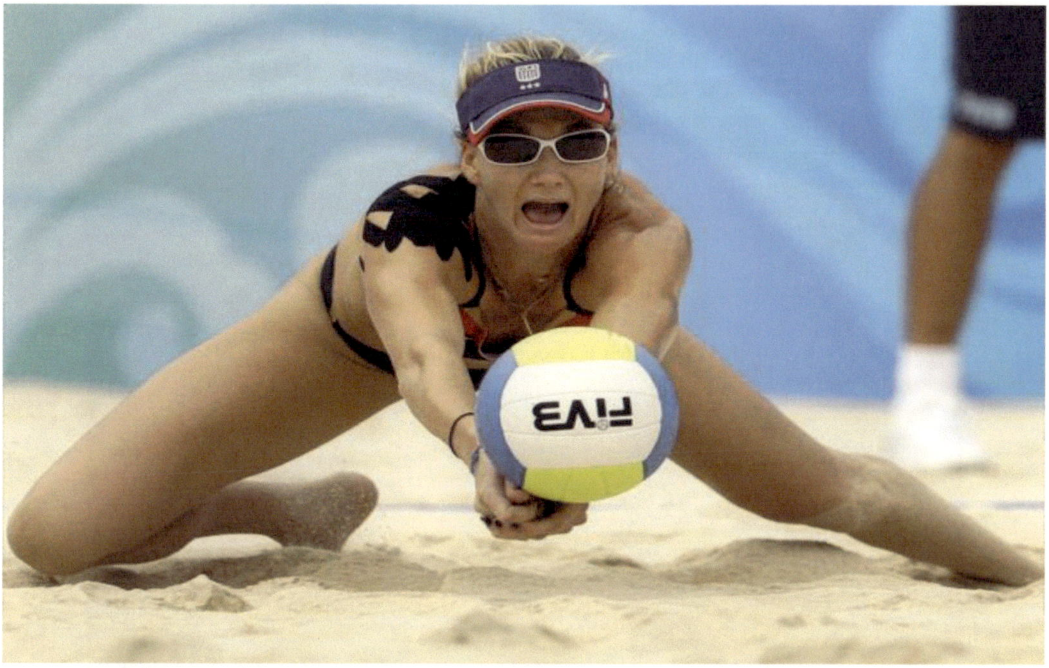

The prevalence of shoulder pain among professional male and female beach volleyball players is considerably lower than that in most other team sports; however, data from a recent cohort study showed the presence of three most common overuse conditions, low back pain (19%), knee pain (12%), and shoulder problems (10%).[103]

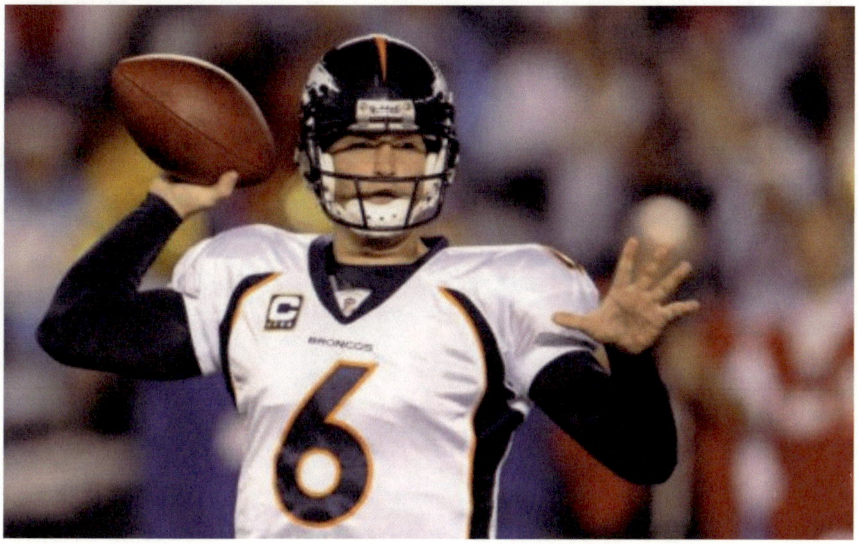

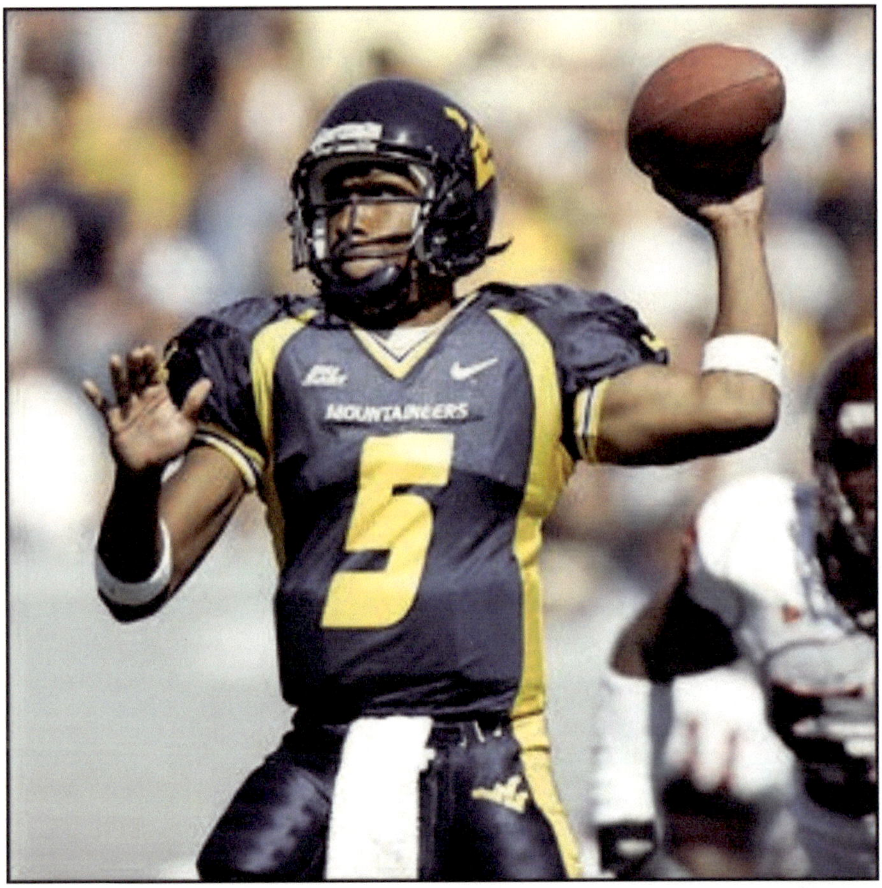
MOUNTAINEERS
5

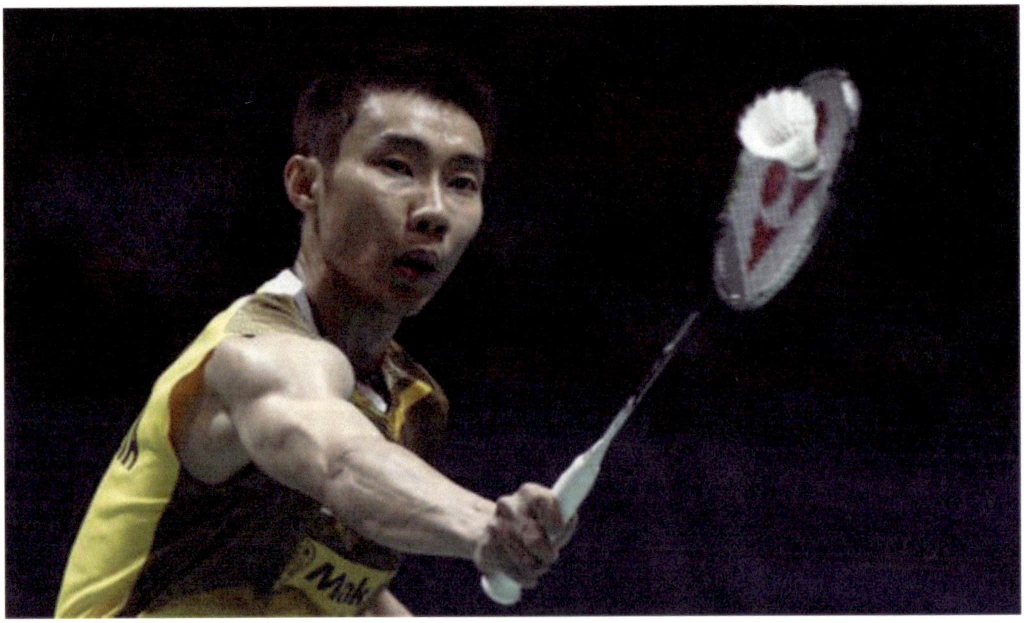

Shoulder injuries are also common in quarterbacks (in American Football) who are at risk for shoulder injury secondary to both the throwing motion as well as from contact injury.[104] Shoulder injuries are the second most common injury reported (15.2%). Overuse injuries were responsible for 14% of the injuries, the most common being rotator cuff tendinitis (6.1%) followed by biceps tendinitis (3.5%).

Previous or present pain in the dominant shoulder was reported by 52% of recreational badminton players,[105] and in a survey of world class players showed that previous or present shoulder pain on the dominant side was reported by 52% of the players.[106] Previous shoulder pain was reported by 37% of the players and ongoing shoulder pain by 20% of the players.

In the professional golfer, the shoulder is the third most commonly injured body area, after the lumbar spine and the wrist or hand, whereby for amateur golfers in the United States, the shoulder has been cited as the fourth most commonly affected site, trailing the lumbar spine, the elbow, and the wrist or hand.[107] The non-dominant shoulder is particularly vulnerable to injury, with most golf injuries occurring as a result of the golf swing, and mostly at impact of the head of the golf club with the turf. The prevalence of golf-related shoulder pain has been demonstrated at 12%.[108] Rotator cuff disease and subacromial impingement involving the lead shoulder are among the most common problems in golfers.[107]

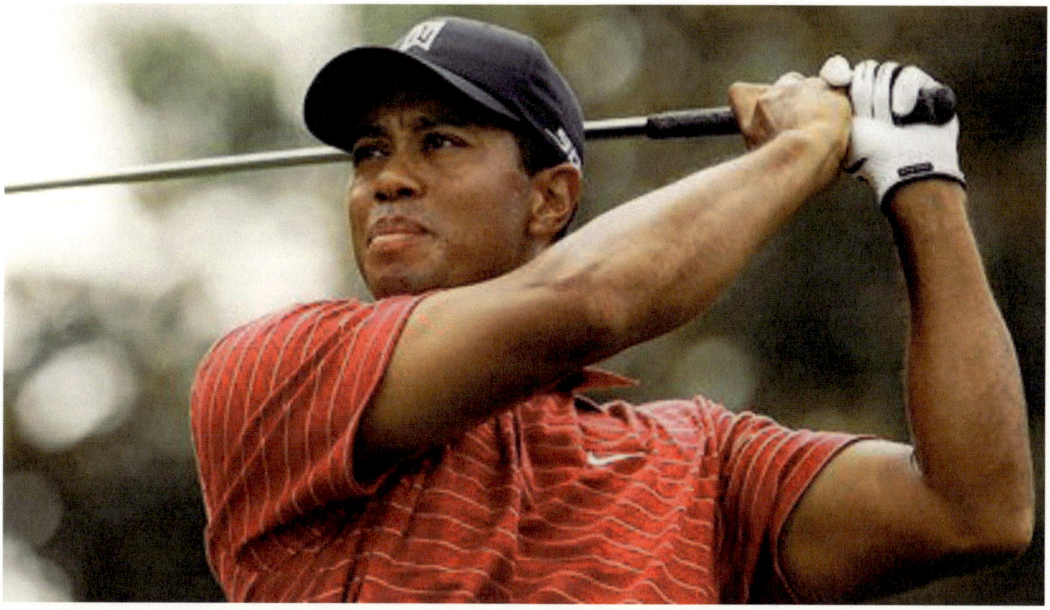

Shoulder pain has a very high prevalence in sports especially overhead sports due to the highly repetitious actions of the glenohumeral joint and high velocity forces transmitted through static and dynamic stabilising structures of the articulation, which eventually leads to breakdown of normal shoulder functioning. Inherently, the glenohumeral joint is capable of exceptional range of motion, however, this leads to a compromise in stability. Hence, when the dynamic stabilisers of the humeral head are placed under repetitive load — as seen in amateur and elite athletes such as swimmers, volleyball, softball or baseball players — this can lead to fatigue and failure of the dynamic stabilising structures, especially the rotator cuff. The net effect is disruption of the glenohumeral force couple leading to humeral superior migration and repetitive impingement of subacromial structures.

Epidemiological research in sports is necessary to determine the prevalence of sports-related injuries, and also to quantify the risk factors for injury inherent to individual sports, and to characterise the injury pattern typical of a sport. Injury to the athletic population leads to time lost from training and competition, and general participation in sports.

Risk factors for the development of a shoulder problem in athletes can be divided into intrinsic and extrinsic.[103] The modifiable intrinsic risk factors include: biomechanical considerations, conditioning and core stability, range of motion deficits, scapula dysfunction; while the non-modifiable factors include anatomy, sex and a history of previous injury that represents a strong risk factor for future injury. Extrinsic risk factors include the competitive situation and load placed on the joint, as seen in sports such as volleyball or tennis. The identification of risk factors will help implement prevention strategies aimed at improving technique, training and rehabilitation.

By improving or modifying technique, loads placed on the shoulder can be minimised, while through modification of training practices tissue overload can also be reduced allowing injured structures to repair and heal. Prevention of further injuries or recurrence of injury depends on providing the athlete with an accurate diagnosis and implementing a structured rehabilitation program so that any underlying biomechanical maladaptations are addressed that might precipitate reoccurrences of injury

When considering the sources of shoulder pain in athletes, most are derived from local structures located within the shoulder. The most common clinical diagnosis involves dysfunction of the rotator cuff with signs of impingement seen in 74% of shoulder pain sufferers.[109–111]

An ultimate goal of future research in the field of sports medicine should be a focus on injury prevention so that the athlete can remain competitive in the sporting arena. More research is needed in the identification of sports specific risk factors, but also effective interventions that may effectively reduce not only the risk of primary injury but also secondary re-injury so that the ability of athletes, whether amateur or elite, to participate and enjoy their sports is not compromised.

7. Conclusions

The findings from this narrative epidemiological review confirm that shoulder pain is a common complaint seen in the population and it is also a common presenting symptom to health care practitioners in clinical practice. The available data is mainly derived from the literature, with no quality descriptive data available on the chiropractic profession.

The prevalence of shoulder pain varies widely across different populations that have been studied (from 1–67%) and is probably due to different definitions used for defining shoulder pain. Using a pain drawing-based definition of shoulder pain restricted to an area in and around the shoulder complex is a recommendation for surveys assessing the prevalence of shoulder symptoms in the general population and clinical practice. To solve the problem of the poor specificity associated with symptom-based definitions it is useful to incorporate an additional classification to restrict the definition to more disabling problems.

Shoulder pain is most prevalent in middle age (45–64 years, from 21–55%), which may be attributed to the normal aging process of shoulder structures including the rotator cuff. This would most likely be due to degeneration, acute injury or pathology. Shoulder pain is also common in the younger age group (adolescents aged 12–18 years, from 12–57%) and can be attributed to a postural relationship associated with increased periods of sitting, advancement of technology with greater usage. In summary, the prevalence of shoulder pain is influenced by a number of factors: it tends to increase with age, has a strong gender relationship and is more common in women, and is particularly prevalent in psychologically stressed populations, especially women and adolescents.

Shoulder pain is common in working populations and is due to a multitude of factors including physical and psychosocial. It is one of the most common musculoskeletal problems seen in workers and demonstrates a strong age and female gender relationship. Physical factors associated with the onset and prevalence of shoulder pain in the working population include physical load and vibration, repetitive movements, work-related posture, and also the duration of computer and mouse use in a work setting. A number of psychosocial variables correlate with shoulder pain in workers including high mental demands, low job satisfaction and poor social support.

Author details

Mario Pribicevic
Faculty of Science, Macquarie University, Australia

8. References

[1] Bjelle A. Epidemiology of shoulder problems. Baillieres Clinical Rheumatology 1989; 3,437–511.

[2] Anderson JAD. Industrial rheumatology and the shoulder. British Journal of Rheumatology 1987; 26: 326–328.

[3] Sommerich CM, McGlothin JD, Maras WS. Occupational risk factors associated with soft tissue disorders of the shoulder: a review of recent investigations in the literature. Ergonomics 1993; 36(6): 697–717.

[4] McBeth J, Jones K. Epidemiology of chronic musculoskeletal pain. Best Practice & Research Clinical Rheumatology 2007; Vol. 21, No. 3, pp. 403–425.

[5] Croft P, Pope D, Silman A. The clinical course of shoulder pain: prospective cohort study in primary care. Primary Care Rheumatology Society Shoulder Study Group. Br Med J 1996; 313:601–2.

[6] Van der Windt DA, Koes BW, Boeke AJ, Deville W, De Jong BA, Bouter LM. Shoulder disorders in general practice: prognostic indicators of outcome. Br J Gen Pract 1996; 46:519–23.

[7] Hasvold T, Johnsen R. Headache and neck or shoulder pain- frequent and disabling conditions in the general population. Scandinavian Journal of Primary Health Care 1993; 11(3): 219–224.

[8] Pope DP, Croft PR, Pritchard CM, Silman AJ. Prevalence of shoulder pain in the community: the influence of case definition. Annals of Rheumatic Diseases 1997; 56: 308–312.

[9] Parsons S, Breen A, Foster NE, Letley L, Pincus T, Vogel S, et al. Prevalence and comparative troublesomeness by age of musculoskeletal pain in different body locations. Fam Pract, 2007. 24(4): p. 308–16.

[10] Elliott AM, Smith BH, Penny KI, Smith WC, Chambers WA. The epidemiology of chronic pain in the community. Lancet 2002; 354: 1248–1252.

[11] Breivik H, Collett B, Ventafridda V, Cohen R, Gallacher D. Survey of chronic pain in Europe: prevalence, impact on daily life and treatment. Eur J Pain 2005; 10(4):287–333.

[12] Picavet HS, Schouten JS. Musculoskeletal pain in the Netherlands: prevalence's, consequences and risk groups, the DMC(3)-study. Pain 2003. 102(1–2): p. 167–78.

[13] Takala J, Sievers K, Klaukka T. Rheumatic symptoms in the middle-aged population in Southwestern Finland. Scandinavian Journal of Rheumatology 1982; 47(Supplement): 15–29.

[14] Cunningham LS, Kelsey JL. Epidemiology of musculoskeletal impairments and associated disability. American Journal of Public Health 1984; 74(6): 574–579.

[15] Bergenudd H, Lindga¨rde F, Nilsson B, Peterson CJ. Shoulder pain in middle age. A study of prevalence and relation to occupational work load and psychosocial factors. Clinical Orthopaedics 1988; 231: 234–238.

[16] Anderson HI, Ejlertsson G, Leden I, Rosenberg C. Chronic pain in a geographically defined general population: studies of differences in age, gender, social class, and pain localization. The Clinical Journal of Pain 1993 Sep; 9(3): 174–182.

[17] Urwin M, Symmons D, Allison T, Brammah T, Busby H, Roxby M et al. Estimating the burden of musculoskeletal disorders in the community: the comparative prevalence of symptoms at different anatomical sites, and the relation to social deprivation. Annals of Rheumatic Diseases 1998; 57: 649–655.

[18] Makela M, Heliovaara M, Sainio P, Knekt P, Impivaara O, Aromaa A. Shoulder joint impairment among Finns aged 30 years or over: prevalence, risk factors and co-morbidity. Rheumatology (Oxford) 1999 Jul; 38(7): 656–662.

[19] Badley EM, Tennant A. Changing profile of joint disorders with age: findings from a postal survey of the population of Calderdale, West Yorkshire, United Kingdom. Annals of Rheumatic Diseases 1992; 51(3): 366–371.

[20] Chard MD, Hazleman R, Hazleman BL, King Rh, Reiss BB. Shoulder disorders in the elderly: a community survey. Arthritis and Rheumatism 1991; 34: 766–769.

[21] Urwin M, Symmons D, Allison T, Brammah T, Busby H, Roxby M et al Estimating the burden of musculoskeletal disorders in the community: the comparative prevalence of symptoms at different anatomical sites, and the relation to social deprivation. Ann Rheum Dis 1998; 57:649–55.

[22] Jones JR, Hodgson JT, Clegg TA, Elliott RC. Self-reported work related illness in 1995. Norwich: HMSO, 1998.

[23] McCormick A, Fleming D, Charlton J. Morbidity statistics from general practice. Fourth national study 1991–92. London: HMSO, 1996:55.

[24] Badcock LJ, Lewis M, Hay EM, Croft PR. Consultation and the outcome of shoulder-neck pain: a cohort study in the population. J Rheumatol 2003; 30:2694–9.

[25] Walker Bone K, Palmer KT, Reading I, Coggon D, Cooper C. Prevalence and impact of musculoskeletal disorders of the upper limb in the general population. Arthritis Rheum 2004; 51:642–51.

[26] Christensen MG, Kollasch MW. Overview of Survey Response. In: Job analysis of chiropractic: a project report, survey analysis and summary of the practice of chiropractic within the United States. Greeley, CO: National Board of Chiropractic Examiners; 2005.

[27] Van der Windt DA, Koes BW, De jong BA, Bouter LM. Shoulder disorders in general practice: incidence, patient characteristics, and management. Annals of Rheumatic Disorders,1995; 54(12) 959–964.

[28] Bot SD, van der Waal JM,Terwee CB, van der Windt DA, Schellevis FG, Bouter LM et al. Incidence and prevalence of complaints of the neck and upper extremity in general practice. Ann Rheum Dis, 2005. 64(1): p. 118–23.

[29] Vechio P, Kavanagh R, Hazleman BL, King RH. Shoulder pain in a community based rheumatology clinic. British Journal of Rheumatology 1995; 34 440–442.

[30] Linsell L, Dawson J, Zondervan K, Rose P, Randall T, Fitzpatrick R et al. Prevalence and incidence of adults consulting for shoulder conditions in UK primary care; patterns of diagnosis and referral. Rheumatology (Oxford) 2006; 45(2): p. 215–21.

[31] Perquin CW, Hazebroek-Kampschreur AAJM, Hunfield JAM. Pain in children and adolescents: a common experience. Pain 2000; 87: 51–58.

[32] Siivola SM, Levoska S, Latvala K, Hoskio E, Vanharanta H, Keinanen-Kiukaanniemi S. Predictive factors for neck and shoulder pain: a longitudinal study in young adults. Spine, 2004. 29(15): p. 1662–9.

[33] Diepenmaat AC, van der Wal MF, de Vet HC, Hirasing RA. Neck/shoulder, low back, and arm pain in relation to computer use, physical activity, stress, and depression among Dutch adolescents. Pediatrics 2006 Feb; 117(2): 412–416.

[34] Vikat A, Rimpela M, Salminen JJ, Rimpela A, Savolainen A, Virtanen SM. Neck or shoulder pain and low back pain in Finnish adolescents. Scand J Public Health, 2000. 28(3): p. 164–73.

[35] Hakala P, Rimpela A, Salminen JJ, Virtanen SM, Rimpela M. Back, neck, and shoulder pain in Finnish adolescents: national cross sectional surveys. BMJ, 2002. 325(7367): p. 743.

[36] van der Windt DA, Croft PR. Shoulder pain. In Crombie IK, Croft PR, Linton SJ, LeResche L & Von Korff M (eds.). Epidemiology of Pain a report of the Task Force on Epidemiology of the International Association for the Study of Pain. Seattle: IASP Press, 1999, pp. 257–281.

[37] Punnett L, Herbert R. Work-related musculoskeletal disorders: is there a gender differential, and if so, what does it mean? Women and Health 2000; 38(6): 474–492.

[38] Walker-Bone K, Palmer KT, Reading I, Cooper C. Soft-tissue rheumatic disorders of the neck and upper limb: prevalence and risk factors. Seminars in Arthritis and Rheumatism 2003; 33(3): 185–203.

[39] Treaster DE, Burr D. Gender differences in prevalence of upper extremity musculoskeletal disorders. Ergonomics 2004; 47(5): 495–526.

[40] Larsson B, Sogaard K. Work related neck–shoulder pain: a review on magnitude, risk factors, biochemical characteristics, clinical picture and preventive interventions. Best Practice & Research Clinical Rheumatology 2007 Vol. 21, No. 3, pp. 447–463.

[41] Unruh AM, Ritchie J, Merskey H. Does gender affect appraisal of pain and pain coping strategies? The Clinical Journal of Pain 1999 Mar; 15(1): 31–40.

[42] Chesterton LS, Barlas P, Foster NE, Baxter DG, Wright CC. Gender differences in pressure pain threshold in healthy humans. Pain 2003 Mar; 101(3): 259–266.

[43] Wijnhoven HA, de Vet HC, Picavet HS. Prevalence of musculoskeletal disorders is systematically higher in women than in men. The Clinical Journal of Pain 2006 Oct; 22(8): 717–724.

[44] Ekberg K, Karlsson M, Axelson O, Bjorkqvist B, Bjerre-Kiely B, Malm P Cross-sectional study of risk factors for symptoms in the neck and shoulder area. Ergonomics 1995, 38: 971–980.

[45] Skov T, Borg V, Orhede E. Psychosocial and physical risk factors for musculoskeletal disorders of the neck, shoulders, and lower back in salespeople. Occupational and Environmental Medicine 1996, 53: 351–356.

[46] Chard MD, Hazleman BL. Shoulder disorders in the elderly (a hospital study). Ann Rheum Dis. 1987 Sep; 46(9):684–7.

[47] Vogt MT, Simonsick EM, Harris TB, Nevitt MC, Kang JD, Rubin SM et al. Neck and shoulder pain in 70- to 79-year-old men and women: findings from the Health, Aging and Body Composition Study. Spine J, 2003. 3(6): p. 435–41.

[48] Bergenudd H, Nilsson B. The prevalence of locomotor complaints in middle age and their relationship to health and socioeconomic factors. Clinical Orthopaedics and Related Research 1994, 308: 264–270.

[49] Marcus M, Gerr F. Upper extremity musculoskeletal symptoms among female office workers: associations with video display terminal use and occupational psychosocial stressors. American Journal of Industrial Medicine 1996, 29: 161–170.

[50] McCracken LM, Matthews AK, Tang TS, Cuba SL. A comparison of blacks and whites seeking treatment for chronic pain. The Clinical Journal of Pain 2001 Sep; 17(3): 249–255.

[51] Jensen C, Borg V, Finsen L, Hansen K, Juul-Kristensen B, Christensen H. Job demands, muscle activity and musculoskeletal symptoms in relation to work with the computer mouse. Scand J Work Environ Health1998;24:418-24.

[52] Andersen JH, Haahr JP, P Frost. Risk factors for more severe regional musculoskeletal symptoms: a two-year prospective study of a general working population. Arthritis Rheum, 2007. 56(4): 1355–64.

[53] Leclerc A, Chastang JF, Niedhammer I, Landre MF, Roquelaure A. Incidence of shoulder pain in repetitive work. Occup Environ Med, 2004. 61(1): p. 39–44.

[54] Malchaire J, Cock N, Vergracht S. Review of the factors associated with musculoskeletal problems in epidemiological studies. International Archives of Occupational and Environmental Health 2001; 74(2): 79–90.

[55] van der Windt DA, Thomas E, Pope DP. Occupational risk factors for shoulder pain: a systematic review. Occupational and Environmental Medicine 2000; 57(7): 433–442.

[56] Bergenudd H, Lindgarde F, Nilsson B, Petersson CJ. Shoulder pain in middle age a study of prevalence and relation to occupational work load and sychosocial factors. Clinical Orthopaedics and Related Research 1987,231 234–237.

[57] Ariens GA, van MechelenW, Bongers PM, Bouter LM, van der Wal G. Physical risk factors for neck pain. Scandinavian Journal of Work, Environment and Health 2000; 26(1): 7–19.

[58] Malchaire J, Cock N, Vergracht S. Review of the factors associated with musculoskeletal problems in epidemiological studies. International Archives of Occupational and Environmental Health 2001; 74(2): 79–90.

[59] Grooten WJ, Mulder M, Josephson M, Alfredsson L, Wiktorin C. The influence of work-related exposures on the prognosis of neck/shoulder pain. Eur Spine J. 2007 Dec; 16(12):2083–91.

[60] Miranda H, Punnett L, Viikari-Juntura E, Heliövaara M, Knekt P. Physical work and chronic shoulder disorder. Results of a prospective population-based study. Ann Rheum Dis. 2008 Feb; 67(2):218–23. Epub 2007 May 25.

[61] Devereux JJ, Vlachonikolis IG, Buckle PW. Epidemiological study to investigate potential interaction between physical and psychosocial factors at work that may increase the risk of symptoms of musculoskeletal disorder of the neck and upper limb. Occup Environ Med 2002; 59:269–277.

[62] Stenlund B, Goldie I, Hagberg M. Shoulder tendinitis and its relation to heavy manual work and exposure to vibration. Scand J Work Environ Health 1993; 19:43–9.

[63] Frost P, Andersen JH. Shoulder impingement syndrome in relation to shoulder intensive work. Occupational and Environmental Medicine 1999; 56, 494–498.
[64] Herbets P, Kadefors R, Hogfors C, Sigholm G. Shoulder pain and heavy manual labour. Clinical Orthopeadics and Related Research 1984; 191 166–177
[65] Hughes RE, Silverstein BA, Evanoff BA. Risk factors for work-related musculoskeletal disorders in an aluminum smelter. Am J Ind Med 1997;32:66–75.
[66] Burdorf A, Van Riel M, Brand T. Physical load as risk factor for musculoskeletal complaints among tank terminal workers. Am Ind Hyg Assoc J 1997;58:489–97.
[67] Johansson JA. Psychosocial work factors, physical work load and associated musculoskeletal symptoms among home care workers. Scand J Psychol 1995;36:113–29.
[68] Jacobsson L, Lindgärde F, Manthorpe R. Effect of education, occupation, and some lifestyle factors on common rheumatic complaints in a Swedish group aged 50–70 years. Ann Rheum Dis 1992;51:835–43.
[69] Sobti A, Cooper C, Inskip H, Searle S, Coggon D. Occupational physical activity and long-term risk of musculoskeletal symptoms: a national survey of post office pensioners. Am J Ind Med 1997;32:76–83.
[70] Sim J, Lacey RJ, Lewis M. The impact of workplace risk factors on the occurrence of neck and upper limb pain: a general population study. BMC Public Health, 2006. 6: p. 234.
[71] Pope DP, Croft PR, Pritchard CM, Silman AJ, Macfarlane GJ. Occupational factors related to shoulder pain and disability. Occup Environ Med 1997; 54:316–21.
[72] Nahit ES, Macfarlane GJ, Pritchard CM, Cherry NM, Silman AJ. Short term influence of mechanical factors on regional musculoskeletal pain: a study of new workers from 12 occupational groups. Occup Environ Med 2001; 58:374–81.
[73] Fredriksson K, Alfredsson L, Ahlberg G, Josephson M, Kilbom A, Wigaeus Hjelm E et al. Work environment and neck and shoulder pain: the influence of exposure time. Results from a population based case-control study. Occup Environ Med 2002; 59:182–8.
[74] Dembe AE. The changing nature of office work: effects on repetitive strain injuries. Occup Med 1999, 14:61–72.
[75] Hakala PT, Rimpelä AH, Saarni LA, Salminen JJ. Frequent computer-related activities increase the risk of neck-shoulder and low back pain in adolescents. Eur J Public Health. 2006 Oct; 16(5):536–41.
[76] Diepenmaat AC, van der Wal MF, de Vet HC, Hirasing RA. Neck/shoulder, low back, and arm pain in relation to computer use, physical activity, stress, and depression among Dutch adolescents. Pediatrics. 2006 Feb; 117(2):412–6.
[77] Eltayeb S, Staal JB, Kennes J, Lamberts PH, de Bie RA. Prevalence of complaints of arm, neck and shoulder among computer office workers and psychometric evaluation of a risk factor questionnaire. BMC Musculoskelet Disord 2007 Jul; 14; 8:68.
[78] Juul-Kristensen B, Søgaard K, Strøyer J, Jensen C. Computer users' risk factors for developing shoulder, elbow and back symptoms. Scand J Work Environ Health. 2004 Oct; 30(5):390–8.

[79] Brandt LP, Andersen JH, Lassen CF, Kryger A, Overgaard E, Vilstrup I, Mikkelsen S. Neck and shoulder symptoms and disorders among Danish computer workers. Scand J Work Environ Health. 2004 Oct; 30(5):399–409.

[80] Andersen JH, Harhoff M, Grimstrup S, Vilstrup I, Lassen CF, Brandt LPA et al. Computer mouse use predicts acute pain but not prolonged or chronic pain in the neck and shoulder. Occup. Environ. Med. 2008; 65; 126–131.

[81] Jones JR, Hodgson JT, Clegg TA, Elliott RC. Self-reported work-related illness in 1995. Results from a household survey. HMSO 1998, London, pp 180.

[82] Aronsson G, Gustafsson K, Dallner M. Sick but yet at work. An empirical study of sickness presenteeism. Journal of Epidemiology Community Health 2000, 54, 502–509.

[83] Stewart WF, Ricci JA, Chee E, Morganstein D, Lipton R. Lost productive time and cost due to common pain conditions in the US workforce. JAMA 2003, 290(18), 2443–2454.

[84] Van Leeuwen MT, Blyth F M, March LM, Nicholas M K,Cousins M J. Chronic pain and reduced work effectiveness: The hidden cost to Australian employers. European Journal of Pain 2006, 10, 161–166.

[85] van den Heuvel SG E, IJmker S, Blatter BM, de Korte EM. Loss of Productivity Due to Neck/Shoulder Symptoms and Hand/Arm Symptoms: Results from the PROMO-Study. J Occup Rehabil (2007) 17:370–382.

[86] Harkness EF, Macfarlane GJ, Nahit ES, Silman AJ, McBeth J. Mechanical and psychosocial factors predict new onset shoulder pain: a prospective cohort study of newly employed workers. Occup Environ Med. 2003 Nov; 60(11):850–7.

[87] Nahit ES, Hunt IM, Lunt M, Dunn G, Silman AJ, Macfarlane GJ. Effects of psychosocial and individual psychological factors on the onset of musculoskeletal pain: common and site-specific effects. Ann Rheum Dis 2003, 62:755–760.

[88] Cole DC, Ibrahim S, Shannon HS. Predictors of work-related repetitive strain injuries in a population cohort. Am J Public Health 2005, 95:1233–1237.

[89] Reilingh ML, Kuijpers T, Tanja-Harfterkamp AM, van der Windt DA. Course and prognosis of shoulder symptoms in general practice. Rheumatology (Oxford). 2008 May; 47(5):724–30.

[90] Bot SD, van der Waal JM, Terwee CB, van der Windt DA, Scholten RJ, Bouter LM et al. Predictors of outcome in neck and shoulder symptoms: a cohort study in general practice. Spine. 2005 Aug 15; 30(16):E459–70.

[91] Van der Heijden GJ. Shoulder disorders: a state-of-the-art review. Baillieres Best Pract Res Clin Rheumatol 1999; 13:287–309.

[92] Kuijpers T, Van der Windt DAWM, Van der Heijden GJGM, Bouter LM. Systematic review of prognostic cohort studies on shoulder disorders. Pain 2004; 109:420–31.

[93] Kuijpers T, van der Windt DAWM, Boeke JP, Twisk JWR, Vergouwe Y, Bouter LM et al. Clinical prediction rules for the prognosis of shoulder pain in general practice. Pain 120 (2006) 276–285

[94] Hoozemans MJ, Kuijer PP, Kingma I, van Dieen JH, de Vries WH, van der Woude LH et al. Pushing and Pulling in Association With Low Back and Shoulder Complaints. Occup Environ Med 2002, 59:696–702.

[95] Jobe FW, Kvitne RS, Giangarra CE. Shoulder pain in the overhand or throwing athlete. The relationship of anterior instability and rotator cuff impingement. Orthop Rev. 1989 Sep; 18(9):963–75.

[96] McMaster WC, Troup J. A survey of interfering shoulder pain in United States competitive swimmers. Am J Sports Med. 1993 Jan-Feb; 21(1):67–70.

[97] Bak K, Faunø P. Clinical findings in competitive swimmers with shoulder pain. Am J Sports Med. 1997 Mar-Apr; 25(2):254–60.

[98] Rupp S, Berninger K, Hopf T. Shoulder problems in high level swimmers—impingement, anterior instability, muscular imbalance? Int J Sports Med. 1995 Nov; 16(8):557–62.

[99] Stocker D, Pink M, Jobe FW. Comparison of shoulder injury in collegiate- and master's-level swimmers. Clin J Sport Med. 1995; 5(1):4–8.

[100] Verhagen EA, Van der Beek AJ, Bouter LM, Bahr RM, Van Mechelen W. A one season prospective cohort study of volleyball injuries. Br J Sports Med. 2004 Aug; 38(4):477–81.

[101] J C Reeser, E Verhagen, W W Briner, T I Askeland, R Bahr. Strategies for the prevention of volleyball related injuries. Br J Sports Med 2006; 40:594–600.

[102] Burkhart SS, Morgan CD, Kibler WB. The disabled throwing shoulder: spectrum of pathology. Part III: the SICK scapula, scapular dyskinesis, the kinetic chain, and rehabilitation. Arthroscopy 2003; 19:641–61.

[103] Bahr R, Reeser JC. Fédération Internationale de Volleyball. Injuries among world-class professional beach volleyball players. The Fédération Internationale de Volleyball beach volleyball injury study. Am J Sports Med 2003; Jan-Feb; 31(1):119–25.

[104] Kelly BT, Barnes RP, Powell JW, Warren RF. Shoulder injuries to quarterbacks in the national football league. Am J Sports Med 2004; Mar; 32(2):328–31.

[105] Fahlström M, Söderman K. Decreased shoulder function and pain common in recreational badminton players. Scand J Med Sci Sports. 2007 Jun; 17(3):246—51.

[106] Fahlström M, Yeap JS, Alfredson H, Söderman K. Shoulder pain—a common problem in world-class badminton players. Scand J Med Sci Sports. 2006 Jun; 16(3):168–73.

[107] Kim DH, Millett PJ, Warner JP, Jobe FW. Shoulder Injuries in Golf. Am. J. Sports Med. 2004; 32; 1324.

[108] McHardy A, Pollard H, Luo K. One-year follow-up study on golf injuries in Australian amateur golfers. Am J Sports Med. 2007 Aug; 35(8):1354–60.

[109] Baring T, Emery R, Reilly P. Management of rotator cuff disease: specific treatment for specific disorders. Best Practice & Research Clinical Rheumatology 2007; 21; 2, 279–294.

[110] Morison DS, Greenbaum BS, Einhorn A. Shoulder impingement. Orthop Clin North Am 2000;31:285–93.

[111] Pink MM, Tibone JE. The painful shoulder in the swimming athlete. Orthop Clin North Am 2000;31:247–61.

[112] Images from google images, www.google.com Date accessed: 10/09/12

Chapter 8

Knee Pain in Adults & Adolescents, Diagnosis and Treatment

Sherif Hosny, W. McClatchie, Nidhi Sofat and Caroline B. Hing

Additional information is available at the end of the chapter

http://dx.doi.org/10.5772/51077

1. Introduction

Knee pain is a common symptom affecting both children and adults [1]. Assessment of pain is important in order to determine the aetiology of the underlying condition which can be investigated with mechanistic studies further in order to assess the response to treatment interventions.

We performed a literature search to identify pertinent review articles investigating advances in knee pain diagnosis and management in humans using the MeSH terms and Boolean operators 'knee' AND 'pain'. We identified 11928 relevant articles and limited our search to review articles on humans in English. The structure of the chapter is divided into subheadings covering definition, incidence, aetiology, classification, diagnosis and management. Within each subheading, further sections address the use of novel imaging to quantify disease progression, operative and non-operative management. A separate section will outline the causes and treatment of knee pain in adolescents. A further section outlines future advances in diagnosis and management.

2. Definition

Knee pain is broadly divided into tibiofemoral and anterior knee pain (AKP). Knee pain can be referred from the hip or present as part of radiculopathy. AKP can refer to a number of symptoms. In the past the terms 'chondromalacia patellae' and 'patellofemoral pain' have been used loosely to describe such symptoms. This is to be avoided, as whilst both conditions are recognised, they may not be the cause of the pain. The term 'anterior knee pain' may be used when no specific diagnosis has been made [2].

Jackson et al (2001) divided the causes of AKP broadly into two groups [1]. The first group includes focal lesions which can be identified clinically or radiologically, and is described as *distinct*. This includes overuse syndromes, trauma related lesions, dysplasias, tumours, and iatrogenic lesions. The second group is described as *obscure* and includes types of knee pain that are dynamic, or are more difficult to define. The symptoms may vary widely between individuals with the same clinical findings. This includes patellar maltracking, chondromalacia, idiopathic pain, reflex sympathetic dystrophy and psychogenic pain.

Tibiofemoral knee pain can be described as *acute* or *chronic*. Acute symptoms are often mechanical in nature and due to a recent injury. Pain may arise from acute injury to the menisci, and / or to the ligamentous stabilisers of the knee. Resultant alteration to the biomechanics of the joint can lead to degenerative change and associated symptoms.

Chronic knee pain is commonly due to arthritic change. Osteoarthritis (OA) is the most common and is a degenerative condition caused by focal cartilage loss. It is often described according to conventional radiological findings as described by Kellgren and Lawrence [3]. These include osteophyte formation, narrowing of joint space, sclerosis of subchondral bone and cyst formation. Utilising these changes as a guide, five grades were used to describe OA: 1. None, 2. doubtful, 3. minimal, 4. moderate and 5. Severe [2]. Ahlbäck [4] described the radiographic changes in terms of joint space narrowing (Grades I-II) and bone attrition (Grades III – V). The American College of Rheumatology's classification of OA mentions knee pain occurring over most days of the previous month, crepitus on joint movement and morning stiffness. The World Health Organisation (WHO) Global Burden of Disease defined OA of the knee as a combination of these clinical criteria in the presence of defined radiological changes [5].

Rheumatoid arthritis (RA) is a destructive chronic inflammatory condition that affects the small joints of the hands and feet, along with larger joints. Symptoms initially include pain and swelling as the synovial lining of the joint is inflamed. Chronic progression of the disease leads to cartilage erosion and joint laxity resulting in deformity. Conversely, crystal arthropathy results from the deposition of monosodium urate (gout) or calcium pyrophosphate (pseudogout) within the knee joint. The precipitation of these crystal induces an inflammatory reaction within the joint.

3. Incidence / prevalence

There is some difficulty in establishing the true incidence of knee pain, as the actual definition of knee pain varies according to its cause. Most data available relates to arthritis, as it is a chronic disabling condition, with a significant impact on health. In a cross sectional study of 3341 residents aged over 65 in Oxfordshire, United Kingdom, the prevalence of knee pain was 32.6%, using the SF-36 questionnaire [6].

There is a paucity of reports on the prevalence of knee pain from developed countries, Haq 2011 [7] reported global findings from the Community Orientated Program for Control Of Rheumatic Disorders (COPCORD). Wide variation in knee pain was seen both between rural and urban settings and also between countries. In all studies the prevalence of knee pain was greater in women than in men. Rural Iran had the highest recorded prevalence of 39.2% across the population.

A cohort study by Ingham et 2011 [8] found the risk of knee pain for people over the age of forty in the United Kingdom was 32/1000 person-years (3.2%) or a 12-year cumulative incidence of knee pain of 34.4% (32% for men, 35% for women). There was an increasing trend observed with increasing body mass index. The incidence in a Bangladeshi rural community recorded through COPCORD was only 6.5%.

The incidence of reported knee pain in older patients is increasing, yet this does not always correlate with radiographic changes associated with arthritis. Nguyen et al 1999 [9] reported on three separate time periods measured by the Framingham Osteoarthritis Study in the US. This showed the prevalence of knee pain in men between 2002 and 2005 was 32.9%, and 27.7% in women. An increasing trend in reported knee pain was observed over three decades in the over 70 age group. Surprisingly this trend did not correlate with an increasing body mass index (BMI), confounding the observation seen elsewhere that increased BMI correlates with an increased incidence of OA.

Symptomatic OA in younger patients was recorded by the 1987 Framingham study. Five percent of those over 26 years of age had pain along with radiological changes, with 6.7% of those over 45 years of age reporting the same symptoms. McAlindon et al 1992 [10] reported the prevalence of symptomatic isolated patellofemoral osteoarthritis of 11% in males over 55 years, and 24% in women over 55 years. In asymptomatic patients 3.8% of both men and women had isolated radiographic patellofemoral OA.

Jarvholm et al 2008 [11] reported that occupational factors are important risk factors for developing OA of the knee. In a population of male construction workers in Sweden the relative risk for surgically treated OA of the knee was 4.7. Those with more labour intensive roles had an increased risk. In a study of Finnish forestry workers the incidence of knee pain was 10% over a one year period [12]. Increased age, being overweight and knee straining activities all increased the likelihood of developing pain. The persistence of symptoms was associated with increased age and job dissatisfaction.

It is difficult to establish the exact incidence of knee pain specifically due to RA, although there appears to be a decreasing trend in knee arthroplasty for these patients. In a study of Californian adults over two decades Louie et al 2010 [13] noted that the demand for knee arthroplasty decreased in younger patients, and paralleled the general population requirements in older patients. The introduction of the use of methotrexate in the 1970s, and more recently the use of Tumour Necrosis Factor α has been attributed to milder forms of the disease and the slowing of radiographic deterioration [14].

4. Aetiology

In order to understand the aetiology of anterior knee pain it is vital to appreciate the biomechanical factors governing normal loading conditions. The weight distribution through the knee is governed by the mechanical axis of the lower limb. Usually this passes through or just medial to the centre of the knee joint in the coronal plane. Deviation of the mechanical axis away from this leads to increased contact stresses at the joint surface.

Morrison et al 1970 [15] showed that the mean maximum joint force at the knee was 3.03 times body weight (range 2.06-4.0) during normal gait cycle. During stance phase the centre of pressure passed through the medial side of the joint, indicating that most of the joint force is centred there.

Understanding the movement of the tibiofemoral joint is aided by magnetic resonance imaging (MRI) studies [16]. As the knee flexes the femoral condyles roll backwards and slide on the tibia. This mechanism, along with the increasing arc of curvature of the posterior aspect of the femoral condyles, allows increased flexion of the knee. Dynamic studies have shown the lateral femoral condyle to have increased backward movement of the contact area relative to the medial femoral condyle. This in effect produces rotation of the tibia internally as the knee flexes.

The patella forms part of the extensor mechanism of the knee and has thick articular cartilage to withstand the joint reaction force. It allows an increased lever arm of the extensor mechanism which enhances its strength. The medial and lateral articular facets enter the trochlear groove of the femur at 20° of flexion and maximum contact is achieved with the femur at 45°. The peak contact pressures within the patellofemoral joint occur between 60° and 90° of flexion. This range corresponds to the areas where degenerative lesions are most commonly seen. In the simple action of rising from a chair the force going through the patellar tendon can reach 3.6 times body weight [17]. The joint reaction force can reach 385 N during walking, and reach 5972 N when landing from a jump [18].

Hip pathology, from childhood through to adulthood may present as femoral or knee pain and must be eliminated as a cause of symptoms, as does neurological pain due to proximal nerve lesions. Pain is transmitted from nociceptors distributed around the knee. Articular cartilage does not contain nerve endings, therefore damage to this layer is not a direct source of pain. Nociceptor fibres, including those transmitting substance P, have been found to be widely distributed in the soft tissues around the knee joint [19], including the retinaculum, synovium and fat pad. Higher concentrations have been found immediately surrounding blood vessels, suggesting a role in vascular tone and extravasation of fluid leading swelling and effusion. Biedert et al 1992 [20] found increased concentration of type IVa nerve fibres were found in the retinaculum, patellar ligament and pes anserinus. Gronsblad 1985 [21] reported the presence of Substance P-immunofluorescent nerves and enkephalin-immunofluorescent nerves in the synovial membrane and the menisci. Dye 1998 [22] underwent arthroscopy of his own knees while conscious, and identified anterior synovium, fat pad and joint capsule as the most sensitive areas to pain. The insertion of the cruciate tendons provokes some pain, as did peripheral meniscus. The articular surface of the patella did not evoke significant discomfort. Hochmann et 2011 [7] looked at the contribution of neuropathic pain in patients with chronic knee pain. Having excluded those with pre-existing neurological conditions, 19% reported symptoms consistent with neuropathic pain.

Arthritic pain is commonly described as a dull ache, which is made worse on movement after a period of rest. While the loss of articular cartilage in osteoarthritis is not a direct source of pain, the resultant changes to the subchondral bone show radiological and histological changes. The loss of the articular cartilage changes the stresses on the underlying subchondral bone, which itself has pain receptors. Subchondral bone may react to increasing shearing forces by becoming reactive and sclerotic [23]. Bone scintigraphy studies have shown an increase in delayed phase tracer in the tibiofemoral compartment in of patients reporting knee pain [24]. This is likely to represent increased metabolic bone turnover in response to the changing physical stress environment of the bone. The increased tracer uptake has been shown to have a sixfold increased risk of progression to OA [25].

The increasing use of MRI in evaluating knee pain has allowed detection of histological changes not previously seen on plain radiographs. Bone marrow oedema, or bone marrow lesions (BML), appear on MRI as increased signal on fat suppressed T2 weighted images. The presence of BMLs has been associated with an increase in reported pain, and have a strong association with progression to radiographic changes of OA. This may help explain the degree of symptoms in patients with only mild radiographic changes associated with arthritis. McAlindon 1992 [10] showed that only 54% of a cohort of patients over 55 years old with knee pain had radiographic evidence of OA. Conversely 17% of asymptomatic patients had radiographic changes consistent with OA, suggesting that radiographic changes alone do not fully explain the symptoms reported. In the presence of OA, Hill 2001 et al [26] found that the degree of synovial thickening and presence of an effusion correlated with the level of pain reported. It is also likely that individuals differ in perception of pain. Valdes et al 2011 [27] has reported an amino acid variant in the TRPV1 gene is associated with lower pain thresholds in radiographic OA.

Rheumatoid arthritis (RA) is a destructive inflammatory arthropathy that affects the small joints of the hands and feet, along with the large joints. An autoimmune reaction targets the synovial lining of the joint, leading to destruction of the cartilage and changes to the soft tissue structures around the knee causing deformity. The altered biomechanics of the joint accelerate the degenerative changes of the cartilage. Without appropriate pharmacological treatment or surgical intervention it can lead to profound disability and pain. The evolution of disease modifying anti-rheumatoid drugs (DMARDs) has had a significant effect on the number of patients requiring surgery [13].

Gout and pseudogout are caused by the deposition of crystals within the joint. The crystals induce the release of mediators resulting in inflammation. Whilst the reaction is usually self-limiting, its course can be shortened with use of anti-inflammatory medication. There has been increased incidence in gout noted over the last three decades [28]. Although genetic factors feature, it is also thought to be related to diet, lifestyle and increased longevity. Gout is the result of deposition of monosodium urate crystals within the joint. Urate is produced in the metabolism of purine, and is excreted in urine. If serum urate levels are elevated' monosodium urate levels in the extracellular fluid become saturated and crystals develop.

Acute soft tissue injuries around the knee cause pain and a variable amount of swelling. The anterior cruciate ligament (ACL) is supplied by the middle genicular artery. Acute rupture of the ligament activates nociceptor fibres, and the ensuing haemarthrosis stretches the joint capsule. While the initial pain subsides, the consequence of the altered biomechanics of the knee leads to chronic symptoms. Lohmander 2004 [29] reported that 12 years after injury of the ACL in young female athletes 75% reported significant knee pain and 42% had symptomatic radiographic knee osteoarthritis, whether a reconstruction was carried out or not.

Meniscal injuries can also be acutely painful at the time of injury. Proposed sources of pain include the resulting synovitis or distortion of the capsule from the meniscal tear. Mine et al 2000 [30] reported the presence of nociceptor fibres, mainly in the more vascular outer third (the red zone) and also at the anterior and posterior horns. This suggests an additional source of pain, although it does not fully explain the discomfort experienced from tears in the avascular inner third (white zone).

Like ACL injuries, meniscal injuries can lead to long term degenerative change. Berthiaume et al 2005 [31] used serial MRI to show that meniscal injury and volume loss was associated with an increased risk of degenerative change. Many people with symptomatic meniscal tears choose to have a partial or total meniscectomy. Roos et al 1998 [32] presented the results of a 21 year follow up study of patients post total open meniscectomy. The relative risk of developing tibiofemoral OA was 14.0 compared controls. Currently modern treatment algorithms have been to conserve healthy meniscus using a minimally invasive approach. Englund et 2004 [33] reported that even with limited resection the relative risk of radiological OA was 7.0 compared to matched controls, and 2.7 for symptomatic OA.

Anterior knee pain can occur in both children and adults. Both groups can be difficult to treat and the exact diagnosis can be elusive. Whilst there are certain terms used to describe the mechanisms by which the pain occurs, there will be cases where a true diagnosis is never made. In the past the term *chondromalacia patella* has been used. This should be avoided as it falsely attributes a pathological process and may lead to incorrect treatment and affect patient expectations.

Wear of the articular cartilage in the patellofemoral joint is associated with chronic knee pain. Like the tibiofemoral compartment not all with radiographic features of arthritis have symptoms [10]. The cause of the articular wear can be mechanical or inflammatory in nature. The even distribution of load across the joint avoids stress concentration, the alignment of the patella is thought to contribute to acute and chronic symptoms. There is some anatomical variation in the shape of the joint [34], which may predispose the early degenerative change. Dye et al [35] reports a shift in thinking away from biomechanical malaligment of the patellofemoral as a cause of acute pain. Instead he proposed that inflammation of synovium and fat pad along with increased metabolic activity in subchondral bone have aetiological importance.

5. Knee pain in children & adolescents

There are recognised pathological changes that are unique to the skeletally immature knee [36]. Overuse of the knee can result in pain that only resolves after a period of rest. This is due to stress injuries from repetitive use, usually because of increased demands placed on the knee. They are also more common during growth spurts. Once the knee has been afforded time to recover from such stress then the symptoms usually resolve. The junction of the patellar ligament at the tibial tuberosity is a common site for such pain. Termed Osgood Schlatter's disease, the pain is in response to repeated stress causing mild avulsion injuries. The natural history is one of spontaneous resolution before adulthood [37]. Sinding-Larsen-Johannson disease presents as pain at the distal pole of the patella and responds to a simple non-operative therapy like Osgood Schlatter similar to the treatment of Osgood Schlatter disease.

5.1. Traction apophysitis

Osgood-Schlatter and Sinding-Larsen-Johansson disease is commonly seen in the male 12-14 age group. Kneeling is painful in Osgood-Schlatter disease and the tibial tubercle is painful to palpation. There may also be a prominence which is visible on the XR knee lateral. In later stages the tubercle will have a fragmented appearance due to the separation of the chondro-osseous fragments [1] Treatment is conservative with reduction in the usually very high level of activity and simple analgesics (NSAIDS) till the symptoms have subsided. Quadriceps strengthening is avoided as this increases stresses across tibial tuberosity. This usually resolves within one to two years although the bony tibial tubercle prominence may persist. If they remain symptomatic there may be an ossicle in the substance of the tendon with an associated bursa of which surgical removal can be curative.

Whereas Osgood-Schlatter disease affects the tibial tubercle Sinding-Larsen-Johansson disease affects the lower pole of the patella. Treatment is the same as that for Osgood-Schlatter, namely conservative.

Osteochondritis dissecans should be considered as a cause if tibiofemoral and anterior knee pain. Most commonly affecting the lateral aspect of the medial femoral condyle, its cause has not been established although repeated trauma and vascular insult are likely to play a role [37]. A multipartite patella may also cause anterior knee pain, and may be detected on plain radiograph. Saupe 1943 [38] described three types: inferior pole, lateral patellar margin, and superolateral pole. Pain usually originates from the junction of the main body of the patella and the fragment.

Idiopathic anterior knee pain in the adolescent is difficult to treat. The cause has not been ascertained and prescribed treatments not always successful. The term chondromalacia patella has occasionally been used in describing such a problem, however this should be avoided as the term describes chondral changes that are not always present in anterior knee pain. Nimon et al [39] carried out a 14-20 year follow up on idiopathic anterior knee pain and determined that no operative intervention provided a better long term outcome than non-operative treatment.

Tumours should be considered as a cause of continuing knee pain, especially when night pain is present. There may also be localised swelling and skin changes. Malignant primary tumours are less common, if there is any doubt as to the diagnosis then at least plain radiographs in two planes should be sought.

5.2. Classification

Knee pain can present as an acute episode or a more chronic course. It is usually described by the causative pathology. The common causes of knee pain change with age of the patient, in children soft tissue and tendon causes are more common while in older adults arthritis is more prevalent.

Knee pain can be classified according to the affected compartments or structures. Anatomically the knee is divided into the tibiofemoral joint, medial and lateral, and its associated soft tissue structures. The patellofemoral joint is described separately, along with the associated tendinous structures that form the extensor mechanism of the knee.

The tibiofemoral joint contains the weight bearing surfaces of the femur and the tibia. The medial and lateral menisci are interpositioned between the two and have a role in load distribution. The anterior and posterior cruciate ligaments and the medial and lateral collateral ligaments provide stability along with the contents of the posterolateral corner of the knee.

The anterior part of the knee includes the patella, which acts to increase the lever arm of the extensor mechanism of the knee. The quadriceps insert into the proximal pole and the patellar ligament (also referred to as patellar tendon) links the inferior pole with the tibial tuberosity. The infrapatellar far pad lies posterior to the patellar tendon and is richly innervated.

Acute episodes may be caused by trauma to the bone, articular surface or soft tissues, but also include localised inflammation or minor injuries due to overuse. Chronic episodes often involve degenerative change to the articular surfaces. Arthritis can be idiopathic, or secondary to trauma. Inflammatory arthritis includes rheumatoid arthritis, gout, reactive arthritis and septic arthritis.

There is no broad consensus on classification of OA of the knee. Radiological findings have been described using the definitions of Kellgren and Lawrence. This has been widely used, including the World Health Organisation (WHO) epidemiological studies. Schiphof 1998 [40] assessed 25 different classification criteria of osteoarthritis which could be broken down into radiological, clinical, and both radiological and clinical criteria. One reason why a consensus does not exist is that radiographic findings may not relate to symptoms.

Post 2005 [41] divided anterior knee pain (AKP) into constant pain not activity related, sharp intermittent pain, and activity related pain. The constant pain may be neurological in nature, whether from sensory nerve pathology or autonomic nerves. Also included is pain reported for perceived secondary gain. Sharp intermittent pain usually relates to unstable structures within the knee or loose bodies. Activity related pain is divided into soft tissue overload with normal patellar alignment, or articular tissue overload and degenerate changes of the chondral surface.

5.3. Knee pain classification

Anterior knee pain	Pain type	Distinct/obscure
Patellar tendonitis	Activity related	Distinct
Bipartitite Patella	Intermittent and sharp	Distinct
Osgood-Schlatter/Sinding-Larsen-Johansson syndrome	Activity related	Distinct
Osteochondritis Dissecans	Activity related	Distinct
Synovial Impingement	Intermittent and sharp	Distinct
Chondromalacia patellae	Intermittent and sharp	Obscure
Patellofemoral osteoarthritis	Constant	Distinct
Patellar maltracking	Activity related	Obscure
Excessive lateral pressure syndrome	Activity related	Obscure
Tibiofemoral knee pain		
Tibiofemoral OA	Constant	
Meniscal tears	Intermittent and sharp	
Ligamentous injuries	Activity related	

Table 1. Knee pain classification

6. Diagnosis and management

6.1. Diagnosis

Whilst history, examination and standard radiographic imaging are important in the determination of the aetiology of knee pain, newer imaging techniques and pain maps can also supplement the investigation of the causes of knee pain. This section will summarise pertinent symptoms and signs in the assessment of knee pain as well as describe advances in pain mapping and imaging.

6.2. Patient history

Several points in the history can yield very important diagnostic information about the cause of knee pain. Pain on sitting or climbing/descending stairs is often secondary to patellofemoral aetiology. Pain on squatting often with symptoms of locking or clicking usually relate to a meniscal tear. ACL tears are often described as a sudden 'pop' with immediate swelling and an inability to continue the activity that preceded it. This is a pivoting injury and can be without significant contact. Conversely the same symptoms with a significant contact force may suggest a collateral ligament tear. In both cases acute swelling will occur. A blow to the anterior tibia such as a dashboard or snowboarding injury can result in a Posterior cruciate ligament (PCL) tear. A sensation of an unstable knee or 'giving way' suggests ligamentous laxity or patellar instability. A history of sharp pain may be related to synovial impingement or loose bodies within the knee. Aching pain or pain after activity is thought to be related to inflammatory disorders whereas pain during activity is associated with structural abnormalities such as patellar subluxation or dislocation [42]. OA knee pain is typically insidious in onset and aggravated by movement and weight bearing and relieved by rest.

6.3. Patient examination

When examining a patient observation of their gait and stance can give valuable clues to their diagnosis. Quadriceps circumference if decreased indicates atrophy from inactivity. A palpable knee effusion is relatively non specific but can suggest a meniscal or ligamentous injury in the acute setting or arthritis in the chronic setting. Joint line tenderness indicates a meniscal tear which can also manifest as a block to full extension if big enough (such as a bucket handle tear). Loose bodies can also cause a locked knee.

Patella apprehension tested by pushing the patella laterally at 20-30° of flexion indicates subluxation or dislocation. Patella grind and crepitus signify patellofemoral pathology. The Q-angle as measured from the angle between a line from the anterior superior iliac spine to the centre of the patella and a line from the centre of the patella to the tibial tubercle is increased with patella malalignment representing the degree of valgus translational force exerted upon the patella with quadriceps contraction.

Varus and valgus stress testing will confirm a lateral collateral ligament (LCL) and medial collateral ligament (MCL) injury respectively. Lachman test will be more sensitive than anterior draw for an anterior cruciate ligament (ACL) injury. A pivot shift test with the knee flexed at 20-30° and internal rotation with valgus stress can also signify an ACL tear. The pivot shift however can only be done under anaesthesia. A posterior draw test is sensitive for a PCL injury although care must be taken in misinterpreting a positive posterior draw test as an ACL rupture if the tibia can be translated anteriorly in the anterior draw test.

To test for a posterolateral corner injury an assistant is needed. With the knees stabilised the feet are externally rotated and the thigh foot angle is compared at both 30 and 90° of knee flexion. If there is asymmetry of greater than 15° at 30° flexion only this represents an isolated posterolateral corner (PLC) injury. If asymmetry is present at both 30 and 90° knee flexion this represents a combined PCL-PLC injury.

6.4. Radiological imaging

Conventional radiography of the knee comprises a standard anteroposterior view and a lateral view. The lateral view allows assessment of the vertical position of the patella such as in patella alta (associated with lateral patella dislocation/subluxation, chondromalacia, patella ligament rupture, and Sinding-Larsen-Johansson) and baja (quadriceps tendon rupture, neuromuscular disorders and achondroplasia). Measurement of patellar tilt on the lateral radiograph with the knee if full extension is more sensitive for patellofemoral joint (PFJ) pain and prior dislocation than measures on the axial view [43]. The axial will show PFJ static alignment. The Insall ratio [44] is used to determine relative patellar height. The congruence and sulcus angles are indices of patellar subluxation. Trochlear depth may be measured using the sulcus angle. The congruence angle is a measure of lateral patellar displacement. The lateral patellofemoral angle on the axial view is a measure of patellar tilt. Abnormalities of these measurements may represent mal-alignment although they may be normal in asymptomatic patients when measured in mild degrees of flexion [45]. Computed tomography (CT) allows axial plane evaluation of the PFJ relationships in varying degrees of flexion for detecting malalignment. Imaging over the range of 5-30° of flexion is the most useful for discriminating between normal and abnormal patellar tracking since beyond 30° the patella centralizes in the trochlear groove. Rapid techniques able to capture images during active knee motion are described. This is now performed using helical CT which allows continuous rotation of the X-Ray tube and detectors during active joint motion. From knee extension to 45° flexion 1 image a second is captured resulting in a total scan time of 10 seconds [46].

Magnetic resonance imaging (MRI) can visualize the components of the extensor mechanism and show lesions of articular cartilage and menisci, plicae and osteoarthritic change. Static MR imaging axial sections are obtained with the knee imaged at 4-8 different angle positions. This can be performed using any MR sequence without motion artifact. The disadvantage however is that joint kinematics and muscle contraction effects cannot be assessed. Kinematic MRI using motion triggered or ultrafast imaging techniques can be used to assess the contribution of associated soft-tissue structures to PFJ function with ultrafast imaging being less dependent on patient cooperation and can be performed even with severe patellar pain yielding fewer motion artifacts and better image quality. Kinematic MR imaging is also superior to axial radiographs in assessing patellar realignment surgery as significant differences between pre and post operative measurements are better demonstrated [47]. Overall MR imaging (especially ultrafast sequences) is felt to be superior to CT imaging in evaluation patellofemoral tracking. Muhle et al [46] feel that it should always be used in such cases in preference to CT unless the patient has contraindications to MR imaging. Different MR sequences are appropriate for imaging specific pathologies. Synovitis is best assessed by gadolinium enhanced MR sequences. Joint effusion is best detected on fat suppressed PD or T2 weighted FSE sequences. BML are best visualized on fat suppressed T2 weighted or STIR images. Menisci are typically visualized on sagittal PD (TE<20) FSE sequences and Ligaments on PD or T2 weighted FSE sequences.

6.5. Functional MRI

How the brain processes noxious stimuli in different disease states has been investigated using functional MRI (fMRI). This is also to map the cortical location to which the pain is mapped. fMRI uses a fast MR imaging method for which the image intensity is sensitive to the variations in magnetic field created in the tissue by the presence of paramagnetic deoxyhaemoglobin [48]. An increase in blood flow due to increased metabolic activity while processing a stimulus leads to decreased deoxyhaemoglobin and a small increase in intensity. Even with a modern 3 Tesla scanner this is only 10% increase in signal. With such low sensitivity several measurements are needed in individual patients or multiple patient datasets. Results from fMRI investigations has revealed that central activation of the brain mediates pain during OA and that non steroidal anti inflammatory drugs (NSAIDs) therapies may be partially acting via a central mechanism [49]. Furthermore in a recent paper by Gwilym et al 2009 [50] suggested that in specific groups of patients addressing central components of central pain processing by fMRI may be important for the treatment of long term OA pain.

6.6. PET

Positron emission tomography (PET) can be used to create two or three dimensional images of blood flow or metabolic processes [48]. Studies have shown arthritic pain is also associated with areas of the brain implicated in affect averse conditioning and motivation as well as the normal pain perception areas. Such findings have important implications for the management of patients with long term OA.

The use of fMRI, Positron emission tomography (PET), Single-photon emission computed tomography (SPECT) and Magnetoencephalography (MEG) are novel imaging modalities that have helped unravel how central pain pathways in the perception of chronic pain function.

6.7. Scintigraphy

This is a diagnostic test used in nuclear medicine. Radioisotopes taken internally emit radiation that is captured by external detectors (gamma cameras) to form a two dimensional image. Radioisotopes such as technetium-99m-MDP are preferentially taken up by bone and the specificity can be increased by performing an indium 111-labeled white blood cell test combined with a Technetium-99m-MDP injection. Conditions that cause increased bone turnover or inflammation can be diagnosed.

As such bone scanning can be used to detect fractures within 24 hours of the injury. This initially presents as increased vascularity and delayed scans can show increased uptake for up to six months after a fracture. Similarly bone bruises or trabecular fractures cause increased vascularity and uptake and are often associated with ligamentous injuries which show as bone bruised patterns in the adjacent site of bone attachment. Bone scanning is sensitive at showing stress fractures. Osteoarthritis causes increased uptake of radio nucleotide around the articular surface of the bone because of increased bone turnover. Increased uptake on both sides of a joint is characteristic of osteoarthritis. Bone scanning can also be helpful in the diagnosis and monitoring of CRPS following treatment [51]. Osteomyelitis shows increased vascularity and increased uptake on a three phase bone scan. Similarly cellulitis can also be diagnosed on a bone scan. Scintigraphy presents physiological features whereas radiography, CT and MRI all give structural information. In recent years, however, MRI scanning has largely replaced bone scanning for the diagnosis of localised knee pain.

6.8. USS

Ultrasound (USS) is a diagnostic imaging technique in the context of orthopaedics to visualize muscles and tendons tendons, nerves, ligaments, soft tissue masses, and bone surfaces. Compared to CT and MRI, USS is relatively inexpensive, portable and safe as it does not use mutagenic ionising radiation [52]. It is however largely operator dependent, and is unable to evaluate bone and other structures.

Although USS can be used for detection of ligament ruptures and meniscal injuries within the knee [53,54], this role has largely been superseded with the use of MRI.

Ultrasound is ideally placed for the assessment of tendon lesions, particularly partial and complete quadriceps rupture and tendinitis of the patellar tendon [55]. USS can also evaluate muscle injury and differentiate between partial and complete tears [54]. It is also very valuable in differentiating between swellings around the knee such as popliteal cysts and other local swellings including aneurysm, nerve sheath tumour and ganglia [56].

Joint effusions and bursae are easily detected by ultrasound. Ultrasound guided aspiration of bursitis can be carried out if necessary.

6.9. Arthroscopy

Arthroscopy is useful for direct visualization of bone, cartilage and soft tissue. Despite advances in non-invasive imaging techniques it is still considered the most reliable method for assessing patellar position and tracking. CT and MRI however, still provide useful augments.

6.10. Bone marrow lesions and osteoarthritis progression

Bone scans of patients with OA have shown increased uptake of tracer in the subchondral bone signifying increased turnover [25]. This was found to be associated with increased joint pain and increased risk of progression to radiographic OA. Similarly this has been demonstrated on MRI as increased signal in the marrow on fat suppressed T2 weighted images and has been dubbed bone marrow lesions [57]. Histological these manifest as bone marrow necrosis, trabecular abnormalities and bone marrow fibrosis and oedema [58]. It has also been reported that in patients with radiographic OA those who also had BM oedema lesions more often had knee pain than those without [59]. BMLs are localized to the subchondral bone. As the subchondral bone is innervated BML are thought to be a potential source of pain. Recent longitudinal studies have demonstrated that bone marrow lesions powerfully predict risk of local structural deterioration in OA knees. The risk of medial progression of OA within the knee was increased sixfold if there were medial BMLs. Similarly the risk was increased laterally if there were lesions laterally. Furthermore varus knees had a very high prevalence of medial bone marrow lesions whereas valgus knees had preferential lateral lesions. What is not clear however is whether the limb malalignment itself causes the progression of OA and development of the BML or whether OA progression is a consequence of the presence of BMLs [25]. Tanamas et al [60] found that the relationship between BML presence and cartilage change was independent of tibiofemoral alignment. Furthermore as there is no treatment for BMLs currently there is no justification for the routine use of MRI in assessing OA patients particularly as it is not clear if the lesions themselves cause structural damage or are a consequence of malalignment.

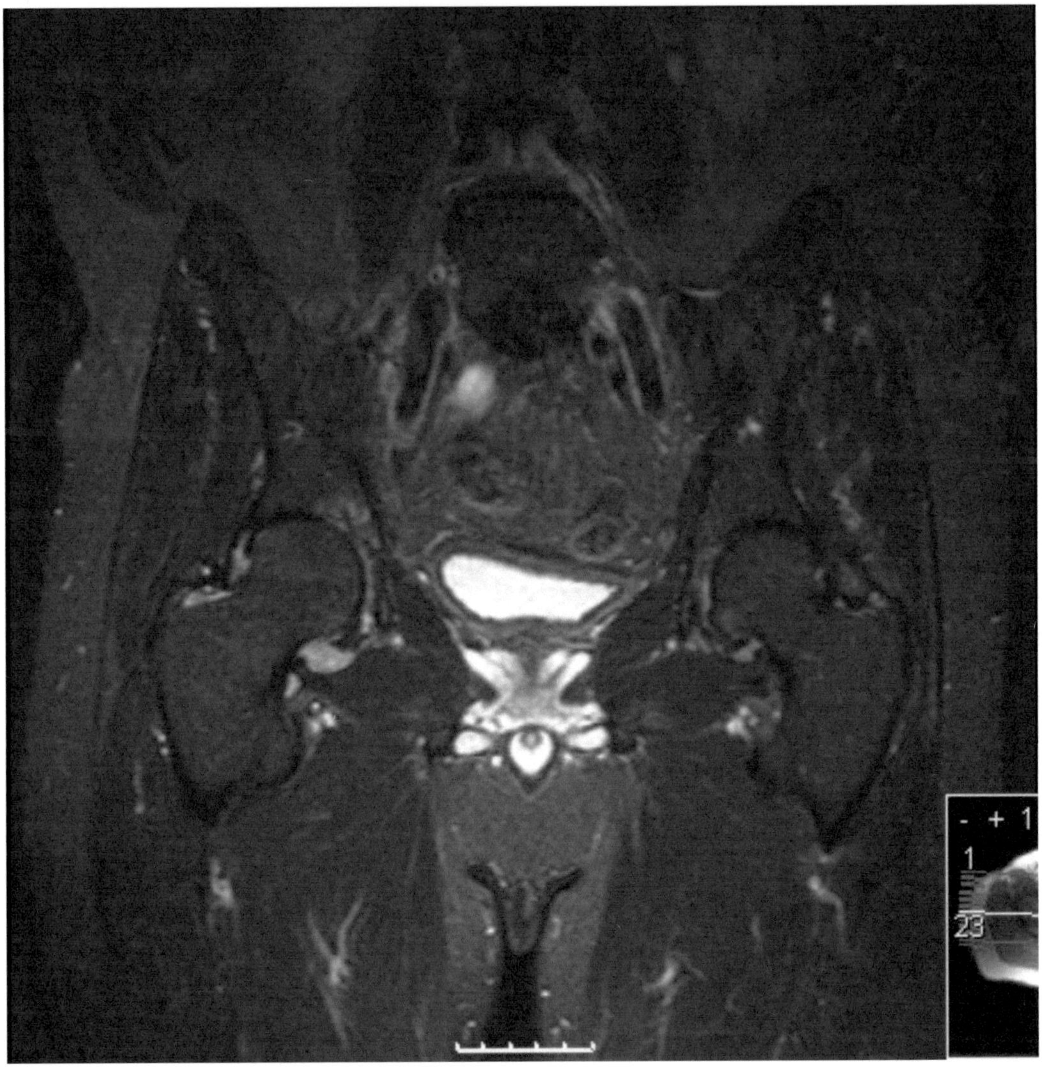

Figure 1. Coronal STIR MRI showing subchondral bone oedema and synovitis

Until recently there has been much focus on articular cartilage in assessing OA severity. There is conflicting data about whether cartilage damage correlates with pain. And recent studies have tied to shift the emphasis to other pathological events such as BML and synovial effusion/synovitis in understanding the cause of OA pain. The clinical implication of BML is not clear. It is present in 78% of patients with knee OA with pain and in 30% of patients in knee OA without pain [59]. BML is not pathognomonic of knee OA but its association is intriguing and not fully understood. This only highlights the need for more research into the matter. It is becoming more evident that pain from OA is multifactorial and that research into such new fields will help predict disease progression and alter improve treatments.

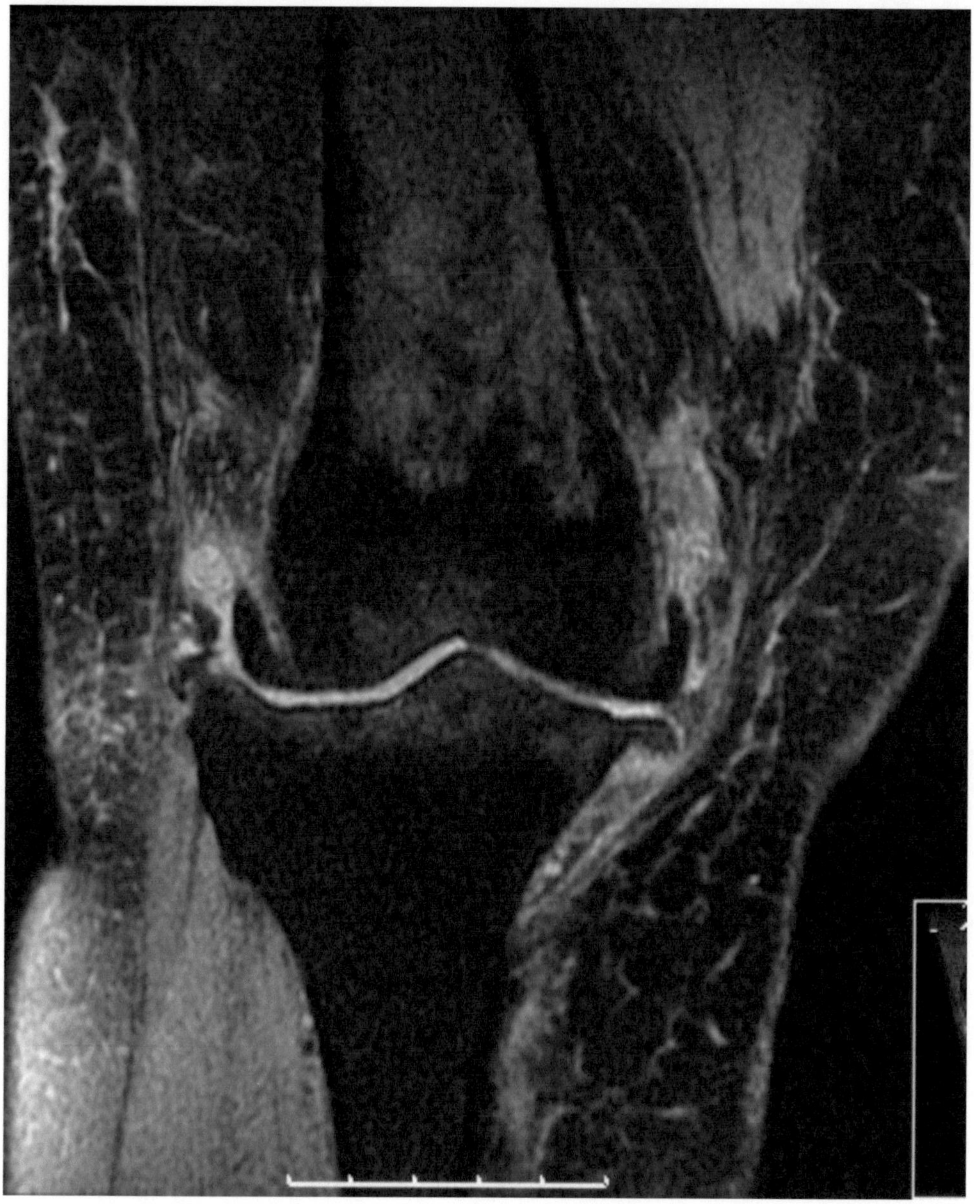

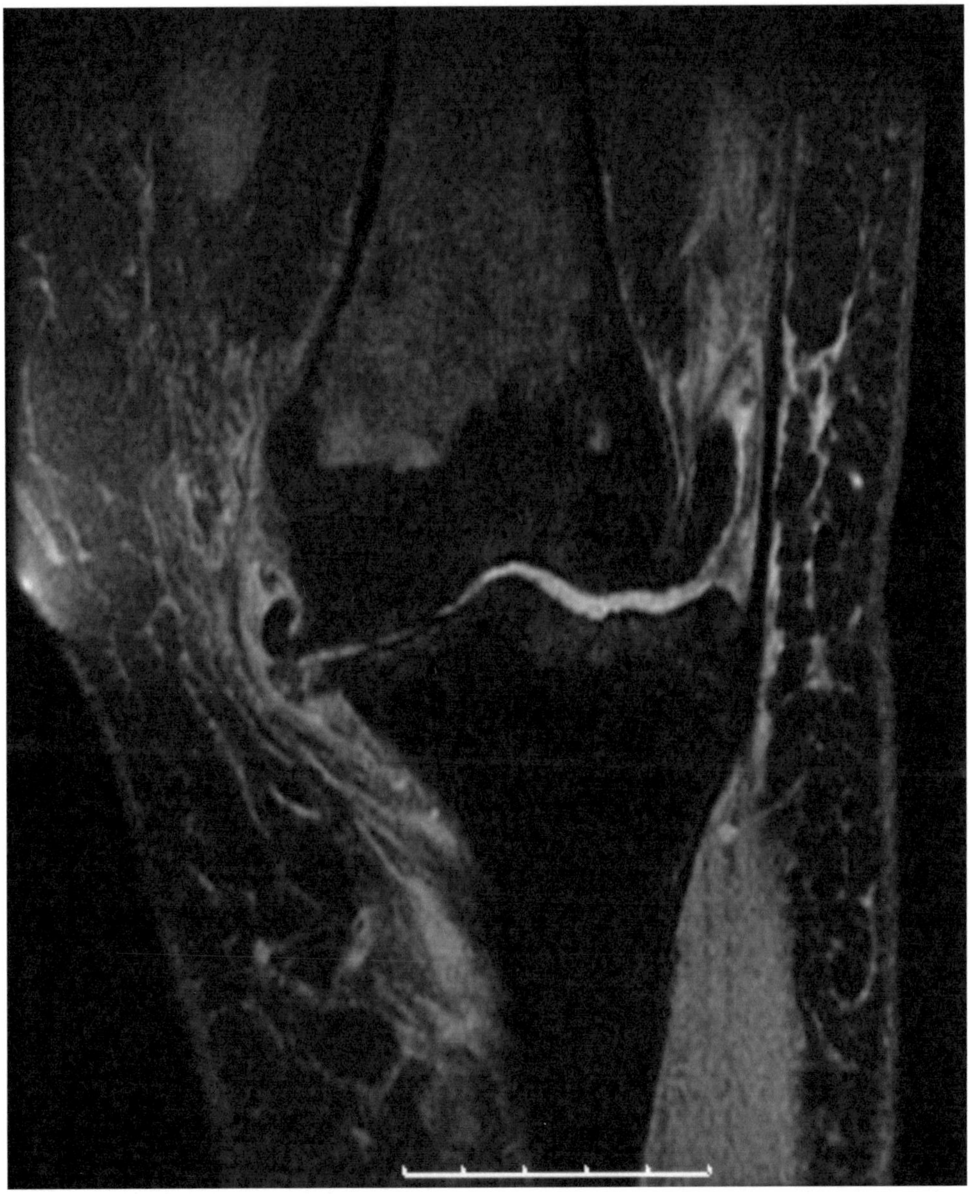

Figure 2. Coronal PD FS images showing severe OA with complete cartilage loss and subarticular tibial plateau bone oedema

7. Anterior knee pain

7.1. Patella tendon tendinitis

Also known as Jumpers knee this is tendinitis at the tendon-bone interface of the lower pole of the patella. This manifests as point tenderness of the lower pole of the patella. The decline squat test will be positive. This can also be confirmed on USS or MRI. The treatment is initially non-operative with physiotherapy and oral anti-inflammatory medications. Steroid injection is contraindicated since this may cause tendon rupture. Cases refractory to conservative management can be managed operatively to try and induce tendon healing by inflicting surgical trauma at the degenerative site [1]. This can vary from simply scrapping away at the site of degeneration to stripping of the deeper half of the tendon if it is affected to drilling the distal pole.

7.2. Bipartite patella

Common in childhood and usually bilateral. The most common site is the superolateral corner and this is the site most likely to be symptomatic. The most effective surgical treatment is simply excision of the fragment

7.3. Osteochondritis dissecans

This presents with pain and crepitus in knee extension against a load. Giving-way can be a result of pain inhibition. Plain XR including 30° skyline view will yield a diagnosis. Classically the majority of lesions are found in the lateral aspect of the medial femoral condyle followed by the lateral femoral condyle and patella. Most commonly seen at the medial patellar facet. Differentiation from chondromalacia patellae may be difficult but chondromalacia tends to be confined to the overlying cartilage whereas osteochondritis involves a fragment of bone. There is a high incidence of contralateral limb involvement 15%-30% [61] and so bilateral knee XR is recommended. Subchondral sclerosis can indicate loosening of the fragment within the crater. CT and MRI will confirm it and show whether separation has occurred. The presence of homogenous high signal beneath the fragment of greater than 5mm in diameter may represent an unstable lesion [62].

Arthroscopy will stage the lesion [1]:

1. Intact lesion with no break in articular cartilage
2. Separated lesion with no break in articular cartilage but beneath the intact layer the bone has separated
3. A trapdoor lesion in which the fragment of osteochondritis dissecans is partially detached
4. Detached loose body.

Stage 1 can be managed with activity modification and cessation of high impact sports especially in patients under 14 who would be expected to heal (the presence of an open physis is encouraging). Separated lesions can be stabilized with biodegradable pins or osteochondral bone pegs. Stage 3 and 4 should be excised leaving stable vertical edges to the crater and microfracture to induce healing within the defect with fibrocartilage.

7.4. Synovial impingement

Pathological plicae are difficult to diagnose as they are a normal finding. Superior, medial and inferior plicae are most common [63]. Identification on arthroscopy does not necessitate excision unless physical examination is abnormal. Pain is worse with knee flexion and relived by extension. There may be a thickened palpable cord [64]. Usually the medial plica. XRs are normal. MRI will identify it but will not necessarily determine if it is pathological. With stronger magnets for MRI this may change however as wear on the medial femoral condyle secondary to a thickened medial plica is identified. Conservative management with activity modification, steroid injections into the plica and physiotherapy is initial treatment followed by arthroscopic excision if necessary.

Hoffa syndrome presents with swelling in the region of the fat pad. Diagnosed with the Hoffa maneuver of applying compression either side of the patella tendon while extending the knee. The test is positive if it elicits pain or apprehension. Diagnosis can be confirmed on MRI as high signal content consistent with irritation of the fat pad [65]. As before treatment is with activity modification then debridement if necessary.

7.5. Chondromalacia

Degenerative condition of the articular cartilage not often seen in skeletally immature. XR are often normal or may show joint space loss if cartilage loss is extensive. Diagnosed on MRI and Arthroscopy. T2 weighted images with fat saturation or fast spin echo intermediate weighted MRI demonstrate good contrast at the interfaces between cartilage and subchondral bone and between cartilage and joint fluid [66]. Usually imaged in the axial plane identifying potential cartilage defects and internal derangement of the cartilage layer before gross morphological cartilage loss. In idiopathic cases with limited damage unrelated to patella subluxation and/or tilt it is acceptable to improve the articular surface arthroscopically. This reduces the amount of debris in the joint and decreases release of proteolytic enzymes and decreases synovitis and delaying osteoarthritis onset [67]. The malacic areas are excised and the subchondral bone is drilled to encourage repair with fibrocartilage. This however will not withstand the large loads and sheer forces hyaline cartilage can. Osteochondral grafting in the form of mosaicplasty can be successful for defects on the femoral condyles but not the undersurface of the patella.

7.6. Patellofemoral osteoarthritis

The standard radiographic features of OA are joint space loss, subchondral sclerosis, cysts and osteophytes. Such radiographic features are also visible on MRI.

7.7. Patellar maltracking

Treatment is dependant differentiating between patients with normal and abnormal anatomy. When examining close attention should be paid to any malalignment including genu valgum, external torsion of the tibia and femoral anteversion which may be associated subluxation or patellofemoral malalignment [68].

Imaging of the patellofemoral instability patient includes weight bearing AP, 45° PA flexion and lateral and axial views. These plain XR provide information about osteochondral fractures patellar height, morphology of the trochlear groove, patellar tilt and sulcus angle. Beyond 45° flexion most patella engage fully with the trochlear groove. As such most imaging studies of the PF tracking should focus on 30-45° flexion.

CT can be helpful in planning a realignment procedure if necessary. MRI will provide information regarding the medial retinacular structures (medial patellofemoral ligament (MPFL) injured in as many as 94-100% of acute patella dislocations [69]. MPFL is extracapsular and can be missed on arthroscopy which is important as MPFL repair is being increasingly advocated to prevent recurrent dislocation, chondral damage and ligament injuries, particularly in cases of acute patella dislocation. Quinn et al [70], described a triad of injuries on MRI consisting of impaction injury to the lateral femoral condyle, osteochondral defect (OCD) of the medial patellar facet and injury of the medial patellar retinaculum. As patellar dislocation can be transient MRI findings provide valuable clues to the pathology and can be the first indication of the diagnosis.

Skyline views provide only static images from which the patellar dynamics cannot be understood. It is important to delineate the pattern of maltracking in before considering management options.

Lateral subluxation in extension is demonstrated clinically by extending the knee against gravity. As the knee extends from 20° flexion to extension the patella can be observed to kick laterally and can be accompanied by crepitus and pain as the patella disengages from a position of stability in the trochlear groove. This is commonly a problem of recurrent dislocations in childhood. The principal cause is malalignment of the quadriceps. This can be managed with physiotherapy or distal realignment of the tibial tubercle by 1.5cm +/- proximal medial advancement of the patellofemoral ligament and lower fibres of vastus medialis. Lateral release and inner range quadriceps exercises are not appropriate.

Conversely maltracking in flexion is easier to see radiologically on skyline views but more difficult to examine for clinically beyond symptoms of instability and pain. With pure subluxation in flexion chondral damage is mild and a simple lateral release will often suffice [1]. However with combined subluxation and tilt the lateral facet is overloaded and the chondral damage can be more severe. Subsequently the threshold for performing a distal realignment is lower.

CT is a very useful imaging modality to study patella tilt and subluxation. Arthroscopy through anterolateral and superolateral portals will allow assessment of patellar tracking between 0-90° and also allow the clinician to observe overhang of the lateral facet.

Chronic patellofemoral instability nonoperative treatment focuses on regaining strength in the quadriceps mechanism and hip abductors. Traditionally for acute dislocation the knee was immobilized in cylinder cast or cricket pad splint. Others prefer early motion controlled with lateral buttress bracing. Operative management in the acute setting is indicated for osteochondral fragment repair or removal. It may also be indicated for repair or reconstruction of the medial retinacular structures.

7.8. Excessive lateral pressure syndrome

Lateral patellar tilt is dominant with little or no subluxation. Imaging shows cartilage loss, sclerosis and cystic change of the lateral patella and trochlear. Dynamic studies show lateral tilt with increasing flexion.

7.9. Patellectomy

Indicated when the articular surface of the patella is so badly damaged over a wide area that it cannot be salvaged and an otherwise relatively normal knee. The patient should rehabilitate in a hinged knee brace back to their activities of daily living but will not be competitive in sports. Quadriceps wasting is inevitable and will not exceed 70% of normal despite extensive rehabilitation. Complications include rupture, subluxation and pain.

7.10. Complex regional pain syndrome

Complex regional pain syndrome (CRPS) manifests as severe pain, swelling and changes in the skin. It is often associated with autonomic dysregulation and can lead to functional loss, impairment and disability. Clinically there must be an initial noxious event that leads to continuing pain, allodynia or hyperalgesia with evidence of oedema and changes in skin blood flow in the area of pain. This must all be in the absence of another condition that could account for such symptoms.

Sweat testing can help in the diagnosis of CRPS. A trial of sympathetic block can also be useful given the aetiology of the condition. Conventional radiographs can also be useful in showing the resultant patchy osteoporosis although a three phase technetium bone scan can detect these changes sooner and will show higher bone density with successful treatment. Nerve Conduction Studies (NCS) are important tests in CRPS as they are very reliable for detecting nerve injury (causalgia).

Treatment is multidisciplinary and involves physiotherapy together with drug treatment such as antidepressants and gamma-aminobutyric acid (GABA) analogues.

7.11. Pain in OA

Pain is the most disabling symptom of OA. Previous work has focused on articular cartilage as the cause although we cartilage is not innervated with nerve fibres. With the advent of widespread MRI use we are no able to investigate the whole joint as an organ to identify the structures that cause pain such that w may develop targeted therapies. In a systematic review by Yusuf et al [71] there was a moderate level of evidence for a positive association for BML and effusion/synovitis with pain in OA. There was limited evidence for an association for knee ligamentous abnormalities and no association with osteophytes and and subchondral cysts. There was conflicting evidence for cartilage defects, meniscal lesions and bone attrition.

7.12. Physiotherapy management of patellofemoral pain

The aims of interventions described are to improve patellar tracking and reduce abnormal stress on the PFJ structures.

Patients respond well to a home exercise program initiated by and regularly followed up with dedicated physiotherapists. General quadriceps exercises are most commonly employed together with specific vastus medialis obliquus (VMO) targeted training. VMO delay or reduction in relation to VL is thought to contribute to lateral patellar tracking. Quadriceps training is the basis of conservative management and studies indicate at least a moderate reduction in pain when performing such exercises including weight bearing and non-weight bearing exercises [72]. Witvrouw et al [73] studied the effects of open kinetic chain exercises (i.e. without weightbearing such as seated knee extension) versus closed chain exercises (such as leg press) in patients with anterior knee pain. Closed chain exercises produced less pain and better functional improvement although both exercises were beneficial.

Maximum compressive load is generated 90° flexion in both types of exercises [74] but open kinetic chain exercises produce higher loads from 45° to full extension. Escamilla et al [75] showed that closed chain exercises produced greatest quads activity at near full knee flexion with more activity in the vasti muscle whereas open chain exercises produced greatest quads activity near full extension with more rectus femoris activation. Further studies [76] confirmed greater VMO activity with closed chain exercises. Whilst closed chain exercises seem to confer more advantages not all patients will tolerate them as well as open chain. It is worth also noting that eccentric strengthening (muscle contraction while lengthening e.g. walking down stairs) produces the highest muscle strains and so may be recommended for the later stages of rehabilitation. Flexibility is important in eccentric loading to help absorb energy [41] and so patients undergoing rehabilitation for anterior knee pain will benefit from hip, quadriceps, hamstring and gastrocnemius stretching.

While an increased Q angle is thought to predispose the patella to excessive lateral tracking this has been disputed in recent literature [72]. This may be related to the static nature of a Q angle measurement that does not reflect real life kinematics. Souza et al et al [77] described the use of a dynamic Q angle and theorized that femoral adduction and internal rotation relative to the pelvis impart a valgus knee force and stress lateral PFJ structures. This has been confirmed on kinematic MRI and has justified the use of targeted hip exercises in treating patients with PFJ pain. Results from studies indicate that those who participated in exercise programs targeting hip abductors and external rotators reported at least a moderate reduction in pain (72) Faulty foot mechanics can also increase the dynamic Q angle [78] and has led to the use of foot orthosis for the treatment of PFJ pain with moderate success [79].

In combination with quadriceps exercise patellar taping is effective. Taping involves applying medially directed adhesive tape to glide, tilt and rotate to the patella to increase patellofemoral contact and reduce pain. Studies have reported a strong reduction in pain [80]. Whether this effect is due to improved patellar alignment or better proprioceptive awareness and neuromuscular control is still debated. The evidence for patellar bracing is less convincing although some studies have shown a moderate improvement [81]. It may be that bracing shifts contact of the patella with the trochlea to areas of non-irritation.

Whitelaw et al [82] found that 87% of patients with PF pain improved with a combination of physical therapy and NSAIDS and that 68% of those patients maintained that improvement at 16 months. Kannus et al [83] followed up patients for 7 years and found that almost three quarters of patients maintained subjective and functional recovery from 6 months to 7 years with quadriceps exercises, rest and NSAIDs.

Based on such high success rates patients with PFJ pain should be managed with non-operative measures till such time that symptomatic improvement has reached an unacceptable plateau.

8. OA management

8.1. Simple analgesics

Current OA treatment guidelines recommend paracetamol as a first line treatment followed by a NSAID. NSAIDS are proven to be better at improving pain and function in osteoarthritis. The combination of paracetamol and ibuprofen is associated with significant improvements in pain relief, function and quality of life as compared to paracetamol use alone for both short and long term use [84] but at the expense of an increase in side effects, primarily GI (PPI) bleeding.

Adjuncts to simple analgesics include weight loss and activity modification and physiotherapy. Opioid analgesics (such as dermal patches) are also used. Beyond that intra articular HA and steroid injections are considered the third step in management followed by surgical referral.

8.2. NSAIDs

Trials show that selective Cox-2 inhibitors are less harmful to the lower GI tract than conventional NSAIDS prescribed together with a proton pump inhibitor gastro-intestinal since PPIs offer no protection to NSAID induced effects on the small bowel and colonic mucosa [85].

8.3. Hyaluronic acid injection

Hyaluronic acid (HA) injections are widely used in the medical management of knee OA. There are a variety of different products available on the market with differing molecular weights, origins, and viscosities. Opinion is divided about the efficacy of HA injections. A recent meta-analysis [86] confirmed a modest efficacy for knee OA just minimally exceeding clinical significance. HA was found to be effective at 4 weeks post injection and reach peak effectiveness at 8 weeks with a residually detectable effect at 24 weeks. When at its peak effectiveness it appeared to be more effective than acetaminophen and NSAIDS and comparable to Cox-2 inhibitors.

8.4. Glucosamine

Controversy exists on the efficacy of glucosamine in the symptomatic treatment of knee OA. Meta-analyses have provided conflicting results. As with HA, conflicting trial results may be due to the use of different formulations. A recent large multicentre double blinded trial testing glucosamine and chondroitin preparations (GAIT) found that overall, there were no significant differences between the glucosamine or chondroitin preparations tested and placebo within the subset of patients with mild knee pain either together or alone. There was a subset of patients with moderate-to-severe pain, in whom glucosamine combined with chondroitin sulfate provided statistically significant pain relief compared with placebo. However, because of the small size of this subgroup these findings should be considered preliminary and need to be confirmed in further studies.

8.5. Biotherapy

Preclinical studies have shown that nerve growth factor regulates the structure and function of responsive sensory neurons including small diameter nociceptive afferents [85]. Tanezumab, an antibody against nerve growth factor (NGF) was clinically trialled as the first biotherapy for knee OA. Early results were impressive for efficacy but trials were halted by the FDA because of an unexpected increase in joint prosthesis in the tanezumab group compared to the placebo group. Schnitzer et al 2011 [87] showed that repeated injections of tanezumab in patients with moderate to severe knee OA provided relief (45-60% reduction of pain) and better function with a low incidence of side effects (parasthesia).

8.6. Pharmacological treatment reference guide

Simple	**Mode of action**	**Typical dose**	**Precautions/Side effects**
Paracetamol	Not fully understood – likely COX inhibitor	500mg-1G QDS	Hepatotoxicity in overdose
NSAIDS	COX inhibitors	Ibuprofen 400mg TDS Naproxen 500mg BD	Gastrointestinal and renal adverse reactions
Opiate alternatives			
Codeine	Acts on opioid receptor	15-60mg QDS	Nausea. Constipation. Itching. Dependence.
Tramadol	Acts on opioid receptor	50-100mg QDS	Nausea. Constipation. Itching. Dependence.
Supplements			
Glucosamine/Chondroitin	Unknown – possible proteoglycan synthesis/cartilage protection	1500mg/1200mg	Generally safe
Hyaluronic acid	Lubricant	Intra-articular injection	Generally safe

Table 2. Pharmacological treatment reference guide

8.7. Weight loss

Weight loss is difficult to achieve and is perhaps even more difficult to maintain. Despite this it is frequently recommended for the treatment of OA. In a study by Bliddal et al [88] reported at 1 year patients allocated to a low fat high carbohydrate and protein diet had reduced pain in the knee due to OA. This result and others indicate that approximately 30% of obese patients with knee OA can achieve significant long term weight loss and improve their pain symptoms. Though studies have shown an improvement in pain levels there is yet no evidence in difference in function or disability. However as pain is the main problem of OA there is good justification for advocating weight loss initially.

8.8. Knee arthroplasty

Knee joint replacement is an effective and cost-effective intervention for people with advanced OA. There are however no clear indications for the use of knee joint replacements and it can be difficult to know when in the course of OA it is best to operate [89]. This is evidenced by the great variability in rates of knee joint replacement [90 Furthermore a minority of patients are made symptomatically worse by surgery. There is also the difficulty of there being a number of different approaches and prosthesis available and the decision on whether to perform a total knee replacement or unicompartmental replacement or even high tibial osteotomy for the young functionally demanding patient with unicompartmental disease.

Ultimately the decision to operate will depend on the best available research evidence in combination with the experience of the surgeon depending on the individual patient's needs and expectations.

8.9. Anaesthesia for knee operations

Most knee operations are now done under a general anaesthetic or a regional anaesthetic or a combination of the two. For arthroscopic procedures theses are usually performed as daycase procedures and so a quick general anaesthetic is generally the rule. This is augmented with a local anaesthetic (such as 10mls 0.5% bupivacaine) injected into the knee joint and port sites to help with post operative pain relief.

Anaesthesia for knee arthroplasty should provide stable intra-operative conditions and allow adequate postoperative analgesia to promote early mobilisation and better surgical outcomes.

Regional anaesthetic techniques can have several advantages over general anaesthesia for knee arthroplasty such as less intra- and post-operative blood loss.

9. Common techniques

9.1. Spinal anaesthesia

Patients will be awake for the procedure. There is a reduced risk of venous thromboembolism and reduced blood loss compared with general anaesthesia. Spinal anaesthesia provides early postoperative analgesia and can be supplemented by patient controlled analgesia (PCA).

9.2. Epidural analgesia

Provides very good pain relief which can be extended postoperatively. However it is dependent on adequate anaesthetic input and training of nursing staff. It has the added requirement of needing urinary catheterisation which may delay postoperative mobilisation. Patients need to be aware that they will feel a sensory and motor disturbance affecting both legs.

9.3. Femoral and sciatic nerve blocks

Do not provide surgical anaesthesia but rather good pain analgesia for to the first 12-24 hrs. They avoid the need for a urinary catheter in most patients and allow mobility in bed.

9.4. Pain coping skills

Patients with chronic pain often develop maladaptive thought patterns known as pain catastrophising and abnormal behavior patterns such as guarding or inactivity that contribute to physical and emotional suffering. In a study by Riddle et al [91] patients receiving psychologist directed pain coping skills training reported significantly greater reductions in pain severity and catastrophising as well as improved function. This provides preliminary evidence that such treatments may be efficient in reducing the number of patients unhappy with the results of knee arthroplasty.

10. Conclusion

The diagnosis and management of knee pain can be challenging. As with most aspects of medicine, a thorough history and careful examination will often lead to the correct diagnosis. Traditionally XR and USS imaging have been the most accessible to the clinician in confirming the diagnosis. With the increased availability of CT and MR it is now possible to investigate knee pain in much greater depth within a shorter period of time without resorting to invasive procedures. With the advances in imaging techniques, particularly in MRI, soft tissue knee pathologies can be much better delineated and appropriate treatment planned. This has transformed the diagnosis and management of anterior knee pain. Nevertheless an experienced physiotherapist is invaluable in treating patients with anterior knee pain with surgery reserved for when a plateau has been reached which is unacceptable for the patient. With the advent of more powerful MR scanners and more sophisticated sequences we can also begin to understand the pathology of knee OA better. Although undoubtedly BMLs have a role in knee OA their exact relationship to progression of knee OA and causality is not yet fully understood. No doubt this is an area of future research and development. The role of analgesics in OA has been proven. As have the surgical options predominantly in the way of arthroplasty, with good proven results. It is the interim steps in between that are not yet proven and need further research and development. The role of biotherapeutic agents whilst temporarily sidelined may become more important if initial discoveries hold true. We know that pain from OA is likely to be multifactorial and with the advent of functional MRI we can begin to understand the central processing of pain in chronic knee OA. This may yield yet more possibilities for the treatment of OA.

Author details

Sherif Hosny, W. McClatchie, Nidhi Sofat and Caroline B. Hing
St George's Hospital NHS Trust, Blackshaw Road, London, UK

11. References

[1] Jackson, A.M., *Anterior Knee Pain.* Journal of Bone and Joint Surgery British, 2001. 83B: p. 937-48.

[2] Cutbill, J.W., et al., *Anterior knee pain: a review.* Clinical journal of sport medicine, 1997. 7: p. 40-45.

[3] Kellgren J, Lawrence J. Radiological assessment of osteoarthrosis. *Ann rheum Dis* 1957;16: 494-502

[4] Ahlbäck S. Osteoarthrosis of the knee: a radiographic investigation. *Acta Radiol Stockholm* 1968; (suppl 277):7-72.

[5] Symmons D, Mathers C, Pfleger B. Global burden of osteoarthritis in the year 2000. Geneva: World Health Organization; 2003.

[6] Dawson J, Linsell L, Zondervan K, Rose P, Randall T, Carr A, Fitzpatrick R. Epidemiology of hip and knee pain and its impact on overall health status in older adults. *Rheumatology* 2004;43:497-504

[7] Haq S, Davatchi F. Osteoarthritis of the knees in the COPCORD world. *Int J Rheum Dis* 2011;14:122-129

[8] Ingham S, Zhang W, Doherty S, McWilliams D, Muir K, Doherty M. Incident knee pain in the Nottingham community: a 12-year retrospective cohort study. *Osteoarthritis Cartilage* 2011;19:847-852

[9] Nguyen U, Zhang Y, Zhu Y, Niu J, Zhang B, Felson D. Increasing prevalence of knee pain and symptomatic knee osteoarthritis: Survey and cohort data. *Ann Intern Med.* 2011;155:725-732

[10] McAlindon T, Snow S, Cooper C, Dieppe P. Radiographic patterns of osteoarthritis of the knee joint in the community: the importance of the patellofemoral joint. *Ann Rheum Dis* 1992; 51:844-849

[11] Jarvholm B, From C,Lewold S, Malchau H, Vingard E. Incidence of surgically treated osteoarthritis in the hip and knee in male construction workers. *Occup Environ Med* 2008;65:275–278

[12] Miranda H, Viikari-Juntura E, Martikainen R, Riihimaki H. A prospective study on knee pain and its risk factors. *Osteoarthritis Cartilage* 2002;10:623–630

[13] Louie G, Ward M. Changes in the rates of joint surgery among patients with rheumatoid arthritis in California, 1983–2007; *Ann Rheum Dis* 2010;69:868–871

[14] Fevang B, Lie S, Havelin L, Engesaeter L, Furnes O. Reduction in Orthopedic Surgery Among Patients With Chronic Inflammatory Joint Disease in Norway, 1994–2004. *Arthritis Rheum* 2007;57:529-32.

[15] Morrison J. The mechanics of the knee joint in relation to normal walking. *J Biomechanics* 1970;3:51-61

[16] Freeman M, Pinskerova V. The movement of the normal tibiofemoral joint. *J Biomechanics* 2005;38:197-208

[17] Amis A Farahmand F. Biomechanics masterclass: extensor mechanism of the knee. *Curr Orthop* 1996;10:102-109

[18] Feller JA, Amis A, Andrish J, Arendt E, Erasmus P, Powers C. Surgical biomechanics of the patellofemoral joint. *Arthroscopy*. 2007;23:542-53.

[19] Witonski, Wagrowska-Danielewicz M. Distribution of substance-P nerve fibres in the knee joint in patients with anterior knee pain syndrome. *Knee Surg Sport Traumatol Arthrosc*. 1999;7:177-83.

[20] Biedert R, Stauffer E, Friederich N. Occurrence of free nerve endings in the soft tissue of the knee joint: A histologic investigation. *Am J Sports Med* 1992;20:430-433

[21] Gronblad M, Korkala O, Liesi P, Karaharju E. Innervation of synovial membrane and meniscus. *Acta Orthop Scand* 1985;56:484-486

[22] Dye, S.F., *The Pathophysiology of Patellofemoral Pain.* Clinical Orthopaedics and Related Research, 2005. NA;(436): p. 100-110.

[23] Bassiouni H. Bone marrow lesions in the knee: the clinical conumndrum. *Int J Rheum Dis* 2010;13:196–202

[24] Kraus V, McDaniel G, Worrell T, Feng S, Vail T, Varju G, Coleman R. Association of bone scintigraphic abnormalities with knee malalignment and pain *Ann Rheum Dis* 2009;68:1673-1679

[25] Felson D, McLaughlin S,Goggins J, LaValley M, Gale E, Totterman S, Li W, Hill C, Gale D. Bone marrow edema and its relation to progression of knee osteoarthritis. *Ann Intern Med.* 2003;139:330-336

[26] Hill C. Knee effusions, popliteal cysts, and synovial thickening: association with knee pain in osteoarthritis. *J* Rheumatol 2001;28:1330-1337

[27] Valdes A, De Wilde G, Doherty S, Lories R, Vaughn F, Laslett L, Maciewicz r, Soni A, Hart D, Zhang W, Muir K, Dennison E, Wheeler M, Leaverton P, Cooper C, Spector T, Cicuttini F, Chapman V, Jones G, Arden N, Doherty M. The Ile585Val TRPV1 variant is involved in risk of painful knee osteoarthritis. *Ann Rheum Dis* 2011;70:1556–1561

[28] Richette P, Bardin T. Gout. Lancet 2010;375:318-328

[29] Lohmander L, Ostenberg A, Englund M, Roos H. High Prevalence of Knee Osteoarthritis, Pain, and Functional Limitations in Female Soccer Players Twelve Years After Anterior Cruciate Ligament Injury. *Arthritis Rheum* 2004;50:3145-3152

[30] Mine T, Kimura M, Sakka A, Kawai S. Innervation of nociceptors in the menisci of the knee joint: an immunohistochemical study. *Arch Orthop Trauma Surg* 2000;120:201–204

[31] Berthiaume M, Raynauld J, Martel-Pelletier J, Labonte F, Beaudoin G, Bloch D, Choquette D, Haraoui B, Altman R, Hochberg M, Meyer J, Cline G, Pelletier J. Meniscal tear and extrusion are strongly associated with progression of symptomatic knee osteoarthritis as assessed by quantitative magnetic resonance imaging. *Ann Rheum Dis* 2005;64:556–563

[32] Roos H, Lauren M, Adalberth T, Roos E, Jonsson K, Lohmander L. Knee osteoarthritis after meniscectomy: Prevalence of radiographic changes after twenty-one years compared with matched controls. *Arthritis Rheum* 1998;41:687-693

[33] Englund M, Lohmander L. Risk factors for symptomatic knee osteoarthritis fifteen to twenty two years after meniscectomy. *Arthritis Rheum* 2004;50:2811-2819

[34] Wiberg G. Roentgenographic and anatomical studies on the patellofemoral joint: With special reference to chondromalacia patella *Acta Orthop Scand* 1941;12:319

[35] Dye S. The pathophysiology of patellofemoral pain: a tissue homeostasis perspective. *Clin Orthop Relat Res* 2005;436:100-110

[36] Stanitski C. Anterior knee pain syndromes in the adolescent. *J Bone Joint Surg Am* 1993;75-A:1407-1416

[37] Kodali, P., A. Islam, and J. Andrish, *Anterior knee pain in the young athlete, diagnosis and treatment.* Sports Medicine, Arthroscopy Review, 2011. 19: p. 27-33.

[38] Saupe E. Primäre knochenmarkseiterung der kniescheibe. *Deutsche Z Chir* 1943;258:386-9

[39] Nimon G, Murray D, Sandow M, Goodfellow J. Natural history of anterior knee pain: a 14- to 20-year follow-up of nonoperative management. *J Pediatr Orthop.* 1998;18:118-22.

[40] Schiphof D, de Klerk B, Koes B, Bierma-Zeinstra S. Good reliability, questionable validity of 25 different classification criteria of knee osteoarthritis: a systematic appraisal. *Journal of Clinical Epidemiology* 2008;61:1205-1215

[41] Post W. Anterior knee pain: Diagnosis and treatment. *J Am Acad Orthop Surg* 2005;13:534-543

[42] Cutbill J, Ladly K, Bray R, Thorne, P, Verhoef M. Anterior knee pain: A review. *Clin J Sports Med* 1997;7:40-45

[43] Murray TF, Dupont JY Fulkerson JP. Axial and lateral radiographs in evaluating patellofemoral malalignment. Am J Sports Med 1999;27:580-4

[44] Insall J, Salvati E. Patella position in the normal knee joint. Radiology 1971; 101:101-4

[45] Egund N. The radiographic axial view of the patellofemoral joint: examination in the supine or standing position. Eur Radiol 2001;11:130

[46] Muhle C. Brossman J. Heller M. Kinematic CT and MR imaging of the patellofemoral joint. Eur Radiol 9 508-18 1999

[47] Brossman J, Muhle C, Bull CC, Zieplies J, Melchert UH, Brinkmann G, Schroder C, Heller M Cine MR imaging before and after realignment surgery for patellar maltracking comparison with axial radiographs. Skeletal radiology 24: 191-6 1995

[48] Sofat N, Hamann P, Barrick TR, Howe FA. Activation of central pain pathways in rheumatic diseases: What we have learned from functional neuroimaging studies. Current rheumatology reviews, 2010,6;3

[49] Baliki M, Katz J, Chialvo DR, Apkarian AV. Single subject pharmacological-MRI (fMRI) study: modulation of brain activity of psoriatic arthritis pain by cycloxygenase-2 inhibitor. Mol pain 2005;2(1):32

[50] Gwilym S, Keltner JR, warnaby CE, et al. Pschyosocial and functional imaging evidence supporting the presence of central sensitization in a cohort of osteoarthritis patients. arthritis rheum 2009; 61(9): 1226-1234

[51] Lee GW, Weeks PM: The role of bone scintigraphy in diagnosing reflex sympathetic dystrophy. J Hand Surg [Am] 1995;20:458-63.

[52] Van Holsbeeck M, Intracaso JH. Musculoskeletal ultrasonography. Radiol Clin North Am 1992; 30:907-925

[53] Ptasnik R, Feller J, Bartlett J, Fitt G, Mitchell A, Hennessy O. The value of sonography in the diagnosis of traumatic rupture of the anterior cruciate ligament of the knee. AJR 1995; 164:1461-1463.

[54] L. Friedman K. Finlay E. Jurriaans Skeletal Radiol (2001) 30:361–377

[55] Bianchi S, Abdelwahab IF, Zwass A et al. Diagnosis of tears of the quadriceps tendon of the knee: value of sonography. Am J Roentgenol 1994; 162:1137

[56] Jacobson JA, van Holsbeeck MT. Musculoskeletal ultrasonography. Orthop Clin N Amer 1998; 29:135-167)

[57] Mcalindon TE, Watt I, McCrae F, Goddard P, Dieppe PA. magnetic resonance imaging in osteoarthritis of the knee: correlation with radiographic and scintigraphic findings. Ann Rheum disease 1991;50:14-9

[58] Zanetti M, Bruder E, Romero J, Hodler J. Bone marrow edema pattern in osteoarthritic knees: Correlation between MR imaging and histological findings. *Radiology* 2000; 215:835–840

[59] Felson DT, Chaisson CE, Hill CL, Totterman SM, Gale ME, Skinner KM, et al. The association of bone marrow lesions with pain in knee osteoarthritis. Ann Intern med 2001;134:541-9

[60] Tanamas et al. Bone marrow lesions in people with knee osteoarthritis predeict progression of disease and joint replacement: a longitudinal study. Rheumatology 2010;49:2413-2419

[61] Hefti F, Beguiristain J, Krauspe R, Möller-Madsen B, Riccio V, Tschauner C, Wetzel R, Zeller R.J Osteochondritis dissecans: a multicenter study of the European Pediatric Orthopedic Society. Pediatr Orthop B. 1999 Oct;8(4):231-45.

[62] De Smet AA, Ilahi OA, Graf BK. Untreated osteochondritis dissecans of the femoral condyles: prediction of patient outcome using radiographic and MR findings. Skeletal Radiol. 1997 Aug;26(8):463-7.

[63] Dupont JY. Synovial plicae of the knee. Controversies and review. Clin Sports Med. 1997 Jan;16(1):87-122.

[64] Medial plica syndrome. Sznajderman T, Smorgick Y, Lindner D, Beer Y, Agar G. Isr Med Assoc J. 2009 Jan;11(1):54-7.

[65] Jacobson JA, Lenchik L, Ruhoy MK, Schweitzer ME, Resnick D. MR imaging of the infrapatellar fat pad of Hoffa. Radiographics. 1997 May-Jun;17(3):675-91.

[66] Elias DA, White LM. Imaging of patellofemoral disorders. Clinical radiology 2004;59: 543-557

[67] Muckle DS, Minns RJ. Biological response to woven carbon fibre pads in the knee. A clinical and experimental study. J Bone Joint Surg Br. 1990 Jan;72(1):60-2.

[68] Kodali P, Islam A, Andrish J. Anterior Knee Pain in the Young Athlete Diagnosis and Treatment. *Sports Med Arthrosc Rev* 2011;19:27–33

[69] Nomura E. Classification of lesions of the medial patello-femoral ligament in patellar dislocation. Int Orthop. 1999;23(5):260-3.

[70] Quinn SF, Brown TR, Demlow TA. MR imaging of patellar retinacular ligament injuries. J Magn Reson Imaging. 1993 Nov-Dec;3(6):843-7.

[71] Yusuf E, Kortekaas MC, Watt I, Huizinga TW, Kloppenburg M. Do knee abnormalities visualised on MRI explain knee pain in knee osteoarthritis? A systematic review. Ann Rheum Dis. 2011 Jan;70(1):60-7.

[72] Bolgla, L.A. and M.C. Boling, *Systematic review of the literature: an update for the conservative management of patellofemoral pain syndrome: a systematic review of the literature from 2000 to 2010.* The International Journal of Sports Physical Therapy, 2011. 6(2): p. 112-125.

[73] Witvrouw E, Lysens R, Bellemans J, Peers K, Vanderstraeten G. Open versus closed kinetic chain exercises for patellofemoral pain. A prospective, randomized study. Am J Sports Med. 2000 Sep-Oct;28(5):687-94.)

[74] Wilk KE, Escamilla RF, Fleisig GS, Barrentine SW, Andrews JR, Boyd ML. A comparison of tibiofemoral joint forces and electromyographic activity during open and closed kinetic chain exercises. Am J Sports Med. 1996 Jul-Aug;24(4):518-27.

[75] Escamilla RF, Fleisig GS, Zheng N, Barrentine SW, Wilk KE, Andrews JR. Biomechanics of the knee during closed kinetic chain and open kinetic chain exercises. Med Sci Sports Exerc. 1998 Apr;30(4):556-69.

[76] Tang SF, Chen CK, Hsu R, Chou SW, Hong WH, Lew HL. Vastus medialis obliqus and vastus lateralis activity in open and closed kinetic chain exercises in patients with

patellofemoral pain syndrome: an electromyographic study. Arch Phys Med Rehabil. 2001 Oct;82(10):1441-5.

[77] Souza RB, Draper CE, Fredericson M, Powers CM. Femur rotation and patellofemoral joint kinematics: a weight-bearing magnetic resonance imaging analysis. J Orthop Sports Phys Ther. 2010 May;40(5):277-85.

[78] Tiberio D. Evaluation of functional ankle dorsiflexion using subtalar neutral position. A clinical report. JOSPT Phys Ther. 1987 Jun;67(6):955-7

[79] Collins N, Crossley KM, Beller E, Darnell R, McPoil T, Vicenzino B. Foot orthoses and physiotherapy in the treatment of patellofemoral pain syndrome: randomized clinical trial.Br J Sports med 2009;43(3):169-171

[80] Crossley KM, Bennell KL, Green S, Cowan SM, McConnel J. Physical therapy for patellofemoral pain. A randomized double blinded, placebo-controlled trial. Am J sports med 2002;30(6):857-865

[81] Lun VM, Wiley JP, Meeuwisse WH, Yanagawa TL. Effectiveness of patellar bracing for treatment of patellofemoral pain syndrome. Clin J sport med 2005;35(4):235-240

[82] Whitelaw GP Jr, Rullo DJ, Markowitz HD, Marandola MS, DeWaele MJ. A conservative approach to anterior knee pain. Clin Orthop Relat Res. 1989 Sep;(246):234-7

[83] Kannus P, Natri A, Paakkala T, Järvinen M. An outcome study of chronic patellofemoral pain syndrome. Seven-year follow-up of patients in a randomized, controlled trial. J Bone Joint Surg Am. 1999 Mar;81(3):355-63.

[84] Doherty M et al. A randomised controlled trial of ibuprofen, paracetamol or a combination tablet of ibuprofen/paracetamol in community-derived people with knee pain. Ann Rheum Dis 2011;70:1534-1541.

[85] Berenbaum F. Osteoarthritis year 2010 in review: Pharmacological therapies. Osteorthritis and cartilage 19 (2011) 361-365.

[86] Bannuru RR, Natov NS, Dasi UR, Schmid CH, McAlindon TE. Therapeutic trajectory following intra-articular hyaluronic acid injection in knee osteoarthritis--meta-analysis. Osteoarthritis Cartilage. 2011 Jun;19(6):611-9.

[87] Schnitzer TJ, Lane NE, Birbara C, Smith MD, Simpson SL, Brown MT. Long-term open-label study of tanezumab for moderate to severe osteoarthritic knee pain. Osteoarthritis Cartilage. 2011 Jun;19(6):639-46.

[88] Bliddal et al. Weight loss as treatment for knee osteoarthritis symptoms in obese patients: 1-year results from a randomised controlled trial. Ann Rheum Dis 2011;70:1798-1803.

[89] Dieppe P, Lim K, Lohmander S. Who should have knee joint replacement surgery for osteoarthritis?. Int J Rheum Dis. 2011 May;14(2):175-80.

[90] T. Dixona, M.E. Shawb, P.A. Dieppe. Analysis of regional variation in hip and knee joint replacement rates in England using Hospital Episodes Statistics. Public Health. 2006;120(1) 83–90

[91] Riddle DL, Keefe FJ, Nay WT, McKee D, Attarian DE, Jensen MP. Pain coping skills training for patients with elevated pain catastrophising who are scheduled for knee arthroplasty: a quasi-experimental study. Arch phys rehabil. 2011 Jun;92(6):859-65.)

Chapter 9

Physical and Psychological Aspects of Pain in Obstetrics

Longinus N. Ebirim, Omiepirisa Yvonne Buowari and Subhamay Ghosh

Additional information is available at the end of the chapter

http://dx.doi.org/10.5772/53923

1. Introduction

Childbirth is said to be a highly joyful experience [1] and a universally celebrated event. Childbirth however fulfilling is a painful experience for the majority of women [2,3] and analgesia is regularly required for relieving pain [4]. In non-human primates, labour is thought to be relatively painless, and of short duration, usually unassisted, although changes in behaviour in the days prior to delivery may suggest some degree of labour pains [5]. Exceptionally, very few women may not feel any pain, others can control their responses to reduce pain [3]. Most women think that pain is going to be a major part of giving birth. Each labour has the personal seal of each woman [6]. For religious, cultural and philosophical reasons many groups have sought to prevent and treat pain. Pain may have adverse effects on the other and foetus. The psychological effects of severe pain should not be over looked particularly where it is associated with an adverse fatal maternal outcome [7]. Childbirth is an emotional experience for a woman and her family. The mother needs to bond with the new baby as early as possible and initiate early breast-feeding, which helps to contract the uterus and accelerate the process of uterine involution in the postpartum period [8]. This is affected by pain after delivery whether the delivery is spontaneous vaginal delivery or operative.

Labour as a life event is characterised by tremendous physiological and psychological changes that require major behavioural adjustments in a short period of time [9, 10]. Pain is an individual and multi-factorial experience influenced by culture, previous pain events, beliefs, moods, and ability to cope. The patients' personality affects pain perception and response to pain relieving drugs. Maternal satisfaction has to be taken into consideration when evaluating quality and planning a maternal and child health care service [11]. Labour presents a physical and psychological challenge for women. The latter stages of pregnancy can be a difficult time emotionally. Fear and apprehension are experienced alongside excitement. There emotions both positive and negative will affect the woman's birth experience.

2. Pain in obstetrics

Maternal comfort is of major importance during and after labour [12]. Pain in obstetrics arises from numerous sources and reasons from labour pain, caesarean section, episiotomy and postpartum. Attention to comfort and analgesia for women during and after labour is important for physical reasons and out of compassion. Pain management in obstetric practice therefore focuses on pain relief in labour, pain control during caesarean section and postpartum pain treatment [13]. Pain related to childbirth may present during pregnancy, during labour when more than 95% of women report pain occasionally during caesarean section if there is a poor quality nerve block or prolonged surgery and after delivery when more than 70% of mothers report acute or chronic pain [14].

2.1. Labour pain

Labour although varies with the individual may be the most painful experience, any women may ever encounter. Concerns about pain in labour are as old as mankind [15]. Pain can make patients feel uncomfortable and become sleepless and agitated. Pain also stimulates the sympathetic nervous system, which causes increase in the heart rate, blood pressure, sweat production, endocrine hyperfunction, and delays the patients prognosis [16, 17]. Pain management makes low priority in many low to middle income countries that are struggling to meet United Nations Millennium Development Goals such as eradication of poverty and hunger, universal primary education and reduction in child and maternal morbidity and mortality [18].

Parturient perception and response to labour pain depends on the intensity of pain, psychological factors, cultural beliefs, previously painful experiences, history of pregnancy, social and marital status [19]. Some other factors influencing labour pain and delivery are the parturient psychological state, mental preparation, family support, medical support, cultural background, primipara versus multipara, size and presentation of the foetus, size and anatomy of the pelvis, use of medications to augment labour (oxytocin) and duration [15]. A long, painful labour may lead to an exhausted, frightened, and hysterical mother incapable of decision-making [20]. The degree of pain experienced during labour is related to the frequency, intensity, and duration of uterine contractions and dilatation of the cervix. In addition, the position of the foetus, decent of the presenting part, stretching of the perineum and pressure on the bladder, bowel, and sensitive pelvic structures also contribute to pain levels [21]. Labour pain is a complex and subjective interaction between multiple physical, psychosocial, environment plus cultural factors and a woman's interpretation of the labour stimuli [22]. Women experience varying degrees of pain in labour and exhibit an equally varying range of responses to it. An individual's reaction to pain of labour may be influenced by the circumstances to her labour, the environment, her cultural background preparations towards her labour and the support available to her [23]. During labour, the woman is dealing not only with the contractions but also with the myths that the culture has created for her. Labour and birth, although viewed as a normal physiological process, can produce significant pain requiring appropriate pain management [24].

Labour pain is caused by stretching of the cervix during dilation, ischemia of the muscle wall of the uterus with the build-up of lactate and stretching of the vagina and perineum in the second stage of labour. Both the experience and perception of pain are regarded as subjective and this remains difficult for an observer to measure objectively [3,21].

There are three stages of labour namely first, second and third stage of labour. The first stage of labour begins with the onset of regular contracts and ends with complete cervical dilation [25, 26]. The second stage of labour commences from full cervical dilation to the delivery of the baby while the third stage is from the delivery of the baby until the delivery of the placenta. Pain during the first stage of labour occurs mostly during contractions and is caused by uterine contractions and cervical dilatations [27, 28]. Pain is carried by the visceral afferent fibres of T10-11 from the uterus, cervix, and upper vagina from the cervical plexus and enters the spinal cord at the T10-11 levels. The visceral afferent fibres also enter the sympathetic chain at L2 and L3 levels [29,30]. Pain at the end of the first stage signals the beginning of foetal descent. Pain in the second stage of labour is due to stretching of the birth canal, vulva, and perineum and is conveyed by the afferent fibres of the posterior roots of the S2 to S4 nerves. In the second stage of labour, expulsion of the foetus activates somatic afferent pain fibres from the mid and lower vagina, vulva, and perineum. These signals are conveyed via the S2 – S4 spinal nerve roots that form the pudendal nerve. The pudendal nerve projects bilateral through the inferior sciatic foramen, where it is accessible for blockade by local anaesthetist. Neuraxial representation of labour pain is not continuous and the interceding segments represent and mediate the sensory and motor innervations of the lower extremities.

Painful contractions may lead to maternal hyperventilation and respiratory alkalosis, which in turn shift the oxygen haemoglobin dissociation curve to the left, decrease delivery of oxygen to the foetus [31]. The pain of labour is associated with reflex increase in blood pressure, oxygen consumption, and liberation of catecholamines, all of which could adversely affect uterine blood flow. Increased carbon dioxide, peripheral vascular resistance, and increased oxygen consumption in turn accompany this. This could be dangerous for women with pre-existing cardiopulmonary problems [15].

2.2. Cultural aspects, beliefs and myths of labour and labour pain

Cultural and religious beliefs can affect the perception and interpretation of labour pain. In some cultures the woman is expected to scream and cry uncontrollable while in others the woman may not externally express much distress in her labour. Cultural influences on labour pain can take many varied forms. Cultural beliefs and ethnicity are known to influence the perception of pain such factors can play a vital role in how a woman copes with pain in labour [18].

In some cultures, solitary, and unassisted births are valued and seen as a source of pride [5]. Considering the mysterious qualities of conception, it's easy to see why it's the subject of so many myths [32]. Some women believe that labour pain is natural and would not accept pain relief in labour. Some feel that it is best to express their pain and let their feelings go. Others may see labour as an opportunity to demonstrate their strength and stoicism in a particular way. They may for example moan, scream, sway, click their fingers or tap rhythmically, shake their heads, chant, pray or call god. As a girl grows up into a woman, she becomes involved through the stories of other women with the female body that suffers agony and pain during labour.

Some Hispanic women may believe that they should not take any pain medications as the indication may not be good for the baby. Screaming during the labour and delivery is considered to be harmful to the baby as the culture considers pregnancy to be a hot stage of life [33].

In rural parts of India and Bangladesh, a common belief is that women should bear the pain of childbirth in silence to demonstrate their courage and character. The Japanese believe that the greatest experience of a woman's life is to hear her baby's cry and this should be the only sound heard during labour [32]. Several African studies have found that many women would desire to have labour analgesia if given the opportunity. In humid Benin, Africa the Bariba women are also expected to give birth in silence and girls are taught that a woman who fusses or cries during childbirth is lower than an ant. In Nigeria, among the Hausa, there is great social pressure not to show any sign of pain. Labouring quietly and patiently is thought to demonstrate proper modesty. The Fulani girls from Nigeria are taught from an early age how shameful it is to show fear of childbirth [32]. The Bonny people of southern Nigeria belief that a woman shouting and crying during labour will cry in subsequent deliveries therefore she is advised by her mother and elder female relatives when pregnant not to shout or cry during labour. They are taught it shows how strong and capable she is as a woman to endure pain that no amount of shouting or screaming can reduce the pain so why not just bear it in silence. This psychological preparedness is handed down from generations to generation. Many of these beliefs are 'myths' because they are untrue, however there are many beliefs and practices that have been used in non-western cultures for years that are effective [32].

3. Physical and psychological aspects of labour

Psychological factors help to explain the efficacy of psychotherapy. People who have painful conditions or injuries are often additionally affected by emotional distress, depression and anxiety [34]. Fear and anxiety are significant influences on pain experiences which is one reason why mothers are accompanied by another person during childbirth. Psychosocial factors have been implicated in the pain experienced during childbirth, which can have both short and long-term consequences on the mother's health and her relationship with her infant [33]. For several decades, childbirth educators have focused on the alleviation or reduction of pain and suffering. During the childbirth experience a wide array of non-pharmacological pain relief measures as well as pharmacological interventions are presently available to woman in labour. Relaxation, breathing techniques, positioning, massage, hydrotherapy, music, are some self-help comfort measures women may initiate during labour to achieve an effective coping level for their labour experience. A woman's reactions to labour pain may be influenced by the circumstances of her labour including the environment and the support she receives [35]. During childbirth in addition to or in place of analgesia women manage pain using a range of coping strategies. Antenatal education provides an opportunity prior to birth to help women to prepare for an often painful event [36]. Loneliness, ignorance, unkind or insensitive treatment during labour, along with unresolved past psychological or physical distress increases the chance that the woman will suffer. The physical sensation of pain is magnified and frequently becomes suffering when it coexists with the negative psychological influences [37]. Maternal satisfaction is influenced by outcome of labour, support and interactions with staff, control over pain rather than amelioration. Good communication and team effort are needed to reap the benefits of pain free labour while minimizing the potential effect of epidural analgesia on labour outcome. Many women in labour each day in sub-Saharan Africa particularly in Nigeria, childbirth is experienced not as a joyful event but as sad experience due to midwives attitude towards the labouring woman who shout and yell at labouring women especially if she screams cries or complains of labour pain.

4. Pain relief in labour

Modern views on pain and influence of western concepts of pain are gradually changing the perception and desires for pain relief in labour [5]. Adequate analgesia is important as pain causes an increase in circulating catecholamines which in turn impair uteroplacental perfusion [38]. Analgesia may mask the signs of early preterm labour and therefore tocometry is useful to detect contractions [39]. The choice of analgesic technique depends on the medical status of the patient, progress of labour and resources at the facility [40,41]. There are a number of different forms of pain relief in labour with differing side effects and efficacious labour pain relief is an important aspect of women's health [42]. Pain relief during labour is desirable in order to reduce maternal distress and enhance the progress of labour as most women wish they had some degree of pain relief during labour [43].

In low income countries, pain relief in labour remains essentially rudimentary. Reasons for this are largely theoretical and include racial differences in pain threshold with some women not minding the pains of labour, religious background which makes some women think that labour pains is a divine will [44, 45]. Good antenatal care in may not be available in some countries, it is important that the few who seek for modern care of the parturient be allowed to derive maximum benefit, so as to encourage others to attend hospital for delivery [46].

5. Non-pharmacological methods of labour pain relief

The non-pharmacological methods avoid the use of drugs for pain relief in labour [47]. Transcutaneous electrical nerve stimulation (TENS), hypnosis and acupuncture to relieve labour pains has been shown in many studies [15,19]. The non-pharmacological approach to pain includes a wide variety of techniques to address not only the physical sensations to pain but also to prevent suffering by enhancing the psychological and spiritual components of care [10]. The non-pharmacological methods of labour pain relief require patient preparation and antenatal education. Psychological and non-pharmacological techniques are based on the premise that the pain of labour can be surpassed by recognising one's thought.

6. Continuous support

Continuous support in labour is associated with shorter labour labours and reduced requirement for analgesia. Traditional cultures have always had the support of experienced women to be with the woman in labour. In some places doulas are available. Continuous labour support provided by a doula, a lay woman trained in labour support, consistently has decreased the use of obstetric interventions. Intermittent labour support does not convey the same benefits as continuous support low income women who otherwise would labour with minimal or no social support receive the greatest benefit from a doula [48]. Continuous support from a partner or caregiver can reduce the frequent use of epidural analgesia and the amount of other analgesia administered to a mother [14].

7. Tens

A low voltage electrical impulse is delivered to the skin via four pads which are placed over the lower back with a boost during uterine contractions. Its mechanism of action is also based on the gate control theory of pain [28].

7.1. Massage

This is commonly used to help reflex tense muscle and soothe an calm the individual. Touching another human being can communicate positive messages such as caring, concern, reassurance or love. Massage is the intentional and systemic manipulation of the soft tissues of the body to enhance health and healing is used during labour to enhance relaxation and reduce pain [44].

Other methods like water immersion and acupuncture are known to reduces labour pain intensity and analgesic use.

8. Pharmacological methods of pain relief in labour

Pain relief in labour is teamwork between the anaesthetist, midwife and obstetrician. In considering analgesia for the woman in labour, it should be borne in mind that whatever the method of pain relief employed it should be safe for both mother and baby [46].

The ideal analgesia for labour should provide rapid onset excellent pain relief in both the first and second stage of labour without risk or side effects to mother or foetus and should also retain the mother's ability to mobilise and be independent during labour [49]. The ideal labour analgesic should also provide effective pain relief, tailored to the changing needs of the parturient throughout the different phases of labour with minimal motor blockade and adverse material, foetal effects so as to provide the parturient with a highly satisfactory birthing process. There is growing awareness of the importance of empowering the parturient in decision making process in labour and delivery [19]. The ideal properties of labour analgesia should produce good analgesia without loss of consciousness, should not prolong or depress the process of labour, should not produce neonatal depression, should not produce maternal cardiorespiratory depression, should not possess unpleasant maternal side effects, should have high technical success rate, be predictable and constant in its effects, be reversible if necessary, be easy to administer, be under the control of the mother, should not interfere with uterine contractions, should not prolong the period of labour [50, 49].

Pharmacological methods of pain relief in labour include parenteral opioids, inhalational and regional techniques [46,47]. Epidural and parenteral opioids are superior to non-pharmacological techniques for relieving pain in labour. Systemic analgesia has become less common, whereas the use of newer neuraxial techniques with minimal motor blockade have become more popular [24].

8.1. Parenteral analgesics

Nearly all parenteral opioids analgesics and sedatives readily cross the placenta and can depress the foetus and reduce foetal heart rate variability due to depression of the central nervous system [19,46]. Systemic analgesics are still widely used around the world, despite being significantly less efficacious than epidural analgesia. Pentazocine is still used in some developing countries where pethidine, morphine are not readily available. Many parenteral opioids have been used to provide obstetric analgesia but the most popular have been pethidine, morphine and diamorphine [20].

8.2. Pethidine

This is an analgesic and antispasmodic drug is usually given intramuscularly. It is decreased in popularity as nausea; vomiting, drowsiness and lack of control are important side effects. It works when given intramuscularly in about twenty minutes given good pain relief for some and sedation for most patients [3]. Pethidine readily crosses the placenta and ionizes in the relative acids foetal circulation, leading to accumulation. It is a neonatal respiratory depressant. Its onset of time is within ten minutes when given intramuscularly and lasts up to two-three hours.

Pethidine causes analgesia, amnesia, dysphonia and sedation with a series of adverse effects like maternal and neonatal respiratory depression, nausea, sedation and hallucinations. It is metabolised to norpethidine which has pro-convulsant properties therefore it should be used with caution in patients with pre-eclampsia, renal failure or uncontrolled epilepsy.

8.3. Morphine

Primary maternal outcomes include maternal satisfaction with pain relief one or two hours after drug administration and characteristic of the labour process, secondary outcomes include subsequent use of epidural analgesia, adverse symptoms (example nausea, drowsiness) inability to urinate or participate in labour, caesarean delivery or instrument assisted vagina delivery and maternal qualitative outcomes such as satisfaction with the overall birth experience. Some of the advantages of systemic analgesia are easy availability, simple to administer. Disadvantages of systemic analgesia less efficacious compared to epidural analgesia. Non-steroidal anti-inflammatory drugs have been used in some centres but this may affect the foetus adversely.

9. Inhalational pain relief in labour

Nitrous oxide is relatively insoluble in blood and has these properties. Entonox is premixed 50% nitrous oxide and 50% oxygen under pressure in a cylinder [47] and is administered usually via on an on-demand valve with a face mask or mouth piece [20]. Nitrous oxide has a low blood gas solubility coefficient [0.47] so it equilibrates rapidly with the blood. There is minimal accumulation with intermittent use in labour as it is rapidly washed out of the lungs. Adverse effects of entonox include drowsiness, disorientation and nausea which results in actual loss of consciousness in 0.4% of cases after prolonged use [46].

10. Regional labour pain relief techniques

Regional analgesia for labour encompasses pudendal nerve block, paracervical block, spinal, epidural and combined spinal epidural block. Regional analgesia is the most effective form of analgesia in labour [27,29]. It reduces maternal pain, cardiovascular work and anxiety with minimal effects on the foetus. Regional analgesia is widely available in the developed world and has changed the labour experience for many women making it much more pleasurable and satisfying and requires dedicated staff and monitoring. The pulse, blood pressure, oxygen saturation and consciousness of the patient must be monitored to check for signs of toxicity of the local anaesthetic being used or adverse effects of the methods of the technique. This is why it is not commonly available in developing countries. It is widely accepted that the most reliable method for labour analgesia is neuraxial analgesia via the conventional spinal and epidural technique [19]. There are relatively few contraindications to regional analgesia, the absolute contraindications are maternal refusal, coagulopathy, infection at the injection site, uncontrolled hypovolaemia and raised intracranial pressure due to a space occupying lesion [27]. Regional analgesia is often performed early in labour to optimise positioning and may be easier in the sitting position since the midline may be identified more easily than the lateral position [51].

Bupivacaine has been the most widely used local anaesthetic for regional analgesia in labour [52]. The use of epidural, spinal and combined spinal epidural techniques for obstetric care has increased dramatically because of the quality and safety of the analgesia and anaesthesia produced the ability to titrate the degree and duration of pain relief and the expanding number of situations for which their use is appropriate. In a randomised, non-blinded controlled trial at a university hospital in the United States of America by Wong et al, in 728 nulliparous women, neuraxial analgesia started in early labour did not increase the risks of caesarean section or instrumental delivery, compared to initial use of systemic analgesia with epidural started later, at 4cm or at least two requests for analgesia [53].

10.1. Single shot spinal

This regional labour analgesia can be provided in low resource settings however care must be taken during ambulation and manpower shortages are significant limitation. Spinal labour analgesia using whitcare needles and bupivacaine [2.5 mg) with or without narcotic.

Spinal anaesthesia is a simple and reliable technique with rapid onset. Spinal (subarachnoid) anaesthesia provides an awake and comfortable patient with minimal risks for pulmonary aspiration of gastric contents. Despite the lower abdominal incision sensory dermatome level is required to prevent referred pain from traction on the peritoneum and uterus [30].

10.2. Epidural pain relief in labour

The epidural technique may enable a lesser incidence and extent of maternal hypotension because of the ability to administer the dose of local anaesthetic in a fractionated manner and allow compensatory cardiovascular medicines to respond to the more slowly developing sympathetic blockade [30]. The epidural technique is the most common neuraxial technique used for labour analgesia because of relative rapid sensory analgesia with minimal motor blockade; uterine affects a maternal or foetal toxicity. Epidural bupivacaine provides excellent pain relief during labour and delivery and is still the most widely used local anaesthetic in obstetric analgesia. However, it is potential for motor blockade and central nervous system and cardiac toxicity by accidental intravenous injection of high dose is clinically undesirable especially for obstetric patients [54]. Many factors such as gestational age, ruptured membranes, cervical dilatation can influence pain intensity. The degree of motor block during epidural analgesia depends not only on the drug used but also on the cumulative dose of the local anaesthetic. Epidural analgesia provides effective pain relief during labour and delivery and has no significant adverse effects on infant and outcome [55]. Epidural analgesia has been safely and effectively used since the 1960s. The introduction of low dose epidural low anaesthetics to maintain labour as well as the use of patient controlled epidural analgesia intra-partum has reduced the use of local anaesthetic and minimised its side effects [56]. In some studies epidural analgesia increases the duration of the second stage of labour rates of instrument assisted vagina deliveries and the likelihood of maternal fever [57]. Though women who receive epidural analgesia during labour are more likely to require instrumental or caesarean delivery there is little evidence to suggest that the epidural itself is to blame. There is an association between epidural analgesia and labour outcome but this is probably not causative. Epidurals have consistently been shown to provide superior analgesia when compared with non-epidural analgesia for labour pain, although this is not always associated with greater maternal satisfaction. Analgesia can be readily converted to anaesthesia by increasing the local anaesthetic concentration, facilitating instrumental or caesarean delivery. Labour analgesia benefits patients with hypertension and some types of cardiac disease example mitral stenosis because it blunts the haemodynamic effects that accompany uterine contraction are increased preload, tachycardia, increase systemic vascular resistance, hypertension and hyperventilation [31]. For mobile epidurals affects motor function leading to weakness of the lower limbs, decrease the concentration and adding an opiate provides good pain relief with sparing of motor function and ambulatory epidural service is not yet available in all centres [3].

Epidurals have some potential disadvantages. The dura may be accidentally punctured and causes severe postural headache. This can be cured in most cases with an autologous epidural blood patch, the blood clots in the epidural space and presumably works by sealing the leak of cerebrospinal fluid, thus restoring intracranial pressure. Urinary retention after an epidural is best prevented by careful attention to bladder emptying. Labour epidural analgesia techniques and medications have progressed to provide more predictable and effective labour analgesia. It is now possible for a parturient to experience pain free labour with minimal side effects to both the mother and the foetus while maintaining maternal autonomy.

The use of a patient controlled modality for labour pain control such as patient controlled epidural analgesia has been shown to confer a greater sense of maternal control over the birthing process and has gained maternal acceptance worldwide [19]. Patient controlled epidural analgesia allows patients to self-administer a pre-set amount of local anaesthetic and/or opioid epidurally to meet their own requirements via a patient controlled analgesia device, thus maintaining the neuraxial block within an effective therapeutic range [56].

10.3. Combined spinal epidural labour analgesia

Combined spinal epidural labour analgesia involves injection of an analgesic agent or local anaesthetic drug or both into the intrathecal space immediately before or after epidural catheter placement. A number of variations in this technique have been described. Nevertheless, it is known that despite these variations this technique results in an immediate and significant reduction in pain during labour [11]. This technique offers some benefits including faster onset of analgesia, decreased incidence of motor blockade, more reliable technique, higher level of patient satisfaction and decreased incidence of accidental dura puncture [57]. Combined spinal epidural or labour analgesia allows for use of smaller doses of local spinal anaesthetic because the block can be supplemented at any time.

10.4. Pudendal nerve block

It is possible for a pudendal nerve block to be sited on each side of the birth canal to provide analgesia for the second stage of labour or a straight forward instrumental delivery [28,29]. The pudendal nerve arises from the sacral plexus of S2 to S4 and supplies the perineum, vulva and vagina [28]. Pudendal nerve block is often combined with perineal infiltration of local anaesthetic to provide perinael anaesthesia during the second stage of labour [29].

11. Anaesthesia for caesarean section

Delivery by caesarean section is becoming more frequent and is one of the most common major operative procedures performed worldwide [59]. It is estimated that some 1-2% of pregnant women undergo anaesthesia during their pregnancy for surgery unrelated to delivery [60,61,62]. The most common surgical procedures include appendectomy, cholecystectomy, ovarian torsion and trauma [60]. Less commonly cardiac and neurological procedures are undertaken during pregnancy [60]. Consideration of possible foetal effects of the maternal disease process is important [62]. Obstetric anaesthesia can be very challenging as the risks are largely related to changes in anatomy and physiology associated with the birthing process or surgical intervention and pharmacological changes that characterise the three trimesters of pregnancy these changes. Anaesthetists who care for pregnant patients undergoing non-obstetric surgery must provide safe anaesthesia for both the mother and foetus. Anaesthetic techniques and drugs administered are modified accordingly foetal well-being is related to avoidance of foetal asphyxia, teratogenic drugs and preterm labour [38]. Left lateral tilt is done to prevent aortacaval compression meticulous pre-oxygenation to prevent hypoxia [38].

The aim in the non-obstetric surgery in pregnancy is to optimise and maintain utero-placental blood flow and oxygen delivery, avoid unwanted drug effects on the foetus, avoid stimulating the myometrium(oxytocic effects), avoid awareness under anaesthesia under general anaesthesia and use of regional anaesthesia if possible [60]. Caesarean section is often said to be the unique situation where the anaesthetist has to deal with two patients under the same anaesthetic. Protection of the mother is paramount but other goals of anaesthetic management include maintenance of uterine blood flow and foetal oxygenation, avoidance of teratogenic changes and prevention of preterm labour [62].

12. Regional anaesthesia for caesarean section

Though general anaesthesia was previously the favoured technique for caesarean section, there has been a move in favour of regional technique in recent years [59]. Regional anaesthesia is preferred in obstetrics because it is safer than general anaesthesia especially for emergency for emergency caesarean section [63]. Regional anaesthesia is promoted in obstetric practice for reasons of safety. Most women also wish to be awake for caesarean section and anaesthetist try to comply with this whenever possible [63]. Absolute contraindications to regional analgesia and anaesthesia are maternal refusal because the woman's wishes should be respected at all times, allergy, sepsis, increased intracranial pressure, clotting abnormalities and lack of appropriate trained staff and or equipment [64].

12.1. Spinal anaesthesia

Single-shot spinal anaesthesia has become the most popular anaesthetic technique for caesarean section [65]. The ease of establishing subarachnoid block, the rapid onset of intense and reliable block without missed segments make subarachnoid block more attractive for caesarean section [59]. Spinal anaesthesia offers a fast profound and high quality sensory and motor block in women undergoing caesarean delivery. The most common complication of spinal anaesthesia for caesarean delivery is hypotension with a reported incidence greater than 80% [66]. Maternal hypotension may have detrimental effects on uterine blood flow, foetal well-being and ultimately neonatal outcome as measured by unilateral arterial pH and APGAR scores [66]. Lateral uterine displacement and intravenous prehydration are commonly used to prevent hypotension but these have limited efficacy and a vasopressor drug is often required [66].

Continuous spinal anaesthesia can provide excellent labour analgesia and surgical anaesthesia if required and is a very reliable technique [67]. Despite its inherent advantages, it is also one of the most underutilised of regional anaesthetic techniques. Following administration of a subarachnoid technique, the patient may complain of dyspnoea. This can occur because of several factors including blunting of thoracic proprioception, partial blockade of the abdomen and intercostal muscle and increase pressure of the abdominal contents against the diaphragm in the recumbent position. Despite these diagnoses, significant respiratory compromise is unlikely as the blockade rarely affects the cervical nerves that control the diaphragm [30].

12.2. Epidural anaesthesia

Epidural block demands high technical skills and is still favoured by many when gradual establishment of block is desired to minimise hypotension, although combined spinal epidural techniques are gaining popularity [65]. The method is still same for establishing epidural labour analgesia.

12.3. Combined spinal epidural anaesthesia

The combined spinal epidural technique consists of epidural needle placement and administration of subarachnoid medications via a spinal needle placed through the shaft of the epidural needle and placement of an epidural catheter appears to combine the best of both techniques with a blockade that is rapid in onset, it reliable and can be prolonged [30].

13. General anaesthesia for caeserean section

A general anaesthesia is often needed for an emergency caesarean section if there is not enough time to put in a spinal anaesthetic or an epidural [68]. There is an increased risk during pregnancy of aspiration of gastric contents and control of gastric acidity and volume and encountering a different airway [69, 70].

Maternal mortality has decreased, thanks to the use of regional anaesthesia and decreased use of general anaesthesia, improved aids for difficult intubation, more precise respiratory and cardiovascular monitoring [69]. Maternal dangers linked to general anaesthesia in obstetrics are typically represented by pulmonary aspiration of gastric contents (known as mendelson's syndrome), hypoxaemia related to difficult or failed intubation and magnified by physiological changes of pregnancy, multifactorial hypotension(aortacaval compression and regional anaesthesia, possible obstetric haemorrhage, uterine relaxation due to inhalation agents and inhalation [70].

Failed endotracheal intubation was the leading cause of anaesthetic related maternal mortality. This result in failure to intubate, ventilate and hypoxaemia, which may eventually lead to brain damage or death [70]. The incidence of failed intubation in the general surgical population is approximately 1, 2303 ≈0.04% and in obstetric population 1: 300 ≈ 0.33%. reasons for this include a broad spectrum of anatomical and physiological changes which occur in women during pregnancy such as the presence of full dentition, increased airway oedema especially in pre-eclamptic patients, enlargement of the breasts may impact on the ability to place a laryngoscope blade into the mouth due to increased difficulty in navigating the blade handle, failure to allow adequate time for paralysis with suxamethonium and incorrectly applied or over enthusiastic cricoid pressure may distort the larynx [70].

14. Local infiltration

Local infiltration of the incision and surgical site may be done for unstable patients especially in developing countries where patients present late. Up to 100 ml of 0.5% lignocaine with adrenaline can be used to raise two weals on each side of the midline from the symphysis pubis to a point 5cm above the umbilicus. The layer of the abdominal wall should be infiltrated with the solution using a long needle. Once the baby has been delivered additional analgesia or sedation can be given to the mother. The advantage is that there are no ill effects on the mother or baby. The disadvantage is that it is unsuitable for nervous patients and needs the surgeons' co-operation. Local infiltration of the surgical sites is used in developing countries and low income countries where patients present late to health facilities and in areas where home delivery is common. It is indicated in patients with deranged electrolytes and patients who cannot withstand general of regional anaesthesia such as eclamptics.

15. Postpartum pain

Pain in the postpartum period could be 'after pain' due to acute uterine contractions which are intense during breast feeding. It could also arise from episiotomy, breast engorgement, cracked nipple or mastitis [71]. After pains made worse by the act of breastfeeding because of the effect of serum oxytocin which is secreted from the posterior pituitary gland primarily as part of the milk let down reflex [71.72]. Reassurance and mild analgesics like acetaminophen and non-steroidal anti-inflammatory drugs are usually sufficient [71].

15.1. Episiotomy

An episiotomy is a surgical incision made on the perineum to increase the diameter of the vulva outlet during childbirth [73]. Pain from episiotomy and perineal tears during childbirth is associated with significant pain in the postpartum period. Pain from episiotomy may be severe and can result in significant discomfort and interference with basic daily activities and adversely impact on motherhood [74]. Episiotomy may increase risk of chronic perineal pain, which is estimated to occur in 13% to 23% of women after episiotomy. Post episiotomy pain has been treated with systemic analgesia including non-steroidal anti-inflammatory drugs and oral or intravenous opioids [74].

15.2. Post caesarean section pain

Prompt and adequate postoperative pain relief is an important component of caesarean delivery that can make the period immediately after the operation less uncomfortable and more emotionally gratifying. Postoperative pain produces adverse physiologic effects, which manifests on multiple organ systems such as hypoventilation, atelectasis, pneumonia, stress induced hypercoagulable state and incidence of deep venous thrombosis [75, 76]. Proper management of postoperative pain can improve patient comfort, decreased peri-operative morbidity, and decreased cost by shortening the time spent in post anaesthesia care units, intensive care units, and hospitals [74]. Uncontrollable pain can impair functions such as ambulation and dietary intake breast feeding and early maternal bonding with the infant and can impair the mother's ability to optimally care for her infant in the immediate postpartum period [76,77,78,79,80]. High quality pain relief is important after delivery to promote early recovery and optimise the mother's ability to care for her new born [81]. Inadequate pain control can also negatively affect the normal development of infants by affecting nursing activities such as breast-feeding [76,79].

The ideal post caesarean section analgesic regimen would be one that is cost effective, simple to implement and which minimally affect staff workload [81].

Currently opioids form the foundation of post caesarean section analgesia with patient controlled techniques being preferred by mothers. A number of non-opioid analgesics have been used in conjunction with epidural and intrathecal opioids to optimise postoperative analgesia [81]. Patient controlled intravenous opioids are popular after caesarean delivery because of convenience, safety, and consistently high patient satisfaction. The epidural analgesia has more analgesic benefit than intravenous analgesia and provides excellent postoperative pain relief [82].

Author details

Longinus N. Ebirim and Omiepirisa Yvonne Buowari
Department of Anaesthesiology, University of Port Harcourt Teaching Hospital, Rivers State, Nigeria

Subhamay Ghosh
Pain Medicine, Kettering General Hospital, Kettering, Northants, United Kingdom

16. References

[1] Vivilaki V, Antaniou E. Pain relief and retaining control during childbirth: a sacrifice of the feminine identity. Health Sci J. 2009. 3(1): 3-9. www.hsj.gr.

[2] Azibaben I, Olayinka AO, Mombel MO, Achi OT. Perceived effects of midwives attitudes toward women in labour in Bayelsa State, Nigeria. Archives Applied Sci Res. 2012. 4(2): 960-964.

[3] James JN, Prakash KS, Ponniah M. Awareness, and attitudes towards labour pain and labour pain relief of urban women attending a private antenatal clinic in Chennai. India J Anaesth. 2012. 56(2):195-198.

[4] Baker A, Ferguson SO, Roach SA, Drawson D. Issues and innovation in nursing practice: perceptions of labour pain by mothers and their attending midwives. J Adv Nurs. 2001. 35(2): 171-179.

[5] Balliere S. The effects of pain and its management on mother and foetus. Clin Obstet Gynecol. 1998. 12(3): 423-41.

[6] Tobi KU. Anaesthesia for the obstetric patient. In. Ebeigbe PN. (Ed). Foundations of clinical obstetrics in the tropics. Fodah Global Ultimate Limited. Benin City. 2012. 305.

[7] Finlay I, Chamberlain G. ABC of labour care. BMJ. 1999. 318: 927-930. www.bmj.com

[8] Audu B, Yahaya U, Bukur M, Aliyu E, Abdullahi H, Kyari O. Desire for pain relief in labour in north-eastern Nigeria. J Public Health Epid. 2009. 1(2): 053-057.

[9] Vernon H, Ross MD. Pilot program to introduce spinal labour analgesia in a West African hospital. Book of abstracts fourth all African anaesthesia congress Nairobi. 2009. 67.

[10] Harries C, Turner M. Non-regional labour analgesia. In. Clyburn P, Collis P, Harries S, Davies S. (Eds). Obstetric anaesthesia. Oxford University Press. New York. 2008. 154-171.

[11] Ogboli-Nwasor E, Adaji SE, Bature SB, Shittu OS. Pain relief in labour: a survey of awareness, attitude, and practice of healthcare providers in Zaria, Nigeria. J Pain Res. 2011. 4: 227-232.

[12] Leeman L, Fontaine P, King V, Klein Mc, Ratcliffe S. The nature and management of labour pain. Part 1. Non-pharmacological pain relief. American Fam Physician. 2003. 68(6): 1109-1112. www.aafp.org/afp.

[13] Baric A, Pescod D. Obstetric anaesthesia. Australian Society Anaesthetists. 101: 59-69. www.developinganaesthesia.org.

[14] Escott D, Slade P, Spiby H. Preparation for pain management during childbirth: the psychological aspects of coping strategy development in antenatal education. Clin Psychol Rev. 2009. 29(7): 617-22.

[15] Iliadou M. Labour pain and pharmacological pain relief practice points. Health Sci J. 2009. 3(4): 197-201. www.hsj.gr.

[16] Fortescue C, Wee MYK. Analgesia in labour: non-regional techniques. Continuing Education in Anaesthesia, Critical Care, and Pain. 2005. 5(1): 219-223.

[17] McGrady E, Litchfield K. Epidural analgesia in labour. Continuing Education in Anaesthesia, Critical Care, and Pain. 2004. 4(4): 113-116.

[18] Wee MYK, Tuckey JP, Thomas P, Burnard S. The IDVIP trial: a two centre randomized double blind controlled trial comparing intramuscular diamorphine and intramuscular pethidine for labour analgesia. BMC Pregnancy and Childbirth. 2011. 1151. www.biomedcentral.com/1471-2393/11/51.

[19] Bamigboye AA, Holfmeyr GJ. Caesarean section wound infiltration. SAMJ. 2010. 100(5): 313-317.

[20] Simkin PPT, Bolding PTA. Update on non-pharmacological approaches to relieve labour pain and prevent suffering.

[21] Global year against pain in women, real women, real pain. Obstetric pain. www.iasp.com.

[22] Flavia A, Renato P, Adriana SOM, Leila K, Isabella CC, Melania MRA. Combined spinal epidural analgesia and non-pharmacological methods of pain relief during normal childbirth and maternal satisfaction: a randomised clinical trial. Rev Assoc Med Bras. 2012. 58(1): 112-117.

[23] Akhideno II, Imarengiaye Co. Incidence, severity and characteristics of postpartum pain in Nigerian women. Book of abstracts. Fourth all African Anaesthesia Congress. 2009: 69.

[24] Imarengiaye C. Pain management in obstetrics. Book of abstracts of the fourth all African anaesthesia congress. 2009: 72.

[25] Hung-Chien WU, Yu-Chi LIN, Keng-Liang OU, Yung-Hsien C, Ching-Liang H, Hsin-Chieh T Et Al. Affects of acupuncture on post caesarean section pain. Chinese Med J. 2009. 122(15): 1743-1748.

[26] Eccleston C. Role of psychology in pain management. Bri J Anaesth. 2001. 87(1): 144-152.

[27] Managing acute pain in the developing world. Clinical updates. Pain. 2011. 19(3): 19

[28] Fun W, Lew E, Sia AT. Advances in neuraxial blocks for labour analgesia: new techniques, new systems. Minerva Anesthesiol. 2008. 74: 77-85.

[29] Rowbotham DJ, Aitkenhead AR, Smith G. Textbook of anaesthesia. Churchill Livingstone. London. Fourth Edition. 2001. 634-649.

[30] Moos DD. Basic guide to anaesthesia for developing countries. Volume 2. 169-196.

[31] Awim-Somuah M, Smyth RMD, Howell CJ. Epidural versus non-epidural or no analgesia in labour (review). The Cochrane collaboration. 2009. www.thecochranelibrary.com.

[32] Lewis E, Harris S. Pain relief in labour. In. Clyburn P, Collis R, Harries S. Obstetric anaesthesia for developing countries. Oxford University Press. New York. 2010. 37-45.

[33] Hawkins JL, Lobo AM. Obstetric analgesia and anaesthesia. In. Dukes J. (Ed). Anaesthesia secrets. Third Edition. Elsevier. Pennsylvania. 2009: 396-402.

[34] Tsen LC. Anaesthesia for obstetric care and gynaecologic surgery. Longnecker DE, Brown Dl, Newman MF, Zapol WM. (Eds). Anaesthesiology. McGraw Hill. New York. 2008: 1417.

[35] Lin Y, Sia ATH. Dispelling the myths of epidural pain relief in childbirth. Singapore Med J. 2006. 47(12): 1096-1100.

[36] Kuczkoski M. Labour pain and its management with the combined spinal epidural analgesia: what does an obstetrician need to know? Book of abstracts of the fourth all African anaesthesia congress. 2009. 94.

[37] Danziger J. Childbirth myths around the world. Midwives Magazine. 2012. 4: 42.

[38] Hispanic cultural views on pregnancy, prenatal through postpartum.

[39] Claudia S. Psychological evaluation of the patients with chronic pain. Guide to pain management in low resource settings. 93.

[40] Lang AJ, Sorrell JT, Rodgers CS, Lebeck MM. Anxiety sensitivity as a prediction of labour pain. Eur J Pain. 2006. 10(3): 263-70.

[41] Supporting women in labour. Midwifery Practice Guideline. 2008. www.rcm.co.uk.

[42] Simkin P, Bolding A. Update on non-pharmacological approaches to relieve labour pain and prevent suffering. J Midwifery Women's Health. 2004. 49(6): 489-504.

[43] Hool A. Anaesthesia in pregnancy for non-obstetric surgery. Anaesthesia Tutorial of the Week. 2010. 185. www.totw.anaesthesiologist.org.

[44] Williams WK. A questionnaire survey on patients attitudes towards epidural analgesia in labour. Hong Kong Med J. 2007. 13(3): 208-215.
[45] Practice guidelines for obstetrics anaesthesia. Anesthesiology. 2007. 10(4): 843-63.
[46] Famewo CE. Lectures in anaesthesia and intensive care for medical students and practitioner. Third Edition. Lovemost Printers Ltd. Ibadan. 2004: 84.
[47] Simkin P, Klein MC. Non pharmacological approaches to management of labour pain. www.update.com.
[48] Manizah P, Leila J. Perceived environment stressors and pain perception during labour among primiparous and multiparous women. Reprod Infertil. 2009. 10(3): 217-23.
[49] Gaiser R. Evaluation of the pregnant patient. In. Longnecker DE, Brown DL, Newman MF, Zapol WM. (Eds). Anaesthesiology. McGraw Hill. New York. 2008: 358-373.
[50] Nwasor EO, Adaji SE. Alleviating the pains of labour health care providers experience in a low-income setting. Book of abstracts of the fourth all Africa anaesthesia congress. 2009. 67.
[51] Tobi KU. Questions and answers in anaesthesia and intensive care. Fodah Global Ultimate Limited. Benin City. 2011. 56-58.
[52] Marenco JE, Santos AC. Anaesthesia for non-obstetric surgery during pregnancy. In. Braveman FR. Obstetric and gynaecologic anaesthesia. The requisites in anaesthesiology. Elsevier. 2006. 11-25.
[53] Norctchiffe SA. Obstetric anaesthesia and obesity. Anaesthesia Tutorial of the Week. 141. www.totw.anaesthesiologists.org.
[54] Wang L, Chang X, Lin X, Hu X, Tang B. Comparison of bupivacaine, ropivacaine, and levobupivacaine with sufentanil for patient controlled epidural analgesia during labour: a randomised clinical trial. Clin Med J. 2010. 123(2): 178-183.
[55] Sharma SK, Alexander JM, Messick G, Bloom S, McIntyre DD, Wiley J, Leverok J. Caesarean delivery. A randomised trial of epidural analgesia versus intravenous meperidine analgesia during labour in nulliparous women. Anaesthesiology. 2002. 96: 546-51.
[56] Analgesia and anaesthesia during labour and birth: implications for mother and foetus. J Obstet Gynecol Neonatal Nurs. 2003. 32(6): 780-93.
[57] Elegbe EO. (Ed). Oduntan and Oduro's handbook of anaesthetic for medical students and general medical practitioners. HEBN Publishers Plc. Ibadan. 2007: 88.
[58] Leeman L, Fontaine P, King V, Klein MC, Ratcliffe S. The nature and management of labour pain. Part II. Non-pharmacological pain relief. American Fam Physician. 2003. 68(6): 1109-1112. www.aafp.org/afp.
[59] Collins C, Gurung A. Anaesthesia for caesarean section. Update in anaesthesia. 7-17.
[60] Giane N, Eliane MG, Ligia MSS, Yara MMC. Effects on mother and foetus of epidural and combined spinal epidural techniques for labour analgesia. Rev Assoc Med Bras. 2009. 55(4): 405-9.
[61] Imarengiaye CO, Ande AB, Obiaya MO. Trends in regional anaesthesia for caesarean section at the University of Benin Teaching Hospital. Nig J Clin Pract. 2001. 4(1): 15-8.
[62] Walton NKD. Anaesthesia for non-obstetric surgery during pregnancy. Continuing Education in Anaesthesia, Critical Care, and Pain. 2006. 6(2): 83-85.

[63] Kinsella SM, Girgirah K, Scrutton MJL. Rapid sequence spinal anaesthesia for category-1 urgency caesarean section: a case series. Anaesth. 2010. 65: 664-669.
[64] Collis R, Harries S, Hussain S, Garry M. In. Clyburn P, Collis R, Harries S, Davies S. (Eds): obstetric anaesthesia. Oxford University Press. New York. 2008. 173-220.
[65] Halperen SH, Soliman A, Yee J, Angle P, Loscouich. A conversion of epidural labour analgesia to anaesthesia for caesarean section: a prospective study of the incidence and determinants of failure. Bri J Anaesth. 2009. 102(2): 240-3.
[66] Levy DM. Anaesthesia for caesarean section. Bri J Anaesth. CEPD Rev. 2001. 1(6): 171-176.
[67] Lee A, Kee WDM, Gin T. Prophylactic ephedrine prevents hypotension during spinal anaesthesia for caesarean delivery but does not improve neonatal outcome: a qualitative systemic review. Can J Anaesth. 2002. 49(6): 588-599.
[68] Obstetrics anaesthesia association. General anaesthesia for unplanned caesarean section information card. www.oaaformothers.info.
[69] Alexander R, Parahore A. Clinical decision making in obstetric patients. In. Gulle A. (Ed). Anaesthesia pain, intensive and emerging medicine. Proceedings of the 22nd postgraduate course in critical care medicine. Springer, Venice-Mestre, Italy. 2007. 132-135.
[70] Scott J, Flood P. Anaesthesia for caesarean delivery. In. Braveman FR. Obstetric and gynaecologic anaesthesia. The requisites in anaesthesiology. Elsevier. 2006. 57.
[71] Al-Hakim NHH, Alidreesi ZMS. The effect of local anaesthetics wound infiltration on postoperative pain after caesarean section. J Surg Pakistan. 2010. 15(3): 131-134.
[72] Fawole AO, Adesina OA. Complaints in the puerperium. In. Ebeigbe PN. (Ed). Foundations of clinical obstetrics in the tropics. Fodah Global Ultimate Limited. Benin City. 2012. 232-236.
[73] Collis R, Rees L. Antenatal Issues Including Pain Management. In. Clyburn P, Collis R, Harries S, Davies S. (Eds). Obstetric anaesthesia. Oxford University Press. New York. 2008. 109-152.
[74] Odusola P. Common obstetric procedures. In. Ebeigbe PN. (Ed). Foundations of clinical obstetrics in the tropics. Fodah Global Ultimate Limited. Benin City. 2012. 208.
[75] Aissaoui Y, Bryere R, Mustapha H, Bry D, Inamili ND, Miller C. A randomised controlled trial of pudendal nerve block for pain relief after episiotomy. Anaesth Analg. 2008. 107(2): 625-629.
[76] Lecing AY. Postoperative pain management in obstetric anaesthesia-new challenges and solutions. J Cli Anaesth. 2004. 16: 57-65.
[77] Carvalho S, Osiorio J, Carreira S, Saldanha L. Post caesarean section analgesia.
[78] Kuczkowski KM. Post-operative pain control in the parturient: new challenges (and their solutions). J Cli Anaesth. 2004. 16: 1-3.
[79] Lim Y, Jha S, Sia AT, Rawal N. Morphine for post-caesarean analgesia: intrathecal epidural or intravenous? Singapore Med J. 2005. 46(8): 392-396.
[80] Gadsden J, Hart S, Santos A. Post-caesarean delivery analgesia. Anaesth Analg. 2005. 101: 562-569.
[81] Momani O. Controlled trials of wound infiltration with bupivacaine for postoperative pain relief after caesarean section. Bri Med Bull. 2001. 23(2): 83-85.
[82] Caveleiro C, Delgado R, Carvalho B, Valentim A, Matires E, martins m et al. comparison of three different epidural analgesic protocols for pain relief after caesarean section.

Chapter 10

A Novel Application of Virtual Reality for Pain Control: Virtual Reality-Mirror Visual Feedback Therapy

Kenji Sato, Satoshi Fukumori, Kantaro Miyake,
Daniel Obata, Akio Gofuku and Kiyoshi Morita

Additional information is available at the end of the chapter

http://dx.doi.org/10.5772/51139

1. Introduction

Virtual reality is state of the art technology, but its concept can be found in many fields even in the past. These technologies, such as computer graphics, simulation, and human-computer interfaces have all led to the evolution of virtual reality technology. The virtual reality technology developed in the 1960s is similar to what we see in the present day. In the fields of computer graphics, Ivan Sutherland created the pioneering virtual reality system, *The ultimate display* in which he used computers for the designing, construction, navigation and habitation of virtual worlds. He also developed a head mounted display which was designed to immerse the viewer in a visually simulated 3D environment. During the 1960s and 1970s, virtual reality technology had been applied to aerospace and military fields. The US Air Force established a laboratory at Wright-Patterson Air Force Base in Ohio and created flight simulators for high speed military aircraft. This resulted in the construction of the Super Cockpit in the 1980s which Tom Furness created as the director of this project. It is widely credited that Jaron *Lanier*, director and founder of *VPL* (*Visual Programming Language*), coined the term virtual reality in 1989 to bring all of the virtual projects of VPL, such as eyephone, dataglove and datasuit under a single term. In 1990 the human machine interfaces for teleoperators and virtual environments conference was held in Santa Barbara, CA and *virtual reality* was given as a general term for all related technologies.

Virtual reality (VR) consists of indispensable elements including a virtual world, immersion, sensory feedback, and interactivity. The distinguishing characteristic of VR is a sense of immersion that occurs from the user interacting with a VE using multimodal stimuli, such as visual, auditory, and tactile stimuli. Another distinguishing characteristic is that VR gives the illusion that objects that do not exist in the real world exist inside a computer-generated VE. Virtual reality technology is used in a variety of fields and possible medical application has attracted keen interest. Potential benefits have been reported in applications such as treatment of post-traumatic stress disorder following the terrorist attack on the World Trade Center [1], rehabilitation following a stroke [2], and disability management following accidents or surgery [3]. Virtual reality technology holds the promise as an analgesic modality in diverse ways. There is growing evidence about the successful application of VR technology to alleviate acute pain during medical procedures. Recently, the application of VR for chronic pain control has also been gaining attention. There are excellent review articles about this issue [4] [5].

This manuscript consists of three chapters. Chapter 1 presents an overview of VR technology applied to pain treatment, especially focusing on the treatment of chronic pain such as phantom limb pain. The scope of the topic in chapter 1 expands into a new approach for the treatment of phantom limb pain. Because technology is advancing rapidly, it is now possible to create a prosthesis that allows patients to control it by their thoughts alone. Perhaps if patients with phantom limb pain could use a high-tech prosthesis that they can directly control with their thoughts, phantom limb pain could be relieved. Chapter 2 introduces the virtual reality-mirror visual feedback (VR-MVF) therapy that we have developed and its analgesic efficacy in patients with complex regional pain syndrome (CRPS). Chapter 3 introduces our VR-MVF system for home use. Although the advanced MVF with VR technology showed increased analgesic efficacy and benefit, few patients can benefit from this treatment. The reason why VR-MVF has not yet become popular for clinical practice is due to the cost and the elusiveness of the technology required for VR. We have been working on two projects to resolve these problems. The drawbacks of virtual reality should be considered, because it will limit the applicability of VR for wide-spread use. Drawbacks of VR can be divided into two categories, technology-related disadvantages and VR-related side effects. Technology-related disadvantages include the high cost and the complexity of the system which requires extensive knowledge of VR for its repair and maintenance. For example, the hardware including the head-mounted displays, data-glove and motion capture system, requires frequent adjustments to be made for maintaining the sense of immersion. Particular concern for VR-related side effects is necessary because these systems are occasionally applied to patients with impairment. These patients may have a higher susceptibility to side effects. There are also concerns about the social impact that virtual environments affect on people, such as the psychological effects of prolonged usage. As an example of social disadvantage, some concerns are raised on desensitization. Although virtual reality technology is applied to systemic desensitization therapy which is a technique used to treat phobias and fear, in extreme cases there are concerns that users could fail to recognize the consequences their actions in virtual environments may cause in the real world. VR-related side effects include *Cybersickness* and *Aftereffects*. Cybersickness is a form of motion sickness. Symptoms include eyestrains, blurred vision, headaches, vertigo, imbalance, nausea and vomiting. Cybersickness is believed to occur as a result of conflicts between visual, vestibular and proprioceptive perception. Symptoms of Aftereffects include disturbed locomotion, postural instability, fatigue and drowsiness. The users adapt to the sensorimotor requirements in virtual environments (VEs), and after leaving VEs they must readapt to the sensorimotor requirements in the real world. Aftereffects is believed to occur as a result of a lag in the sensorimotor response recalibration.

1.1. Virtual reality and pain management

Virtual reality technology as an analgesic modality was initially applied to attenuate pain perception during painful medical procedures. Hoffman *et al.* first reported that VR could alleviate pain perception during painful burn care in adolescent patients [6]. The application of VR for pain control during burn care has been the most intensively studied application [7-8]. Other procedures to which VR has been applied include dental procedures [9] and intravenous placement [10]. Virtual reality technology with a head-mounted display allows the user to feel as if they are present in the VE, and interaction with the VE through manipulation strengthens the user's immersion. With strong immersion, the user's attention is focused on the VE, which subsequently can take the user's attention away from pain. This is the distraction theory, which is one of the hypotheses of the mechanism of VR analgesia. Virtual reality analgesia has been speculated to be the result of distraction. Recently, advancement in neuro-imaging studies has revealed how VR distraction modulates pain processing in brain regions known as the pain matrix [11][12]. Neuroimaging studies have identified several brain regions that are consistently activated during nociceptive stimulation. These brain regions are referred to as the pain matrix which includes the anterior cingulate cortex (ACC), the insula, the thalamus, and the primary (S1) and secondary (S2) somatosensory cortices. Hoffman et al conducted a study using fMRI in healthy volunteers to investigate the associated changes in pain-related brain activation during nociceptive thermal stimulation and compared these results under conditions of no analgesia, opioid (hydromorphone) analgesia alone, VR distraction alone, and opioid analgesia combined with VR distraction [12]. VR distraction alone significantly reduced subjective pain and significantly reduced pain-related brain activity in the insula, thalmus, and S2. Combined opioid with VR distraction reduced pain reports more effectively than did opioid alone for subjective pain.

Although interests and expectations in the application of VR for the treatment of chronic pain are growing, few studies about the analgesic efficacy of VR in patients with chronic pain have been reported. The application of VR to chronic pain treatment has not progressed further due to the lack of complete understanding about the mechanism of VR analgesia. We still do not know how we can use VR technology to build a system for providing analgesic efficacy for patients with chronic pain. However, a novel approach is to enhance the existing treatment, which is already known to have some analgesic efficacy for chronic pain, with VR technology. In this context, VR technology has been successfully applied as VR-hypnosis [13], VR-MVF therapy for phantom limb pain [14], and treatment for CRPS [15]. Hypnotic analgesia has gained special attention as an analgesic modality [16]. Oneal *et al.* integrated hypnotic analgesia with VR technology and applied the combination in the treatment of chronic neuropathic pain [13]. A patient with a 5-year history of C4-quadriplegia and upper extremity neuropathic pain received an audio recording of a hypnotic induction, i.e., suggestions for pain relief. After a 6-month trial of VR-hypnosis, the patient's rating for pain and discomfort dropped more than 30%. Another example of the application of VR to pain treatment has been shown by Sarig-Bahat *et al.* [17]. They developed a VE in which the cervical range of motion (CROM) of a patient with neck pain was assessed during a simple but engaging gaming scenario and compared with that of individuals with no neck pain. The participants' task in the VE was to spray a fly with a spray canister. Once a fly was sprayed, it vanished and a new target appeared within a larger ROM. The results of a single session revealed increasing CROM and decreased neck pain. They speculated that VR may play a role in overcoming the fear of motion via pain distraction, which subsequently improves CROM and results in pain reduction. Patients with chronic pain avoid moving the affected part of the body for fear that it will exacerbate the pain; this is the so-called fear-avoidance model [18]. Lowering fear-avoidance has been shown to be effective for the treatment of chronic back pain [19]. This type of approach is also known as cognitive behavioral therapy, the beneficial effects of which have been shown in patients with chronic pain [20]. The graded exposure of cognitive behavioral therapy *in vivo* can improve disability through reducing anxiety, which results in decreased pain in patients with CRPS [21].

1.2. Virtual reality for phantom limb pain

Virtual reality allows the user to experience a computer-generated VE by using advanced technology such as a head-mounted display with tracking systems. Interestingly, the application of VR to chronic pain treatment was initially made without the help of these cutting-edge technologies. Ramachandran and Roger–Ramachandran introduced mirror visual feedback (MVF) therapy with a virtual mirror box for the treatment of phantom limb pain and reported its promising analgesic efficacy [22]. A vertical mirror was placed and an upper limb amputee was asked to place his normal hand on one side (the reflecting side) of the mirror and to look at the reflection of the hand optically superimposed on the felt location of the phantom. If the subject moved his normal hand, he not only saw his phantom move but felt it moving as well. In some cases, this relieved painful cramps in the phantom limb. A distinguishing characteristic is that the VR gives the illusion as if objects that do not exist in the real world exist inside a computer-generated VE. This outstanding characteristic of VR makes it possible for missing extremities to emerge inside the virtual world. Thus, it seems reasonable to integrate Ramachandran's MVF therapy for phantom limb pain with VR technology. Murray *et al.* developed an immersive VR system that transposes movements of an intact limb onto that of a virtual limb in a computer-generated VE [14]. Their system contains a head-mounted display, data glove and sensors for an upper limb, sensors for lower limb, and a Fastrak tracking device for monitoring the movements of head, arm, and legs. Three patients with phantom limb pain, two with upper limb and one with lower limb amputation, who participated in two or five treatment sessions over a 3-week period, reported a reduction in their pain.

Mirror visual feedback therapy including VR-MVF is not always able to induce beneficial analgesic effects for patients with phantom limb pain. Although most patients feel reduced phantom limb pain during the therapy, pain relief could be sustained in only a limited number patients after the therapy. It is speculated that MVF decreases phantom limb pain by restoring the shrunken somatosensory area (reorganization) that formally corresponded with the deafferentiated limb. Because technology is advancing rapidly, if patients with phantom limb pain had a prosthesis that they could directly control, and, moreover, if patients could feel feedback sensations such as haptic or proprioceptive feelings in response to their motor commands, it would help to restore the normal cortical map and phantom limb pain would be dramatically relieved. Moreover, unlike with MVF, patients with phantom limb pain could wear the high-tech prosthesis and use it in their daily life, which has the advantageous effect of restoring the normal cortical map sooner and subsequently providing long-lasting pain relief. This means that such a high-tech prosthesis could be a new approach for the treatment of phantom limb pain.

It is known that different mechanisms are underlying phantom limb sensation and phantom limb pain. Blakemore *et al.* explained phantom limb sensation using a forward model [23]. A forward model uses an efference copy to predict the sensory consequences of the motor commands and compares this with the actual sensation of the movement. They suggested that the normal experience of the limb is based on this predicted state, rather than the actual state. Even in the case of missing limbs, motor commands lead to the prediction of the movement that results in phantom limbs sensation. Approximately 50-80% of all amputees have phantom limb pain [24]. Both peripheral and central mechanisms and even psychological factors have been implicated as the mechanisms of phantom limb pain [25]. Flor *et al.* especially focused on the pain memory established before the amputation as a powerful elicitor of phantom limb pain. They explained that if a somatosensory pain memory has been established with an important neural correlate in the spinal and supraspinal structures, such as in the primary somatosensory cortex, subsequent deafferentation and an invasion of the amputation zone by neighboring input may preferentially activate cortical neurons coding for pain [25]. Meanwhile, reorganization in the primary somatosensory motor cortex has been strongly correlated with phantom limb pain [26]. However, no conclusive explanation about why reorganization in these brain regions causes phantom limb pain has been made. The adult brain was formerly recognized as a hard-wired organ but recent neuroscientific evidence revealed that substantial plastic changes can occur. It is also known that this plasticity can be reversed. Birbaumer *et al.* showed that suppression of afferent input from the amputation stump by brachial plexus anesthesia eliminated both cortical reorganization and phantom limb pain in half of the subjects [27]. In the other half, both cortical reorganization and phantom limb pain were unchanged during upper extremity anesthesia. The authors suggested that in some amputees, cortical reorganization and phantom limb pain may be maintained by peripheral input, whereas in others, intracortical changes might be overriding. The approach for restoring this reorganization into a normal state is expected to be a promising analgesic modality [28]. Lotze *et al.*, using functional magnetic resonance imaging, investigated the effect of prosthesis use on phantom limb pain and cortical reorganization [29]. Patients who used a myoelectric prosthesis that provides sensory, visual, and motor feedback showed decreasing phantom limb pain that was subsequently correlated with less cortical reorganization compared with patients who used a cosmetic prosthesis or no prosthesis.

1.3. A new treatment approach for phantom limb pain: A brain-controlled prosthesis

The idea of direct brain control of a prosthesis is mainly aimed to improve the functionality of a prosthesis rather than to treat phantom limb pain, which subsequently helps the disability of amputees. However, because phantom limb pain tremendously impairs the amputees' quality of life, the analgesic efficacy provided with a brain-controlled prosthesis on phantom limb pain has also gained keen interest. However, if a high-tech brain-controlled prosthesis can only make movement in response to patients' motor intention and no sensory feedback other than visual feedback can be obtained, there may be no significant difference between MVF therapy and a brain-controlled prosthesis in terms of analgesic efficacy. However, even if this were the case, a brain-controlled prosthesis still might have some advantage over MVF. To construct the image of the missing limb with the reflection of a mirror image in MVF therapy, an amputee makes a motor command of the healthy limb. However, with a brain-controlled prosthesis, only the motor-related brain region for the side of the missing limb is activated. Because there is communication between the two brain hemispheres, activity on one side is known to inhibit activity on the opposite side [30]. In this context, brain activity in the case of a brain-controlled prosthesis might be more strongly activated than that in MVF, which subsequently may be favorable from the point of view of restoring normal brain state. Because delivering sensory feedback as a consequence of motor commands improves the functionality of a prosthesis, researchers working on a brain-controlled prosthesis have been trying to deliver effective feedback. This will give tremendous beneficial effects on the analgesia that a brain-control prosthesis is expected to provide.

To make a brain-controlled prosthesis move, the first step is to extract voluntary commands. Once motor commands are extracted, the next step is to deliver the extracted information (motor commands) to the artificial limb (prosthesis). Ideally, the last step is to deliver the haptic and proprioceptional information as sensory feedback that the patient expects to feel as a consequence of motor commands. Sensory feedback is expected not only to improve the functionality of a prosthesis but also to decrease phantom limb pain. There are several approaches for the extraction of motor commands, incuding electromyographic (EMG)-based controls with targeted reinnervation [31] [32], a brain (cortical)-controlled neuroprosthesis [33] [34], and a longitudinal intrafascicular peripheral interface [35].

For example, an EMG-based control as a recording modality of motor commands has the advantages of simplicity and noninvasiveness because of its surface electrodes. The current detectable by an EMG-based control is larger than that detectable by a brain (cortical)-controlled prosthesis. Meanwhile, a brain-controlled prosthesis needs an invasive intracranial electrode. Hochberg *et al.* have implanted intracranial electrodes in the human motor cortex as a prosthetic control and also reported that a patient with quadriplegia could use neural control to open and close a prosthetic hand [34]. There are considerable problems, including complexity and biocompatibility, which have to be solved before a brain (cortical)-controlled prosthesis can be used as a modality for prosthesis control.

The EMG-based prosthesis which is controlled with myoelectrical signals from a remaining pair of agonist-antagonist muscles in the amputated limb, provide very limited motion. To overcome this drawback, Kuiken *et al.* have developed targeted reinnervation for enhanced prosthetic arm function [31]. Surgery is performed on a patient with a traumatic amputation. Residual peripheral nerves of the brachial plexus are transferred to the patient's pectoral and serratus muscles. When the patient thinks about closing his hand, for example, the amplified myoelectrical signal from the pectoralis muscle causes constriction that is used to control the closing movements of the computerized prosthesis. The targeted muscle reinnervation technique allows an amputee to intuitively control a prosthesis. Another outstanding characteristic of Kuiken's technique is targeted sensory reinnervation that can provide sensory feedback as a result of motor intention. The anterior chest skin that was overlying the targeted muscle reinnervation site is denervated and reinnervated with the ulnar and median nerves. A patient's intention to move the prosthetic hand causes constriction of the anterior chest muscle and simultaneously, the skin on the surface of the constructed muscle activates the reinnervated nerves that subsequently provide the feeling that the patient's hand was touched. Kuiken's technique can allow amputees to directly control a prosthesis with their intentions and delivers sensory feedback as a consequence of motor commands. Before the targeted reinnervation surgery, one amputee had severe phantom limb pain but it resolved after 4 weeks of treatment following the surgery. Motor commands can be extracted by interfaces with the peripheral nervous system. Horch *et al.* implanted longitudinal intrafascicular peripheral interfaces (LIFEs) into the median nerve of three amputee subjects [36]. They reported that the motor signals recorded using LIFEs can be used to control a robotic system. These LIFEs also seem to be able to provoke sensory feedback. In a preliminary study on amputees conducted by Horch *et al.*, they reported that stimulating different afferent nerves using LIFEs could provide sensory feedback [37].

Micera pointed out that the peripheral nervous system-based control of a prosthesis using LIFEs may help to modify the plastic reorganization after the amputation and restore brain areas to a normal state, which subsequently is expected to decrease phantom limb pain [35]. Dietrich *et al.* reported that sensory feedback prosthesis reduced phantom limb pain [38]. In their system, the pressure information measured by a sensor located in the bend between the thumb and index finger of a myoelectric prosthesis was transformed into electrical stimulation patterns by a microcontroller. Then electrocutaneous stimulus was delivered as sensory feedback to the skin of the subject's stump. Two-week training with this system provided significant improvement in the functionality of the prosthesis and reduced phantom limb pain. Although the sensory feedback in Dietrich's system was not exactly haptic or proprioceptive sensation in response to the motor intention, it still could provide considerable analgesia. Thus, if real sensory feedback such as haptic or propriocetive sensation could be provided in the near future, phantom limb pain could be completely relieved. However, both peripheral and central mechanisms and even psychological factors have been implicated as the mechanism of phantom limb pain, so some patients may still not have pain relief from a brain-controlled prosthesis.

2. Application of virtual reality for chronic pain treatment of patients with complex regional pain syndrome

Complex regional pain syndrome includes a variety of pain conditions with both motor and autonomic symptoms [39]. The underlying pathogenesis is not yet fully understood, which makes it difficult to establish effective treatments. Alternative analgesic modalities have been actively sought for the treatment of CRPS. Ramachandran introduced MVF therapy [22]. CRPS type 1 shares many strikingly similar characteristics with phantom limb pain [26] [40] [41]. Mirror visual feedback therapy is expected to provide analgesic effects for patients with CRPS. The advanced MVF system with virtual reality technology (VR-MVF) contains very specific target-oriented motor control tasks and enables subjects to feel engaged and rewarded, thus encouraging them to repeat the exercise with intensity. In this regard, VR-MVF has tremendous potential as a non-invasive alternative analgesic modality for CRPS.

2.1. Virtual reality-mirror visual feedback system

A personal computer-based desktop VR system was developed for MVF therapy. The system contains a personal computer (operating system: Windows XP Professional SP2; central processing unit: Intel Core 2 Duo 3.16 GHz; graphics: Radeon HD 4679), a CyberGlove (Immersion Co.) as a hand input device, a Fastrak device (POLHEUMS Co.) as a real-time position and motion tracker, and a 20-inch desktop monitor (EIZO FlexScan SX2761W, EIZO Nanao MS Corp. Japan). A VE was developed using commercially available software, Autodesk 3DS Max. The system is shown in Figure 1. In the VE, three objects of different sizes and shapes are initially located on the table with a back shelf. The forearm and hand on the affected side appears on VE and every movement or any laterality of the real arm can be precisely reproduced. The movement of the fingers and wrist of the virtual hand is simulated by the CyberGlove, which is attached on the non-affected side because pain is induced if the affected hand is used. The Fastrak position tracker that determines the position and orientation of the virtual arm is mounted on the affected side. In the VR-MVF system, a virtual forearm moves in the same manner as the affected side, but the hand and finger motions are simulated by the non-affected side. This is the biggest difference between MVF therapy with a mirror box and VR-MVF therapy. Recently, we renovated our VR-MVF system (Figure 2). A 50-inch Panasonic TH-P50VT5 display monitor and 5DT Data Glove 5/14 Ultra hand input device were used. A VE was developed using OpenGL (Silicon Graphics) as the application program interface and a three-dimensional model was constructed by Metasequoia. The most distinguishable change was made in the physics simulation. Havok Physics (Havok Co.) was used as the physics engine that makes objects in the VE roll and bounce in a very realistic manner on the screen.

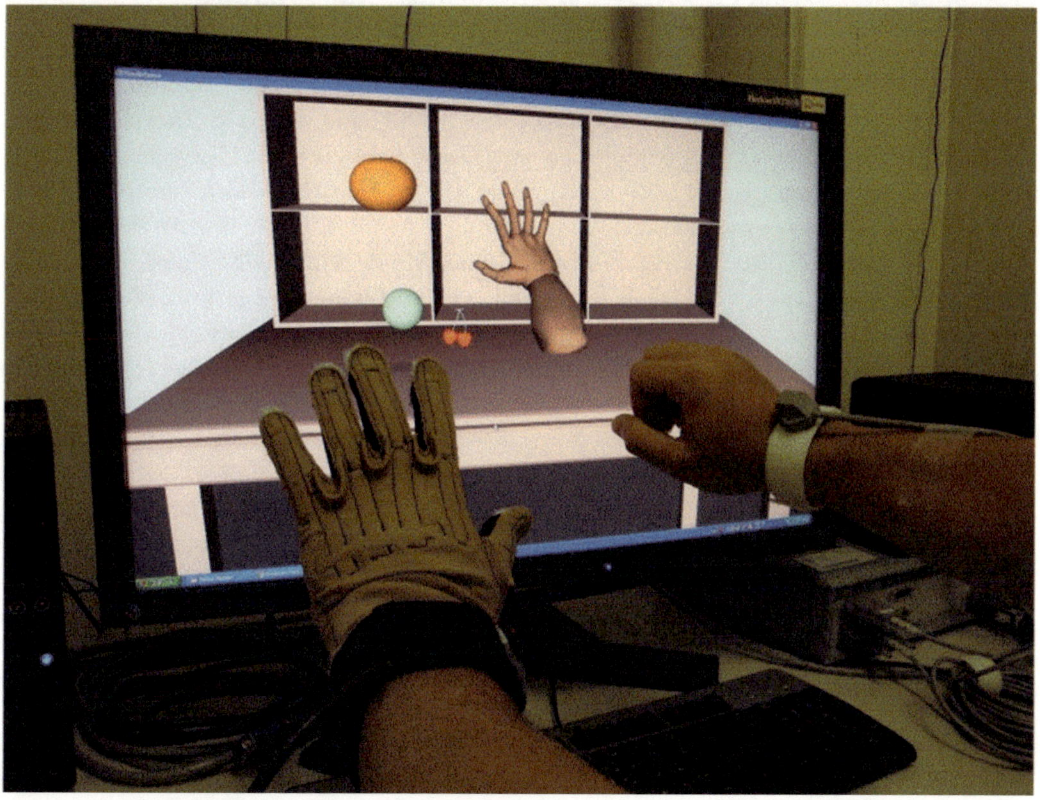

Figure 1. Virtual reality-mirror visual feedback therapy in Okayama University Hospital

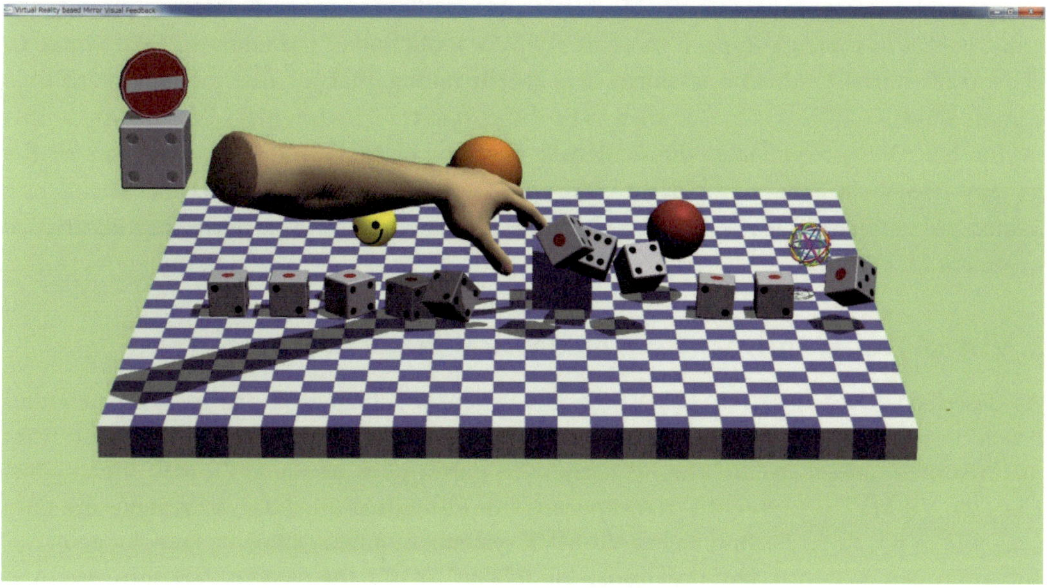

Figure 2. The renovated version of virtual reality-mirror visual feedback therapy

2.2. Application for patients with complex regional pain syndrome

Virtual reality-mirror visual feedback exercises are target-oriented motor control tasks. The sequences of hand exercises consisted of the movements of reaching out, grasping, transferring, and placing. Five patients with CRPS of the hand attended VR-MVF therapy. The therapy was given once a week at an outpatient pain clinic in Okayama University Medical Center, where the VR-MVF system was set up. In each therapy session, no time limit was set. Analgesic medications were continued at the same regimens as before the therapy. If patients reported an increase in pain intensity or related side effects of VR-MVF therapy, treatment was immediately cancelled and additional drugs or treatment were administered. However, if patients reported decreased pain intensity, medication was adjusted or stopped as directed by the patient. Subjective pain was evaluated according to a visual analogue scale (0 = no pain, 100 = worst pain) before and after each treatment session. All patients reported spontaneous pain in the affected limb that increased with movement. The pre-treatment score on the visual analogue scale (64 ± 14) (mean ± SD) decreased to 31 ± 26 after consecutive treatment sessions. Four of the five patients (80%) showed 50% reduction of the pre-treatment visual analogue scale value. The analgesic effect provided by VR-MVF therapy in five cases of CRPS is shown in Figure 3. All cases showed a short-term reduction in pain intensity (before-and-after comparison of the visual analogue score in each session) and four of the five cases showed consecutive decreases of visual analogue scale score, which led to a 50% reduction of the pre-treatment value after respective treatment sessions.

Effective pain reduction (50% reduction) was accomplished after the third treatment session in Cases 1 and 2, the fourth session in Case 3, and the eighth session in Case 5.

In this preliminary work, our VR-MVF therapy was able to provide successful analgesic efficacy: 80% of patients showed more than a 50% reduction of pain intensity after three to eight consecutive treatment sessions. It is worth noting that all five patients were in a chronic state of CRPS, which is known to be difficult to treat by original MVF therapy with a mirror box. In two patients, the analgesic effect continued even after cessation of the therapy. Moreover, none of the five patients in the present study reported experiencing any related side effects. Our result showed that VR-MVF therapy is a promising alternative treatment for CRPS.

3. Virtual reality-mirror visual feedback therapy for home use

As described in Chapter 2, VR-MVF treatment showed increased analgesic efficacy and benefit in patients with CRPS. However, only a limited number of patients can benefit from this treatment and there are several barriers to performing frequent VR-MVF treatments. First, the VR-MVF equipment is too expensive for individual purchase, so systems are only available in hospitals. Second, using VR-MVF systems requires extensive knowledge of VR and computer systems. The user must be able to set up the system, VR software, and treatment tasks. Third, treatment records, such as the hand and finger movement data and visual analogue scale evaluations before and after treatment, are hard to obtain without the help of doctors or medical staff. These problems restrict treatment time and frequency. We have been working on two projects to resolve the problems.

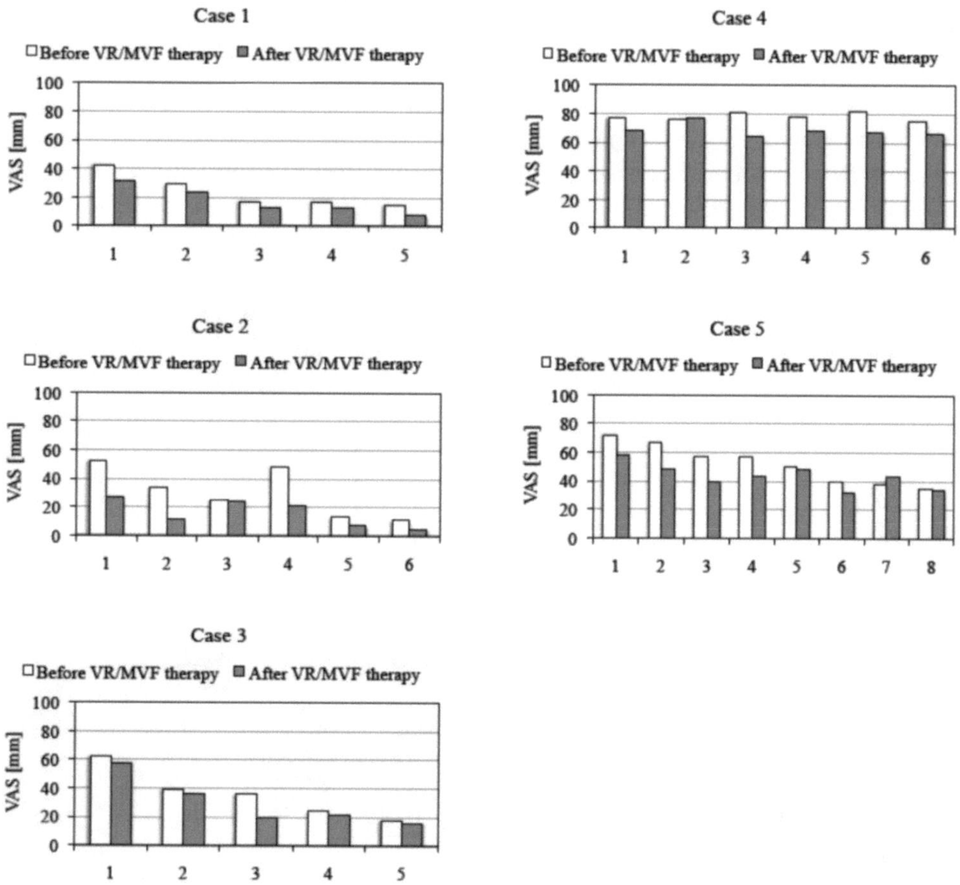

Figure 3. Analgesic effect provided by VR-MVF therapy

A plausible solution for these problems is a remote personal VR-MVF system. This system is composed of an internet-connected personal computer with videophone application software and an inexpensive input device for measuring movements of the non-affected forearm, hand, and fingers. The VE treatment programs are sent through the internet from a server at a hospital. The treatment data, such as pain levels before and after treatment, treatment time, and movement data, are temporarily stored in the personal computer and sent back to the server after treatment sessions. The authors have developed a prototype personal VR-MVF system and plan to expand the prototype to a remote version. This expansion will be accomplished by adding a server and developing data communication and treatment data management software. In a personal VR-MVF system, it is important that the patient be able to observe the virtual hand and forearm movement of the affected side on a display without actually moving the hand and forearm of the affected side. As shown in Figure 4, this system is composed of a computer with a display, an input device, a web camera with an infrared filter, and processing software for the VE and movement data of the non-affected hand. Another web camera is prepared for videophone communication with a doctor at the hospital. The system measures hand movements and grasping actions on the non-affected side by processing the image data collected by six infrared light-emitting diodes (LEDs) in the input device, as shown in Figure 5. The infrared LED on the palm of the hand detects grasping actions and the infrared LEDs around the hand measure hand location and direction. The system then displays the hand and forearm of the affected side in the VE according to these movement measurements. When the LED in the hand is hidden and the input device receives no infrared light, a grasping motion is detected. A prepared animation of a grasping motion is then played. Conversely, when the infrared light from the LED in the hand is received by the input device, a hand-opening motion is detected. The prepared animation of the grasping motion is then played in reverse. The input device does not measure the motion of each finger. These measurements are not necessary because treatment tasks include grasping an object, moving it, and placing it at a specified position.

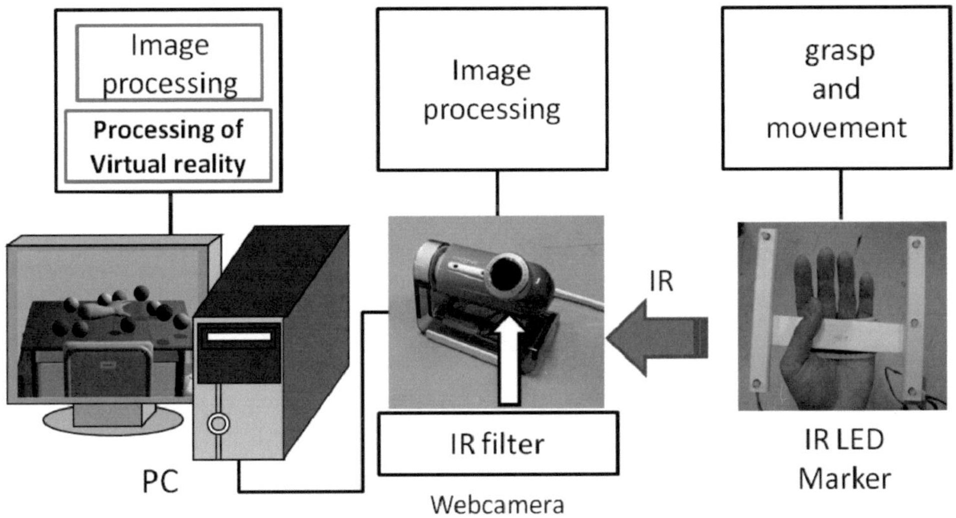

Figure 4. Composition of a personal virtual reality-mirror visual feedback system

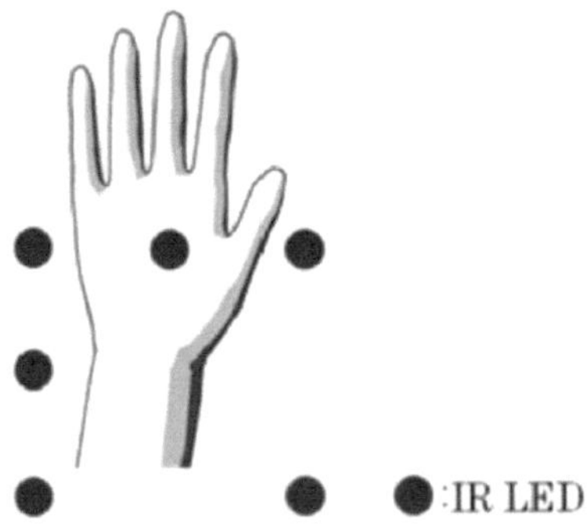

Figure 5. Arrangement of infrared light-emitting diodes in the input device

The applicability of the personal VR-MVF system was evaluated by indices of control and realism by the presence questionnaire [42]. The presence questionnaire is a test for measuring the presence of a VE. Each question is related to one or more categories pertaining to control, sensory, realism, and distraction factors of the VE. Each question is evaluated on a scale of fitness from 1 (completely unfit) to 7 (good fit). The control factor measures how easily the user is able to control an object in the VE. The sensory factor measures how well the user perceives the VE. The realism factor measures how authentic the VE feels to the user. The distraction factor measures the user's level of distraction during the session.

Five men and one woman evaluated the system. All subjects were healthy and right-handed, with an average age of 22.6 years. Because sound was not utilized in the original VR-MVF or the personal VR-MVF systems, questions related to auditory stimuli were omitted.

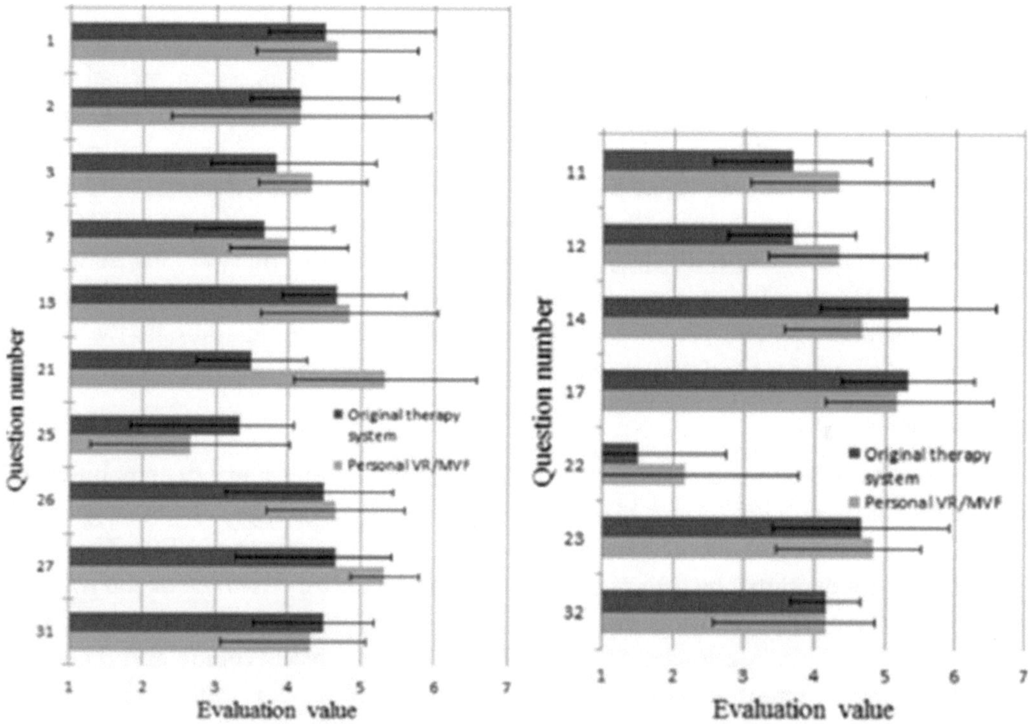

Figure 6. Comparison of presence questionnaire evaluations for the original and personal virtual reality-mirror visual feedback systems (a) Control factor (b) Realism factor

The results of these evaluations are shown in Figure 6. A detailed description of the questionnaire was reported by Witmer [42]. A dark bar indicates the average evaluation of the VR-MVF system and a light bar indicates that of the personal VR-MVF system. The fine lines indicate standard deviations of the evaluation points. For Questions 11 and 25 in Figure 6, lower values indicate better system performance. The personal VR-MVF system received relatively better evaluations than the original system for the questions related to the control factor and comparable evaluations for the questions related to the realism factor. From these results, the personal VR-MVF system was confirmed to be applicable for patients with chronic pain such as CRPS.

Another approach to VR-MVF for home use is based on the idea of transforming the procedure of VR-MVF into sounds (music) in which data are stored in mobile MP3 players that could then be taken home. Hearing the music reminds the patients of images of VR-MVF that are expected to activate the same brain networks activated during VR-MVF. It is intended to provide some kind of analgesia in patients with chronic pain including CRPS.

4. VR-MVF therapy with sound therapy system

Components of the therapy system

The VR-MVF with a sound therapy system is composed of the following components in a virtual environment: data glove, magnetic sensor, virtual upper limb, several virtual square objects, and a 10 × 10 matrix of square white switches to turn objects on and off. The object is pressed once and turned on and then pressed again and turned off like a switch of an illumination lamp. When an object is turned on, the white switch changes to blue and signals to emit a sound (Figure 7). To develop this system, we consulted the Yamaha Corporation on the tenori-on [43] because this electronic musical instrument is comparatively easy for the average person who has never played music to perform on. Playing music that a patient prefers contributes largely to therapy; in addition, the patient would continue treatment with enjoyment.

How to perform music

To use a tenori-on, the user pushes buttons with his or her finger. In our system, however, a user does not press buttons with his or her finger to switch the signal, because grasping virtual objects and moving them are important activities in the therapy of CRPS. Therefore, a patient changes the signal by dropping a spherical object onto a switch he or she wants to turn on or off. As with VR-MVF, the objects behave as real objects by means of simple physics simulation, making it easy to create music. Several objects collide and then each object moves in a different direction. As a result, each object presses a button and the user does not need to drop objects on all buttons that he or she wants to switch. When a button is pressed, no sound is emitted, but a point of emission is set. A pressed button emits its defined sound at a constant frequency when a time line is exceeded. The time line represents the frequency of an emission and moves from right to left. The time line is at the right edge in Figure 7. Each button in a single row produces a different sound. Sounds are allocated to each button from back to front in a row. The sound is ranked from lower to higher in a scale of musical notes. Ten rows having the same sounds are put on the virtual table in Figure 7.

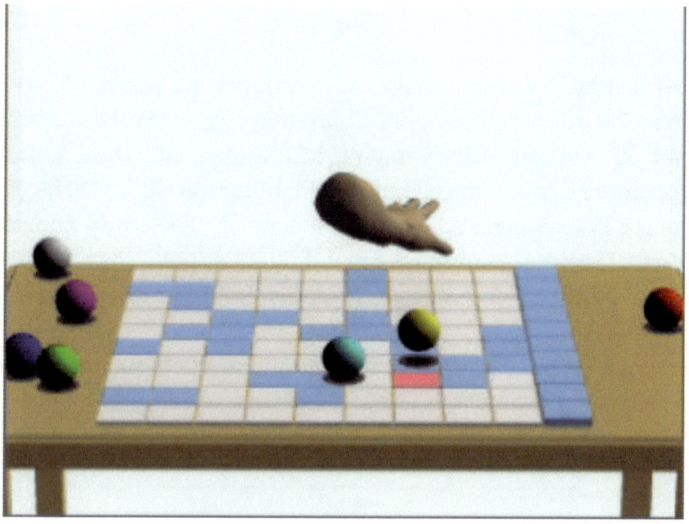

Figure 7. The VR-MVF with a sound therapy system

5. Conclusion

Virtual reality technology has tremendous potential to provide alternative analgesic modalities to patients with chronic pain conditions such as phantom limb pain and CRPS. Virtual reality-mirror visual feedback therapy is a successful example of applying virtual reality technology to pain treatment, especially for patients with chronic pain. In our preliminary study, we showed its beneficial analgesic effects on patients with CRPS. Although VR-MVF is a promising analgesic modality, there are several barriers to VR-MVF becoming a widely used treatment, including its high initial cost. To resolve this problem, we have been working on VR-MVF for home use. Our strategies are intended to provide analgesia for many patients who need an alternative non-invasive analgesic modality.

Author details

Kenji Sato*
Department of Anesthesiology and Resuscitology,
Okayama University Graduate School of Medicine and Dentistry, Okayama City, Japan

Daniel Obata and Kiyoshi Morita
Department of Anesthesiology and Resuscitology,
Okayama University Graduate School of Medicine and Dentistry, Okayama City, Japan

Satoshi Fukumori, Kantaro Miyake and Akio Gofuku
Graduate School of Natural Science and Technology, Okayama University, Okayama City, Japan

* Corresponding Author

6. References

[1] Difede J, Hoffman HG. Virtual reality exposure therapy for World Trade Center post-traumatic stress disorder: a case report. *CyberPsychology & Behavior* 2002;5:529-35.

[2] Jack D, Boian R, Merians AS, Tremaine M, Burdea GC, Adamovich SV, Recce M, Poizner H. Virtual reality-enhanced stroke rehabilitation. *IEEE* 2001;9:308-18.

[3] Shing CP, Fung CP, Chuang TY, Penn IW, Doong JL. The study of auditory and haptic signals in a virtual reality-based hand rehabilitation system. *Robotica* 2003;21:211-8.

[4] Mahrer NE, Gold JI. The use of virtual reality for pain control: a review. *Curr Pain Headache Rep* 2009;13[2]:100-9.

[5] Li A, Montano Z, Chen VJ, Gold JI. Virtual reality and pain management: current trends and future directions. *Pain Manag* 2011;1[2]:147-57.

[6] Hoffman HG, Doctor JN, Patterson DR, Carrougher GJ, Furness TA, 3rd. Virtual reality as an adjunctive pain control during burn wound care in adolescent patients. *Pain* 2000;85[1-2]:305-9.

[7] Das DA, Grimmer KA, Sparnon AL, McRae SE, Thomas BH. The efficacy of playing a virtual reality game in modulating pain for children with acute burn injuries: a randomized controlled trial [ISRCTN87413556]. *BMC Pediatr* 2005;5[1]:1.

[8] Carrougher GJ, Hoffman HG, Nakamura D, Lezotte D, Soltani M, Leahy L, Engrav LH, Patterson DR. The effect of virtual reality on pain and range of motion in adults with burn injuries. *J Burn Care Res* 2009;30[5]:785-91.

[9] Furman E, Jasinevicius TR, Bissada NF, Victoroff KZ, Skillicorn R, Buchner M. Virtual reality distraction for pain control during periodontal scaling and root planing procedures. *J Am Dent Assoc* 2009;140[12]:1508-16.

[10] Gold JI, Kim SH, Kant AJ, Joseph MH, Rizzo AS. Effectiveness of virtual reality for pediatric pain distraction during i.v. placement. *Cyberpsychol Behav* 2006;9[2]:207-12.

[11] Gold JI, Belmont KA, Thomas DA. The neurobiology of virtual reality pain attenuation. *Cyberpsychol Behav* 2007;10[4]:536-44.

[12] Hoffman HG, Richards TL, Van Oostrom T, Coda BA, Jensen MP, Blough DK, Sharar SR. The analgesic effects of opioids and immersive virtual reality distraction: evidence from subjective and functional brain imaging assessments. Anesth Analg 2007;105[6]:1776-1783, table of contents.

[13] Oneal BJ, Patterson DR, Soltani M, Teeley A, Jensen MP. Virtual reality hypnosis in the treatment of chronic neuropathic pain: a case report. *Int J Clin Exp Hypn* 2008;56[4]:451-62.

[14] Murray CD, Pettifer S, Howard T, Patchick EL, Caillette F, Kulkarni J, Bamford C. The treatment of phantom limb pain using immersive virtual reality: three case studies. *Disabil Rehabil* 2007;29[18]:1465-9.

[15] Sato K, Fukumori S, Matsusaki T, Maruo T, Ishikawa S, Nishie H, Takata K, Mizuhara H, Mizobuchi S, Nakatsuka H, Matsumi M, Gofuku A, Yokoyama M, Morita K. Nonimmersive virtual reality mirror visual feedback therapy and its application for the treatment of complex regional pain syndrome: an open-label pilot study. *Pain Med* 2010;11[4]:622-9.

[16] Montgomery GH, DuHamel KN, Redd WH. A meta-analysis of hypnotically induced analgesia: how effective is hypnosis? *Int J Clin Exp Hypn* 2000;48[2]:138-53.

[17] Sarig-Bahat H, Weiss PL, Laufer Y. Neck pain assessment in a virtual environment. *Spine* (Philadelphia PA 1976] 2010;35[4]:E105-12.

[18] Vlaeyen JW, Linton SJ. Fear-avoidance and its consequences in chronic musculoskeletal pain: a state of the art. *Pain* 2000;85:317-32.

[19] Boersma K, Linton S, Overmeer T, Jansson M, Vlaeyen J, de Jong J. Lowering fear-avoidance and enhancing function through exposure *in vivo*. A multiple baseline study across six patients with back pain. *Pain* 2004;108:8-16.

[20] Turk DC, Swanson KS, Tunks ER. Psychological approaches in the treatment of chronic pain patients--when pills, scalpels, and needles are not enough. *Can J Psychiatry* 2008;53:213-23.

[21] de Jong JR, Vlaeyen JW, Onghena P, Cuypers C, den Hollander M, Ruijgrok J. Reduction of pain-related fear in complex regional pain syndrome type I: the application of graded exposure *in vivo*. *Pain* 2005;116:264-75.

[22] Ramachandran VS, Roger-Ramachandran D. Synaesthesia in phantom limbs induced with mirrors. *Proceedings of the Royal Society*, London 1996;263:377-86.

[23] Blakemore SJ, Wolpert DM, Frith CD. Abnormalities in the awareness of action. *Trends Cogn Sci* 2002;6[6]:237-42.

[24] Sherman RA, Sherman CJ, Parker L. Chronic phantom and stump pain among American veterans: results of a survey. *Pain* 1984;18[1]:83-95.

[25] Flor H. Phantom-limb pain: characteristics, causes, and treatment. *Lancet Neurol* 2002;1[3]:182-9.

[26] Flor H, Elbert T, Knecht S, Wienbruch C, Pantev C, Birbaumer N, Larbig W, Taub E. Phantom-limb pain as a perceptual correlate of cortical reorganization following arm amputation. *Nature* 1995;375[6531]:482-4.

[27] Birbaumer N, Lutzenberger W, Montoya P, Larbig W, Unertl K, Topfner S, Grodd W, Taub E, Flor H. Effects of regional anesthesia on phantom limb pain are mirrored in changes in cortical reorganization. *J Neurosci* 1997;17[14]:5503-8.

[28] Flor H, Denke C, Schaefer M, Grusser S. Effect of sensory discrimination training on cortical reorganisation and phantom limb pain. *Lancet* 2001;357[9270]:1763-4.

[29] Lotze M, Grodd W, Birbaumer N, Erb M, Huse E, Flor H. Does use of a myoelectric prosthesis prevent cortical reorganization and phantom limb pain? *Nat Neurosci* 1999;2[6]:501-2.

[30] Daskalakis ZJ, Christensen BK, Fitzgerald PB, Roshan L, Chen R. The mechanisms of interhemispheric inhibition in the human motor cortex. *J Physiol* 2002;543(Pt 1]:317-26.

[31] Kuiken TA, Miller LA, Lipschutz RD, Lock BA, Stubblefield K, Marasco PD, Zhou P, Dumanian GA. Targeted reinnervation for enhanced prosthetic arm function in a woman with a proximal amputation: a case study. *Lancet* 2007;369[9559]:371-80.

[32] Kuiken TA, Marasco PD, Lock BA, Harden RN, Dewald JP. Redirection of cutaneous sensation from the hand to the chest skin of human amputees with targeted reinnervation. *Proc Natl Acad Sci U S A* 2007;104[50]:20061-6.

[33] Schwartz AB. Cortical neural prosthetics. *Annu Rev Neurosci* 2004;27:487-507.

[34] Hochberg LR, Serruya MD, Friehs GM, Mukand JA, Saleh M, Caplan AH, Branner A, Chen D, Penn RD, Donoghue JP. Neuronal ensemble control of prosthetic devices by a human with tetraplegia. *Nature* 2006;442[7099]:164-71.

[35] Micera S, Navarro X, Carpaneto J, Citi L, Tonet O, Rossini PM, Carrozza MC, Hoffmann KP, Vivo M, Yoshida K, Dario P. On the use of longitudinal intrafascicular peripheral interfaces for the control of cybernetic hand prostheses in amputees. *IEEE Trans Neural Syst Rehabil Eng* 2008;16[5]:453-72.

[36] Dhillon GS, Horch KW. Direct neural sensory feedback and control of a prosthetic arm. *IEEE Trans Neural Syst Rehabil Eng* 2005;13[4]:468-72.

[37] Dhillon GS, Kruger TB, Sandhu JS, Horch KW. Effects of short-term training on sensory and motor function in severed nerves of long-term human amputees. *J Neurophysiol* 2005;93[5]:2625-33.

[38] Dietrich C, Walter-Walsh K, Preissler S, Hofmann GO, Witte OW, Miltner WH, Weiss T. Sensory feedback prosthesis reduces phantom limb pain: proof of a principle. *Neurosci Lett* 2012;507[2]:97-100.

[39] Veldman PH, Reynen HM, Arntz IE, Goris RJ. Signs and symptoms of reflex sympathetic dystrophy: a prospective study of 829 patients. *Lancet* 1993;342:1012-6.

[40] Swart CMA, Stins JF, Beek PJ. Cortical changes in complex regional pain syndrome (CRPS) *Eur J Pain* 2009;13:902-7.

[41] Maihöfner C, Handwerker HO, Neundörfer B, Birklein F. Patterns of cortical reorganization in complex regional pain syndrome. *Neurology* 2003;61:1707-15.

[42] Witmer BG, Singer MJ. Measuring presence in virtual environments: A presence questionnaire. *Presence* 1998;7 [3], 225-40.

[43] http://usa.yamaha.com/en/products/musical-instruments/entertainment/tenori-on/tnr-w/?mode=model